All We Have to Fear

ALL WE HAVE TO FEAR

Psychiatry's Transformation of
Natural Anxieties into Mental Disorders

Allan V. Horwitz, PhD

Board of Governors Professor of Sociology
School of Arts and Sciences
Rutgers University
New Brunswick, NJ

Jerome C. Wakefield, PhD, DSW

University Professor
Professor of Social Work
Professor of the Conceptual Foundations of Psychiatry
New York University
New York, NY

OXFORD
UNIVERSITY PRESS

OXFORD
UNIVERSITY PRESS

Oxford University Press, Inc., publishes works that further
Oxford University's objective of excellence
in research, scholarship, and education.

Oxford   New York
Auckland   Cape Town   Dar es Salaam   Hong Kong   Karachi
Kuala Lumpur   Madrid   Melbourne   Mexico City   Nairobi
New Delhi   Shanghai   Taipei   Toronto

With offices in
Argentina   Austria   Brazil   Chile   Czech Republic   France   Greece
Guatemala   Hungary   Italy   Japan   Poland   Portugal   Singapore
South Korea   Switzerland   Thailand   Turkey   Ukraine   Vietnam

Published by Oxford University Press, Inc.
198 Madison Avenue, New York, New York 10016
www.oup.com

Oxford is a registered trademark of Oxford University Press

Library of Congress Cataloging-in-Publication Data

Horwitz, Allan V.
All We Have to Fear: Psychiatry's Transformation of Natural Anxieties into
Mental Disorders/Allan V. Horwitz, Jerome C. Wakefield
      p. cm.
Includes bibliographical references and index.
ISBN 978-0-19-979375-4 (acid-free paper)
1. Anxiety disorders—Diagnosis. 2. Psychiatry—Methodology.
I. Wakefield, Jerome C. II. Title.
RC531.H68 2012
616.85'22—dc23   2011043999

This material is not intended to be, and should not be considered, a substitute for medical or other
professional advice. Treatment for the conditions described in this material is highly dependent on the
individual circumstances. And, while this material is designed to offer accurate information with respect to
the subject matter covered and to be current as of the time it was written, research and knowledge about
medical and health issues is constantly evolving and dose schedules for medications are being revised
continually, with new side effects recognized and accounted for regularly. Readers must therefore always
check the product information and clinical procedures with the most up-to-date published product
information and data sheets provided by the manufacturers and the most recent codes of conduct and safety
regulation. The publisher and the authors make no representations or warranties to readers, express or implied,
as to the accuracy or completeness of this material. Without limiting the foregoing, the publisher and the
authors make no representations or warranties as to the accuracy or efficacy of the drug dosages mentioned
in the material. The authors and the publisher do not accept, and expressly disclaim, any responsibility for any
liability, loss or risk that may be claimed or incurred as a consequence of the use and/or application of any of
the contents of this material.

9 8 7 6 5 4 3 2 1
Printed in the United States of America on acid-free paper

To the memory of my mother and father
—AVH

To Lisa, Joshua, and Zachary
—JCW

PREFACE

Evolutionary accounts of human activities have become fashionable. We are told that such varied phenomena as religious beliefs, storytelling, conceptions of beauty, generosity, the impact of sex hormones, or rape stem from traits that facilitated survival and reproduction in prehistoric hunter–gatherer bands thousands of generations ago. These explanations have been met with a torrent of criticism asserting that such theories are "just-so" stories that are unfalsifiable and, therefore, unscientific. Critics say that whatever features of ancient groups led some behaviors to be more adaptive than others can never be known, but only the subject of unproductive speculation. Astronomers can use telescopes that allow them to view patterns of light that existed many thousands of years ago; archaeologists can glean evidence from fossils about the physical features of creatures in long-past eras—but emotions leave no tangible traces. Therefore, critics claim, we just can't know what emotions were like in the past. Mental fossils and emotional telescopes that let us look back in time do not exist.

However, when it comes to fear and anxiety, perhaps there is an "emotional time machine" that does allow us to uncover what anxious emotions were like thousands of years ago in a different environment from the one we confront daily. If there is any emotion that would have been heavily shaped by our survival needs, it would be fear, which compels us to avoid dangerous situations. Yet many of our current fears make no sense. For example, consider how many people develop symptoms of extreme anxiety before they give talks, even when they are well prepared and confident and even when a disastrous talk would incur no great personal harm; or, consider how many people become terrified when they must ascend to some great height even while knowing there is no danger of falling. Despite the lack of real danger, many people feel intensely afraid under such circumstances; for example, their heart rates increase, their hands shake or become sweaty, their mouths become dry, their stomachs seem to be tied in knots, and they experience dizziness or even faintness. Such responses don't seem in any way rational or proportional responses to the actual danger present in the current situation. Even individuals themselves typically know this, yet their fear remains.

There are two views one might take of such reactions. One view, dominant within American psychiatry today, is that such disproportionate distress must be a mental disorder, where something has gone wrong with mental functioning. This book defends and explores another view—that such feelings of anxiety are often the mental equivalent of the astronomer's views of ancient patterns of light or the archaeologist's fossils. Perhaps the most common current fears, which include speaking in public, heights, snakes, darkness, strangers, and thunderstorms, are living fossils within our own minds, vestiges of what we were more appropriately biologically designed to feel in long-past eras. Such feelings made sense in distant times, when they were naturally selected as adaptive responses to genuine dangers such as bands of strangers or falls from high places. Perhaps our social anxieties about others' negative opinions of us within our own group, which seem so bewildering in a mass culture of endless relationship possibilities, also made sense in a small and cohesive human group where disapproval by even a few others could be quite dangerous. In prehistoric circumstances, such fears could allow people to focus their minds on real threats or to avoid risky situations altogether. Many of our current puzzling and irrational fears thus might be living mental fossils that reflect how humans appropriately felt in the circumstances that existed when emotions were naturally selected and became a part of human nature. We might possess an emotional time machine in the very irrational fears that are inexplicable in terms of our current environment—fears that our distant ancestors experienced quite usefully in response to the sorts of dangers that existed in prehistoric environments.

If such intuitions were our only source of knowledge regarding the ancient origins of many contemporary fears, they might understandably be dismissed as another "just-so" story, yet many different types of evidence indicate that skepticism regarding the evolutionary origins of current human characteristics, while justifiable in some instances, is unwarranted in the case of anxiety. One body of research indicates that not just our closest evolutionary relatives—non-human primates—but all living creatures display avoidance behaviors in the face of danger. Another source of support for the natural basis of anxiousness stems from the responses pre-socialized infants make to threatening situations such as heights, darkness, being left alone, or an angry face. A third reason for thinking that anxiety is a genetically programmed disposition lies in its ubiquitous presence in the earliest written literary and medical documents as well as from the universal recognition of emotions of fear across cultures. Finally, contemporary neuroscientific studies demonstrate that the brain circuitry related to anxiety activates instantaneously in response to evolutionarily threatening objects that are presented too quickly for conscious processing to occur, suggesting that its sources go deeper than rational judgment.

The central question this book confronts is the implications of the fact that anxiety is a naturally designed emotion for conceptions of normality and abnormality. Are natural emotions that are functioning as they were designed to function, but that are currently not only useless and unreasonable but also sources of intense discomfort, mental disorders? Or are such irrational and seemingly out-of-place emotions normal, if mismatched, expressions of our biologically shaped natures that no longer suit our human-reshaped environments? Even as we have reshaped our environments to be congenial to us in remarkable ways, we have also constructed them to be places where many of our natural fears are no longer rational or adaptive. If so, clinical attempts to alter these common emotions might be more related to enforcing conformity to current social norms than to correcting defects within individuals. Calling natural fears that aren't suitable to modern circumstances "mental disorders"—except for certain of the most severe and impairing variants, for every human feature can "go wrong" and become disordered—might mislead us about the sources, nature, and appropriate responses to emotions of anxiety.

ACKNOWLEDGMENTS

For Horwitz: This book was conceived while I was a Fellow-in-Residence at the Netherlands Institute of Advanced Study. This Institute provided an unsurpassed, almost utopian, scholarly environment in which to write. I am grateful to the then-Rector, Wim Blockmans, the staff, the librarians, and the other Fellows of the Institute for the incomparable year I spent there. At Rutgers, I've had the good fortune to have been surrounded by superb scholars and administrators. As always, David Mechanic—the Director of the Institute for Health, Health Care Policy, and Aging Research—has been a constant source of wisdom, guidance, and support. The faculty at the Health Institute and Sociology Department—in particular Deborah Carr, Gerald Grob, Ellen Idler, Jane Miller, Sarah Rosenfield, Kristen Springer, and Eviatar Zerubavel—have constituted a special group of colleagues and friends. Douglas Greenberg, the Executive Dean of the School of Arts and Sciences, has been an exceptional academic leader whose highest priority is to facilitate the research of his faculty. I am grateful to these institutions and individuals for all their help in completing this work.

For Wakefield: My interest in exploring anxiety and its disorders was sparked by my grappling in another book project with Freud's oedipal theory of anxiety neuroses in his case study "Analysis of a Phobia in a Five-Year-Old Boy," known as the case of "Little Hans." I came to believe that anxiety posed novel conceptual challenges regarding how normality and mental disorders are defined and how these categories are used socially—problems that went beyond those that Allan and I addressed in our earlier book on depression, *The Loss of Sadness*. I thank Allan for inviting me to undertake this journey with him. I am grateful to my wife, Lisa, and my sons Joshua and Zachary, for their enthusiastic encouragement throughout my work on this project, and to my mother, Helen Sherman, for her love, which, internalized, makes the anxieties involved in all my work tolerable. My brother Marc contributed his helpful and judicious perspective. The Silver School of Social Work at New York University provided an ideal environment in which to pursue my clinical theory interests; I thank our superb dean, Lynn Videka, for her support of this and many other scholarly endeavors. I also wish to express my appreciation to the NYU Humanities Initiative and its director, Jane Tylus, as well as NYU's provost, David McLaughlin, for a Faculty Fellowship that enabled me to spend a wonderful year focusing on the humanistic implications of psychiatric nosology. Among professional colleagues, I must single out Robert Spitzer and Michael First for many years of illuminating discussion and debate.

Finally, our editor at Oxford University Press, Craig Panner, has been a constant source of encouragement and assistance. We also greatly appreciate the editorial help that Steve Holtje, Kathryn Winder, and Karen Kwak have provided us.

CONTENTS

CHAPTER 1
The Puzzle of Anxiety Disorders

Fears, worries, and apprehensions are painful and ubiquitous aspects of human existence, whether they are common or idiosyncratic, specific or diffuse, rational or irrational. Studies of the U.S. population indicate that the most common forms of psychiatric disturbances by far are various fears that, when intense, psychiatry currently classifies as "anxiety disorders": fear of public speaking, heights, or meeting new people; fears of snakes or rodents; and many other conditions where people experience intense anxiety.[1]

Moreover, it might seem as if a startling increase in the number of anxiety disorders has occurred in recent years. Consider that in 1980, the third edition of the authoritative *Diagnostic and Statistical Manual of Mental Disorders* (*DSM*) of the American Psychiatric Association stated: "It has been estimated that from 2 to 4% of the general population has at some time had a disorder that this manual would classify as an Anxiety Disorder."[2] Then, the first large community study conducted after the publication of this manual, the Epidemiologic Catchment Area Study, found that about one out of ten people had an anxiety disorder in any given year and that roughly 15% of individuals experienced these conditions at some point in their lives.[3] Just two decades later, a similar and equally rigorous study, the National Comorbidity Study Replication (NCS-R), yielded the shocking result that almost one out of five people had had an anxiety disorder over the past year, and more than a quarter of the population (28.8%) had had one at some point in their lives.[4]

Even the NCS-R actually *underestimates* the frequency of anxiety disorders, as measured by psychiatry's current criteria for diagnosing mental disorder. Because it asks people to remember years later what anxieties they had earlier in life, many respondents forget past episodes. A recent New Zealand study with substantially improved methodology that involved repeated interviews of participants established that in any given year between ages 18 and 32, nearly a quarter of all young adults (22.8%) experience an anxiety disorder and that virtually half (49.5%) report at least one such disorder during the entire period.[5] Obviously, the study would have yielded even higher estimates if it had included disorders emerging after age 32 or before age 18.

So, according to current psychiatric criteria, well over half the population suffers from anxiety disorders at some point in their lives. This estimate is roughly *twenty times* as high as the *DSM* assertion just 30 years ago. A change of this magnitude calls for an explanation—one that is lacking in the current psychiatric literature.

The very commonness of anxiety and its disorders raises many perplexing questions not just for psychiatry but also for individuals who confront their own anxieties and try to understand them and to decide what to do about their suffering. Among the questions such a person might ask are:

- How does psychiatry distinguish normal fears from disordered anxieties, and has it got the distinction right?
- If anxiety makes no rational sense, does that mean it is a psychiatric disorder?
- Is the seeming rise in anxiety disorders a real epidemic of medical disorder, a normal response to our increasingly stressful lifestyles, or perhaps an artifact of the way psychiatry's understanding of anxiety has been evolving?
- When my anxieties keep me from doing socially or personally desirable activities such as performing in a theater club, going to a party alone, or making presentations at work—or if I'm afraid of heights and won't go hiking on cliffs or won't travel by air—is there something wrong with me?

This book explores the varieties and subtleties of anxiety and grapples with the question of what distinguishes normal feelings of anxiety from disordered types of anxiousness. Most of all, we try to place the understanding of anxiety within the history and current framework of the psychiatric study of anxiety disorders. We attempt to evaluate how psychiatry confronts an amorphous, variegated human phenomenon such as anxiety and attempts to carve it into normal and disordered conditions and into a variety of distinct types of disorders. We believe that such an investigation of psychiatry's approach to anxiety can teach us much about not only anxiety itself but also how our culture takes a phenomenon and tries to classify it into normal and disordered types in order to study and control it. We also hope to learn something about how correctly or incorrectly—or ambiguously—the definitions of normality and pathology are applied in such a classificatory process.

VARIETIES OF NORMAL FEAR AND ANXIETY

Philosophers have long emphasized that much anxiety results from pondering life's mysteries and uncertainties, as in *angst* about the inevitability of death and the meaning of existence. For most people, however, far more mundane situations— and ones much less immediately threatening than, say, a car rapidly bearing down on one in the street—create anxiousness. They become worried when they might be late for a meeting, miss a plane, park in a no-parking zone, see a police car approaching, or give a public talk. Such everyday occurrences as leaving a middle-school child at home can lead to intense worry among parent and child alike: "All the while I was out, I kept looking at my watch and listening for my phone. He called me four times in an hour: 'When are you coming home? Where are you? Are you on line yet? Did you leave the store yet?' It made me so nervous, I just browsed and left."[6] These worries are built into the structure of modern life, emerging daily or even hourly, especially among people with nervous temperaments.

Sometimes such common occurrences are powerful enough to lead to extraordinarily intense, albeit normal, periods of acute anxiety that resemble what people experience when they suffer from serious anxiety disorders. Consider the experience of the eminent psychiatric researcher Kenneth Kendler,[7] a mountain climber who has had incidents of slipping and sliding until he is literally on the edge of a precipice. At such times, he reports, he experiences feelings of fearfulness and terror along with shortness of breath and heart palpitations; these are indistinguishable from the criteria for panic disorders. Yet, Kendler observes, due to the context in which they arise, his panic symptoms do not indicate a genuine disorder but rather are an intense normal response to a genuinely threatening situation. It is only the context of Kendler's symptoms, and their transient appearance and resolution as his circumstances changed and his safety was restored, that make it possible to differentiate his normal reactions from those of a panic attack. Once Kendler's expectation of a dire outcome receded and his feet were back on the ground, his anxiety naturally disappeared.

Whenever people face life-threatening situations, their resulting fear can be severe—think of the immediate reactions of New Yorkers in the area of the 9/11 attacks and how they ran in panic from the collapsing World Trade Center towers. Soon after the 9/11 attacks, large numbers of people reported symptoms of intense anxiety, but the number of people with anxiety symptoms subsided dramatically over the months following the attacks as people again came to feel a sense of safety. By six months after the attacks, only a negligible proportion still met criteria for an anxiety disorder.[8] The initial responses of the majority seem analogous to Kendler's symptoms and likely did not indicate a disorder at all, but instead were natural reactions to an extremely threatening situation.

Life-endangering contexts can generate a degree of normal anxiety that leads to extreme actions. One example (immortalized in a recent motion picture, *127 Hours*) is that of a hiker in a remote area whose arm got caught under a fallen rock—and who, fearing his eventual death, amputated the arm with his hunting knife in order to escape.[9] Another poignant case is that of an Israeli woman who, when terrorists attacked her house, hid with two of her children—one a 2-year-old—and watched from her hideout as the terrorists killed her husband and older son. Her young daughter started to cry, and the woman, terrified that the girl's cries would give away their hiding place and thus lead to all their deaths, placed her hand over the child's mouth to stifle any sounds. The terrorists left, but the woman's child died of suffocation as a result of the mother's actions—actions that saved two family members from dying along with the child.[10] The intense fears that provoked these extraordinary actions were nevertheless normal-range expressions given the unusually threatening situations that evoked them.

Unlike such responses to immediate—but brief—risks of death, many threatening situations are enduring. The resulting anxiety might also be chronic, yet still normal. For example, many survivors of the Hurricane Katrina disaster in New Orleans experienced anxiety symptoms that, unlike those following the 9/11 attacks, did not subside quickly because the effects of the disaster were not corrected. The lack of adequate housing, schooling, policing, and employment continued for substantial numbers of people long after the hurricane itself was gone.[11] Six months after the disaster, nearly half the residents of the New Orleans metropolitan area still reported high levels of anxiety symptoms. For most of these individuals, this persistent anxiety likely resulted from the continuing uncertainties of their living situations, not from internal psychiatric conditions. Other enduring anxiety conditions, whether they are part of an adolescent's identity crisis or an adult's midlife or empty-nest crisis, involve more amorphous and indefinable yet still powerful senses of anxiety resulting from important life challenges that may initially seem irresolvable.

At other times, it is neither immediate nor chronic dangers and uncertainties that create intense normal anxiety. Instead, some feature of the present situation triggers memories of a terrifying event that provoked such fear in the past. Such normal processes of recollecting terrifying events can quickly arouse intense anxiety and even panic. For example, the features of the 9/11 attacks, such as the roar of jet engines from low-flying aircraft, could years later still create acute feelings of anxiety in New Yorkers. Eight years after 9/11, the Pentagon allowed a low-altitude flyover of Manhattan near the World Trade Center site for the purpose of taking publicity photos of the presidential airplane. *The New York Times*, under the headline "Jet Flyover Frightens New Yorkers," reported that the sight of the low-flying Boeing 747 speeding in the shadows of skyscrapers, trailed by two fighter jets, "awakened barely dormant fears of a terrorist attack, causing a momentary panic that sent workers pouring out of buildings on both sides of the Hudson River. . . . Some sobbed as they made their way to the street."[12] A 36-year-old brokerage worker explained, "We all ran to the window, and I thought, that's it, we're all dead. It brought back all the memories of 9/11. I said, 'I have to get out of here now!'"[13] These responses were intense, but normal, fear responses to a foolishly terrifying act that should have been predicted to trigger such memories and anxieties, given the meaning that such events would inevitably have for those who experienced 9/11.

Clearly, there are many reasons for normal fears and worries to arise and persist. "If you're not nervous," jazz musician Miles Davis reputedly said, "you're not paying attention."[14] Certain fears are appropriate responses to threatening contexts; when these contexts are severely threatening, the resulting anxiety symptoms may be intense. Other fears seem biologically prepared to be triggered easily, but only if one first experiences particular kinds of frightening events. Some fears are more cognitively acquired, such as when we learn information that some object poses a danger to us. Still other fears, such as of heights, darkness, or strangers, seem to be innate. All these varieties of normal fear and worry can arise in people who have no disorder whatsoever, but all these processes can occasionally go wrong and lead to anxiety disorders.

DISORDERED ANXIETY

Many anxiety conditions do not seem to be related in any comprehensible way to external situations, to previous terrifying experiences, or to our biological nature as a species. Take the example of the poet Emily Dickinson who, by the time she was 40, would not leave her home and hid in her room, unwilling to see even her long-time friends.[15] Nothing about Dickinson's circumstances could account for her refusal to walk outside or to meet with people she had known for extended periods of time. A great number of people ranging from Isaac Newton—who spent several years inside his house—to actress Kim Basinger have shared the fear of going out in public.[16]

Other people compulsively engage in ritualistic behaviors that seemingly have no purpose and that make them intensely anxious when their routines are disturbed: "Ms. Johnson can tell you why she needs to chew her food in sets of three bites or drink her beverages three sips at a time. Three is her magic number."[17] Such people may have no desire to engage in their obsessions and may realize they are irrational, but they nevertheless are unable to stop their behaviors.

A more unusual set of compulsions and obsessions beset one of Freud's most famous cases, known as the "Rat Man." Freud reported the patient's presenting symptoms as follows:

> A youngish man of university education introduced himself to me with the statement that he had suffered from obsessions ever since his childhood, but with particular intensity for the last four years. The chief features of his disorder were fears that something might happen to two people of whom he was very fond—his father and a lady whom he admired. Besides this he was aware of compulsive impulses—such as an impulse, for instance, to cut his throat with a razor; and further he produced prohibitions, sometimes in connection with quite unimportant things. He had wasted years, he told me, in fighting against these ideas of his, and in this way had lost much ground in the course of his life.[18]

The patient reported that he had heard a captain in his military unit describe a particularly horrifying torture in which hungry rats were placed in a pot that was overturned onto the buttocks of a man and allowed to eat into his anus. He subsequently had obsessive thoughts that this torture was being perpetrated on his girlfriend and his father (who had already passed away). The patient developed elaborate ritualized statements and gestures to defend against these thoughts.

Although normal anxiety can be terribly uncomfortable, disordered forms of anxiety have the capacity to be some of the most painful and intolerable of all human experiences. Indeed, the sixteenth century philosopher Michel Montaigne famously noted, "The thing I fear most is fear. Moreover it exceeds all other disorders in intensity."[19] Fifteen hundred years before Montaigne, the renowned ancient physician Galen described patients who are so afraid of death that they paradoxically want to kill themselves.[20] Indeed, intense and unremitting anxiety is a risk factor for suicide.[21] Andrew Solomon, who presented his severe depressive sufferings to the public in his best-selling book *Noonday Demons*, observed that the anxiety he experienced as part of his depression in some ways frightened him more than the depression itself:

> Then the anxiety set in. If someone said to me that I had to be depressed for the next month, I would say that as long as I knew it was temporary, I could do it; the most acute hell of depression is the feeling that you will never emerge, and if you alleviate that, the

state, though miserable, is bearable. But if someone said to me I had to have acute anxiety for the next month, I would kill myself, because every second of it is so intolerably awful. It is the constant feeling of being absolutely terrified and not knowing what it is that you're afraid of. It resembles the sensation you have if you slip or trip, the feeling when the ground is rushing up at you before you land. That feeling lasts about a second-and-a-half. The anxiety phase of my first depression lasted six months. It was incredibly paralyzing.[22]

Sometimes memory, or even second-hand information, leads to fear of such intensity and duration that it seems inexplicable as a normal response. For example, some veterans returning from Iraq experience powerful flashes of terror from memories triggered by stimuli most people would perceive as harmless, but that remind them of combat experiences. There is nothing abnormal about situations that trigger such memories also triggering anxiety—in fact, one would assume this power of emotionally salient memories is an adaptive mechanism for keeping us from re-experiencing certain threats. However, sometimes the re-experiencing of the fear becomes so intense and endures so far beyond the immediate circumstances that trigger it that it renders combat-scarred vets unable to carry on with other aspects of their lives—for example, they may experience the crowds of people in a mall as a threat that triggers intense anxiety and hypervigilance, and this feeling may stay with them in a way that makes routine life tasks and relationships impossible.[23] As to the power of second-hand information when it is sufficiently unsettling, Hans Christian Andersen, after hearing about the death of a close friend in a fire aboard a ship, suffered from such an intense lifelong fear of fire that he would carry a rope with him at all times so as to make his escape should a fire trap him.[24]

But not all disordered states of anxiety involve fear of a particular action, event, or object. Sudden panic attacks when there is no obvious context or trigger, in which people not afraid of anything in particular experience heart palpitations and other symptoms that make them think they are having a heart attack and are going to die, can cripple a person's life. Generalized anxiety of a lesser intensity, where one feels anxious or worries disproportionately about various not-very-threatening concerns in contexts that do not truly explain the level of anxiety, can also make an individual miserable.

Unlike natural fears, these unfathomable symptoms—sometimes relatively harmless affectations, sometimes devastatingly distressing and impairing—cannot be explained by consideration of their context or by understandable reactions to memories of past dangers. They seem to indicate that something has gone wrong in the way our fears are aroused and sustained.

MISMATCHES BETWEEN HUMAN NATURE AND THE MODERN ENVIRONMENT

If some anxiety conditions seem to be contextually appropriate and emotionally proportionate to the direness of the situation and others seem inexplicable within their circumstances, a third type of anxiety doesn't quite seem to fit either of these categories. These anxieties are out of proportion to the actual danger in the present environment yet seem understandable as reactions that came down to us as part of our biological inheritance of fears that did make sense in the prehistoric past.

Early hominids had much to fear. The most ancient stages of human evolution featured environments where people without powerful weaponry faced numerous predators, could do little to protect themselves from harsh climates and natural disasters, and were defenseless against disease. Food was often scarce and in many environments was impossible to preserve for long periods of time. Dangers were everywhere at the same time that security from threats was weak and often unavailable. Small bands of just one or two hundred people faced other hostile groups of humans and other predators, without any government to protect them. Although a range of strategies could be adaptive for dealing with some specific circumstances, on average, vigilance, caution, and readiness to flee at a moment's notice would probably have had the greatest evolutionary payoff.

Many fears that do not seem helpful today were useful at the time that they became part of the biological nature of our species. A good example is snake phobia, a common and often intense fear. Charles Darwin recounted an incident that indicates the powerful instinctual nature of snake phobias:

> I put my face close to the thick glass-plate in front of a puff-adder in the Zoological Gardens, with the firm determination of not starting back if the snake struck at me; but, as soon as the blow was struck, my resolution went for nothing and I jumped a yard or two backwards with astonishing rapidity. My will and reason were powerless against the imagination of a danger which had never been experienced.[25]

Much evidence shows that snake fear is biologically programmed to be easily triggered in us, and the reason is not hard to see. Intense fear of snakes was valuable in the ancestral environments where snakes posed serious dangers.

Snake fear might seem outdated and useless to urban dwellers, but its value remains in those modern locations that still feature considerable numbers of snakes, such as the desert terrain of Arizona. One news story under the headline "Rattlesnakes Bite 4 Over Weekend; One Man Wanted To Pet Snake, Doctors Say," reported that snakes bit eight people in the Phoenix area over the previous week.[26]

One victim, Patrick Hotchkiss of Quartzsite, AZ, "had just stepped off his porch Sunday afternoon when he was struck. . . . 'I should've been more vigilant. Usually I am,' said Hotchkiss. . . . Some of the other victims were gardening or hiking. One child was playing in a yard." Some of the bites occurred under odd circumstances that vividly illustrate the danger of having no fear of snakes:

> But others got closer than they should have. Doctors said one man was bitten on the
> hand after trying to pet a snake. They said the man had been drinking prior to the inci-
> dent. "We've seen several people who've tried petting the snakes, and even on occasion
> people trying to kiss the snake. Any of those things usually result in the patient getting
> bitten," said Dr. Michael Levine, a toxicologist at Banner Poison Control Center.

Obviously an innate tendency to develop a fear of snakes might still be a good thing in those environments that snakes inhabit. No matter how inexplicable a fear of snakes might seem at first in an apartment dweller in Manhattan, the fear is quite understandable when placed within the context of our development as a species and the biological nature that evolutionary shaping imparted to us. Some of these natural fears are rooted in immediately perceived real dangers, others in our memories of past dangers that influence our present expectations, and still others in our species' history of natural selection that shaped our fear for dealing with dangers that existed in ancestral times but that no longer pose threats.

But some emotions that were adaptive during this evolutionary period were genetically transmitted to future generations for whom, rather than being protective, they might instead be a constant source of needless distress, suffering, and impairment. Consider the anxiety of the popular former sports announcer John Madden, who, like many people, is terrified of air travel. Despite having to travel long distances almost every week, Madden would never fly but always used buses that were far more inconvenient and time-consuming. Given that flying is many times safer than driving, Madden's intense fear might seem to be as inexplicable as Emily Dickinson's unwillingness to see her friends, but many people tend to be afraid of flying, and their fear seems to make a certain amount of sense in terms of human nature, though not in terms of what is currently rational. Of course, air travel is an invention that did not exist at the time humans evolved, so fear of air travel in and of itself is not a biologically shaped fear. Rather, air travel happens to have several features that human beings were shaped to fear. Intense fear of being at extreme heights where falling would mean death and of entering enclosed spaces where escape is impossible might have been adaptive in ancient periods when such places were genuinely dangerous and to be avoided. Fear of being passive and out of control while facing such anxieties might additionally be naturally anxiety-provoking. People who had fears that motivated them to stay away from such situations might have avoided the occasional disaster and thus passed on to their descendants genes that made them more fearful of entering enclosed spaces, climbing to higher altitudes, and not being in control. Madden's fear could thus reflect the natural, if no longer constructive, operation of such biologically designed psychological mechanisms. Its evolutionary origin would explain why a substantial percentage of the population shares this fear, even if many people manage to overcome it and, unlike Madden, continue to fly.

Air travel is extremely unlikely to pose the risk of falling from a height or finding oneself trapped by a predator in an enclosed space. Such fears are at the same time natural and yet no longer adaptive in most modern environments. They are an unfortunate mismatch between anachronistic but natural emotions that once were functional and our modern, technologically transformed environment.

Yet, sometimes the manifestation of archaic fears in current circumstances does indicate a dysfunction. For example, some snake fears are so great and so beyond a level of rationality or control that they must be considered disorders. Some urban dwellers have such an intense fear of snakes that the phobia may impair their lives despite hardly ever coming into contact with a snake. Images of snakes in movies or magazines, or mere thoughts of snakes, may be intensely anxiety-provoking, and overwhelming fear of encountering a snake may cause such people to avoid situations in which there is even the smallest chance of seeing a snake. This may keep them from traveling or enjoying outdoor activities such as hiking or swimming in ponds, or even gardening in their own backyards. Arguably these are cases of a natural fear going wrong in some way so as to become a disorder that undermines basic functioning.

INDIVIDUAL VARIATION

The ubiquity of innate fears that are not necessarily adaptive in modern life provides one answer to the question of why anxiety disorders seem to be so common. When fears of crawling animals, flying, strangers, or public speaking are considered to be pathological, rates of anxiety disorders will soar because humans were naturally designed to have such fears. A second reason why so much fearful behavior can readily be classified as disordered is that individual tendencies to express anxiety vary continuously. People who are naturally at the high end of this temperamental continuum can be mistakenly classified as having anxiety disorders.

While it is easy to talk in generalities about anxiety, as if all people share the same basic anxieties, the fact is that the sources and intensity of anxiety vary to a remarkable degree from person to person, constituting individualized "fear maps." Different individuals make different kinds of fear assessments of environmental contexts and have different thresholds that activate fear responses.[27] Moreover, people differ in their ability to exert control over their anxious emotions. The great amount of individual variation in emotionality creates a source of ambiguity in distinguishing between normal and pathological psychological states. One might ask regarding biologically designed fears: Why, if it was selected, isn't everyone equally afraid? If such fears are "part of human nature," then why doesn't everyone experience such anxiety? Why didn't evolution converge on one optimal value or a narrow range of values for everyone?

Consider the remarkable normal human variation around one of the most universal fears: height. Indeed, some major tourist attractions capitalize on people's desires to experience the intense anxiety of being at extreme heights while standing on glass surfaces that provide the impression of great instability. For example, one website describes the Sears Tower (currently the Willis Tower) in Chicago as:

> . . . new glass enclosures that extend 4.3 feet beyond the side of the building. Beneath peoples' feet lies the sprawling Illinois city—103 stories, or 1,353 feet, below. Just an inch-and-a-half of glass separates the visitor from the street underneath.

In fact, it is unreasonable to be afraid of walking on such glass surfaces, which are completely safe marvels of engineering (see Figure 1.1).

The comments about this attraction posted on a website that displayed a picture of one of these new transparent spaces demonstrate both the naturalness of fear of heights and the stark individual differences in this fear in reaction to the photo or to their actual experiences. While many people are terrified by the idea of walking on solid glass over an abyss under their feet, even though it is secured by steel, many others are comfortable hanging in the air with no apparent protection:

> I can barely even look at the picture. I certainly couldn't stand on it. It gives me vertigo just thinking about it.
> Its [sic] awesome, but I near crapped myself when the cube moved.
> Now that's scary.
> HA! Not a chance in hell you'd get me out on that thing.
> That would scare me to death as well.
> Never in a million years would I dare to do that.

However, scattered among the overwhelmingly fearful comments were other less terrified and even positive feelings:

> Oooh, I would like to stand there!
> cool image, cool idea.

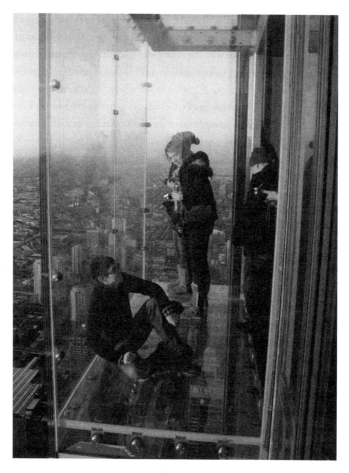

Figure 1.1: Picture of Willis Tower, used with permission from Free Software Foundation.

But even some who had tried it out expressed some degree of cautiousness at the same time:

> I did eventually, and very carefully[,] ease my way out onto the glass abyss.
> I stood on the one in the CN Tower in Toronto. Just be ready.

These thoroughly diverse reactions show how many of our most intense fears, even those that are innate, affect individuals to a greater or lesser degree. While all people have certain innate fears, the diversity of their temperaments and experiences leads to great diversity in how much they are able to suppress these fears over time.

The basic challenge humans face is not to avoid acquiring fears—they are largely part of our nature—but rather to learn how to overcome the many currently useless innate fears that we experience. "It is less a matter of acquiring fears of the dark and of strangers," according to psychologist Stanley Rachman, "than of developing the necessary competence and courage to deal effectively with the existing predispositions or actual fears."[28] Adequate criteria for anxiety disorders must take into account normal human variation in anxiousness and must separate genuine pathology from both high-end anxious temperaments and low-end skilled suppression or endurance of natural fears.

CULTURAL VARIATION

An additional source of variation in anxiety—and correspondingly a source of difficulty in setting boundaries between normal and pathological anxiety—has to do with cultural variation. The capacity to experience emotions is biologically given; the architecture of the brain sets the general parameters for psychological functions. Yet, evolution has also designed humans to be sensitive to culture: people are, in essence, hard-wired to be attuned to processes such as valued cultural goals, social comparisons and evaluations, and social hierarchies.[29] Consequently, recognizing what is a normal-range emotional response often requires a knowledge of the individual's cultural context.

While evolution programmed anxious emotions to arise in threatening and uncertain situations, culture helps define what particular objects and situations people consider to be dangerous, what cues activate their fear responses, and what sorts of things they worry about as well as the degree of intensity or duration with which one should respond. For example, while witchcraft is a common source of anxiousness in many African societies, it is unlikely to be a source of fear in modern Western cultures.[30] Witch fear is seen as reasonable in the former but not the latter. Fears of being buried alive dominated nineteenth century consciousness in the United Kingdom and United States but would be extremely rare at present [31]; conversely, food allergies, a rare source of anxiousness in the past, are a dominant source of worry in the contemporary United States. Criteria for anxiety disorders face the challenge of avoiding pathologizing culturally appropriate fears that result from normal human emotional malleability in response to cultural environments.

Moreover, social structures and values shape the degree of harm that any given state of anxiousness produces, or is considered to produce. For example, the impairments of social and occupational functioning that psychiatry uses to demarcate social phobias from intense shyness emerge only when group norms reward social engagement and outgoing styles of interaction.[32] Social phobias are less likely to be harmful in groups that value restrained styles of sociability. When impairment is the criterion used to distinguish normal shyness from social phobia, identical conditions that are viewed as normal in one context can be judged as disordered in another. Indeed, a culture may simultaneously subject its members to naturally anxiety-provoking experiences and then judge as disordered those who cannot adequately suppress the resulting natural anxiety. For example, our own culture frequently demands that people in certain occupations engage in public speaking to groups of strangers; if this activity provokes intense anxiety, as it is probably biologically shaped to do, our culture then judges that anxiety to be a form of social phobia.

What is appropriate or inappropriate psychological functioning is thus partly biological but also partly cultural. Cultural definitions influence what emotions are considered to be suitable and unsuitable, excessive or deficient, and balanced or unbalanced in given situations. This is why it is difficult and perhaps impossible to define mental disorders without using terms such as "excessive," "unreasonable," "inappropriate," and the like to reflect deviation from sociocultural standards that vary substantially across different cultural contexts. Such terms are not just placeholders until more knowledge is obtained; they are inherent aspects of definitions of anxiety disorders because cultural definitions are an irreducible component of the contextual factors that partially determine whether a fear or anxiety is likely normal or disordered.

We began this chapter by asking the question of how rates of anxiety disorders could have risen by as much as twentyfold over the past thirty years to encompass as much as over half the population. The discussion above indicates some preliminary answers. For reasons later chapters explore in depth, the psychiatric profession developed diagnostic criteria that did not adequately distinguish evolutionarily natural fears from true anxiety disorders. Moreover, these criteria lent themselves to pathologizing people with high-end, but naturally anxious, temperaments that are within normal range rather than disordered. Finally, the criteria did not sufficiently grapple with how culture can shape definitions and expressions of anxiety. The seeming pervasiveness of anxiety disorders results from considering evolutionary normal but currently maladaptive fears, high-end anxious temperaments, and culturally appropriately triggered expressions all as signs of anxiety disorders.

DSM CATEGORIES OF ANXIETY DISORDERS

A central task of this book is to consider whether the current criteria the psychiatric profession uses to diagnose anxiety disorders are adequately separating pathological from natural anxiety. These criteria are found in the *Diagnostic and Statistical*

Manual of Mental Disorders, 4th Edition, Text Revision (DSM-IV-TR). In abbreviated form, the eight primary categories of anxiety disorder are as follows[33]:

> *Specific phobia* is a "marked and persistent fear that is excessive or unreasonable, cued by the presence or anticipation of a specific object or situation (e.g., flying, heights, animals, receiving an injection, seeing blood)."[34]
>
> *Social phobia* or *social anxiety disorder* is "a marked and persistent fear of one or more social or performance situations in which the person is exposed to unfamiliar people or to possible scrutiny by others. The individual fears that he or she will act in a way (or show anxiety symptoms) that will be humiliating or embarrassing."[35]
>
> *Agoraphobia* is "anxiety about being in places or situations from which escape might be difficult (or embarrassing) or in which help may not be available in the event of having a Panic Attack or panic-like symptoms. Agoraphobic fears typically involve characteristic clusters of situations that include being outside the home alone; being in a crowd or standing in a line; being on a bridge; and traveling in a bus, train, or automobile. The situations are avoided (e.g., travel is restricted) or else are endured with marked distress or with anxiety about having a Panic Attack or panic-like symptoms, or require the presence of a companion."[36]
>
> *Panic disorder* is characterized by "recurrent unexpected Panic Attacks about which there is persistent concern. A Panic Attack is a discrete period in which there is the sudden onset of intense apprehension, fearfulness, or terror, often associated with feelings of impending doom. During these attacks, symptoms such as shortness of breath, palpitations, chest pain or discomfort, choking or smothering sensations, and fear of 'going crazy' or losing control are present. . . . The attack has a sudden onset and builds to a peak rapidly (usually in 10 minutes or less) and is often accompanied by a sense of imminent danger or impending doom and an urge to escape"; accompanying symptoms may include "palpitations, sweating, trembling or shaking, sensations of shortness of breath or smothering, feeling of choking, chest pain or discomfort, nausea or abdominal distress, dizziness or lightheadedness, derealization or depersonalization, fear of losing control or 'going crazy,' fear of dying, paresthesias, and chills or hot flushes."[37]
>
> *Posttraumatic stress disorder* is the development of characteristic symptoms following exposure to an extreme traumatic stressor involving direct personal experience of an event that involves actual or threatened death, serious injury, or other threat to one's physical integrity; witnessing an event that involves death, injury, or a threat to the physical integrity of another person; or learning about unexpected or violent death, serious harm, or

threat of death or injury experienced by a family member or other close associate (Criterion A1). The person's response to the event must involve intense fear, helplessness, or horror (Criterion A2). The characteristic symptoms resulting from the exposure to the extreme trauma include persistent re-experiencing of the traumatic event (Criterion B), persistent avoidance of stimuli associated with the trauma and numbing of general responsiveness (Criterion C), and persistent symptoms of increased arousal (Criterion D).[38]

Acute stress disorder is "the development of characteristic anxiety, dissociative, and other symptoms that occurs within 1 month after exposure to an extreme traumatic stressor. . . . [T]he individual has at least three of the following dissociative symptoms: a subjective sense of numbing, detachment, or absence of emotional responsiveness; a reduction in awareness of his or her surroundings; derealization; depersonalization; or dissociative amnesia"; In addition, "the traumatic event is persistently reexperienced (e.g., recurrent recollections, images, thoughts, dreams, illusions, flashback episodes, a sense of reliving the event, or distress on exposure to reminders of the event). Second, reminders of the trauma (e.g., places, people, activities) are avoided. Finally, hyperarousal in response to stimuli reminiscent of the trauma is present (e.g., difficulty sleeping, irritability, poor concentration, hypervigilance, an exaggerated startle response, and motor restlessness)."[39]

Obsessive-compulsive disorder consists of either obsessions or compulsions. Obsessions are "recurrent and persistent thoughts, impulses, or images that are experienced, at some time during the disturbance, as intrusive and inappropriate and that cause marked anxiety or distress," that "the person attempts to ignore or suppress," but are "not simply excessive worries about real-life problems." Compulsions are defined as "repetitive behaviors (e.g., hand washing, ordering, checking) or mental acts (e.g., praying, counting, repeating words silently) that the person feels driven to perform in response to an obsession, or according to rules that must be applied rigidly," where "the behaviors or mental acts are aimed at preventing or reducing distress or preventing some dreaded event or situation; however, these behaviors or mental acts either are not connected in a realistic way with what they are designed to neutralize or prevent or are clearly excessive."[40]

Finally, *generalized anxiety disorder* (GAD) consists of "excessive anxiety and worry (apprehensive expectation), occurring more days than not for a period of at least 6 months, about a number of events or activities," where "the individual finds it difficult to control the worry. . . . The anxiety and worry are accompanied by at least three additional symptoms from a list that includes restlessness, being easily fatigued, difficulty concentrating, irritability, muscle tension, and disturbed sleep."[41]

The *DSM* employs several typical strategies that attempt to distinguish pathological anxiety disorders from normal anxiety. First, the criteria for each condition list a variety of symptoms that indicate the possible presence of the disorder. Second, they require the presence of a sufficient number of symptoms from the defined group, mandate that the anxiety is "marked" and thus possesses a sufficient degree of severity, and indicate a necessary duration of symptoms. Third, in order to exclude trivial, transient, and innocuous anxiety states from disordered status, they indicate that only symptoms that have distressing or impairing consequences are disorders. Finally, the anxiety disorder criteria commonly contain qualifiers such as "excessive," "unreasonable," "inappropriate," or "unexpected" that attempt to differentiate disordered symptoms from natural fears and worries. For example, phobic disorders involve "unreasonable" or "excessive" symptoms, obsessions in obsessive-compulsive disorders are "intrusive" and "inappropriate," and obsessive-compulsive symptoms generally are "excessive or unreasonable." These terms indicate a clear recognition that symptoms alone cannot separate anxiety disorders from natural concerns but must be placed in their contexts.

Despite the *DSM*'s extensive efforts to separate normal from pathological anxiety, the criteria sets raise many questions about how to best draw the lines that distinguish normal and pathological conditions. The remaining chapters of this book will consider a number of general issues about the great complexity involved in establishing boundaries between natural and abnormal states of anxiety.

SOME QUESTIONS ABOUT ANXIETY

Anxiety's ubiquity, diversity, variety of etiological pathways, widely varying levels of intensity in the population, and complex relationship to personal and species histories raise a number of challenging questions about the nature of the normal and the pathological and how we should respond to them. These questions include the following:

1. *What is the basis for distinguishing between natural fears and anxiety disorders—that is, what is the definition of "normal" when it comes to anxiety?* Sometimes anxiety symptoms are natural, designed responses to dangerous situations, but at other times they indicate mental disorders. Definitions of disorder must clarify what distinguishes anxiety disorders from realistic worries, concerns, and fears. We strive to understand whether there is a sharp boundary

(so that in principle we can always tell whether anxiety is normal or disordered), or if the distinction is essentially fuzzy and indeterminate, with vague borders and some gaps. If there is considerable fuzziness, are there nevertheless clear cases on both sides, or is the distinction between normal and disordered anxiety basically arbitrary?

2. *Should anxiety that is grounded in evolutionarily normal fear mechanisms but that is maladaptive in current environments be seen as a disorder or as an unfortunate but normal aspect of human nature?* This is a question about how we should think about "mismatches" between what we fear and what is rational to fear in our current environments. Fears of darkness, wild animals, heights, enclosed spaces, or public speaking are neither reasonable nor particularly useful to most people at present but might nevertheless be programmed into the human genome. Can distinguishing presently irrational natural fears from disorders enhance our understanding of the causes, prognoses, and treatments of both kinds of conditions, or should they be lumped together as disorders?

3. *Do current conceptions of anxiety disorders have misleading implications for research about the causes of anxiety disorders?* The DSM categories of anxiety disorders might poorly reflect genuinely disordered types of brain states: They could lump together people with dysfunctional fear mechanisms, those whose fear mechanisms are normal but who become anxious in situations that are no longer dangerous in modern environments, and some who are higher than average in their normal anxiety responses. Conflating natural and pathological conditions into a single category might make it difficult for research into the causes of anxiety disorders to reach valid or useful conclusions.

4. *Given the ambiguous boundaries between normal fears, anxiety disorders, and environmental mismatches, how do social groups actually come to determine the dividing lines between these conditions?* Nature might not set any distinct lines between normal and pathological anxiety conditions. This would create opportunities for interested social groups to set distinctions among various categories along a wide range of possibilities. What kinds of social and diagnostic considerations influence such decisions?

5. *To what extent do current official psychiatric diagnostic criteria get the distinction between normal and disordered anxiety right, and how do they classify the ambiguous cases?* If the current criteria are flawed, can evolutionary theory help improve current diagnoses of anxiety disorders so that they can better distinguish true anxiety disorders from normal fears and worries?

6. *Can statistics about the number of people in the community with untreated anxiety disorders that stem from these criteria be believed, or are they the result of*

pathologizing natural emotions? Community studies might be especially prone to mistakenly classify both proportionate and mismatched anxious states as anxiety disorders. An evolutionary view can help avoid inflated estimates of disordered conditions.

7. *Can more adequate definitions of anxiety disorders help resist the pathologization of natural emotions?* Drug companies and other interests can exploit the ambiguity and inadequacy of the *DSM* anxiety criteria to maximize the perceived amount of pathology. Their advertisements use widespread worries and concerns that naturally develop in families, schools, and workplaces as examples of anxiety disorders. This might entice viewers to see these conditions as needing pharmaceutical correction. An evolutionary approach to natural versus disordered anxiety can offer a conceptual basis to help restrain such excesses.

8. *Does the medicalization of anxious emotions have more benefits than costs?* It is especially important to distinguish disordered from natural anxiety because threatening situations and consequent anxiousness are omnipresent aspects of human existence. In the absence of a good definition of anxiety disorders, the pervasiveness of anxiety can potentially lead to a massive pathologization of normal emotions when anxiety symptoms are equated with disease. Yet, setting boundaries that enlarge the range of pathology also encourages people to seek medical treatment for their anxiety conditions and, possibly, to get relief from them. Do these benefits override the costs of viewing natural emotions as pathologies?

9. *To what extent does the disordered status of a condition affect the desirability and type of treatment that is warranted?* Normal worries and mismatched emotions, as well as anxiety disorders, create distress and impairment. Does separating these conditions suggest different therapeutic options? In particular, do mismatched but natural anxieties that are not disorders—but that are currently maladaptive—warrant treatment?

The remainder of this book explores the nature of anxiety and the anxiety disorders in order to address these perplexing questions about the distinctions between normal fears and anxiety disorders and to better understand the varieties of maladaptive anxiousness.

TERMINOLOGY

To avoid confusion in subsequent discussions, a comment is necessary about the challenging issue of terminology when speaking of fear, anxiety, and their disorders.

"Fear," which derives from the Old English word *faer*, indicating a sudden calamity or danger, is the term typically used to refer to an emotion that arises in response to a particular danger in the environment.[42] Fear is generally assumed to have some object: if someone is afraid, he or she is afraid of something, as in fear of snakes, flying, or strangers. Fear consists of an unpleasant state of bodily arousal, presumably serving to prepare the individual for quick and vigorous action to elude the danger, accompanied by a focusing of the mind's attention on the perceived danger. Thus, the fear of a certain danger is directed at the danger. When it seems appropriate, we use terms such as "worry" or "concern" as rough synonyms for less intense fears. All of these terms share the same presupposition that they have some content that refers to an object; one fears or is worried or is concerned about something.

The distinction between fear and anxiety has been drawn in a variety of ways. Sometimes, it is based on the immediacy of the situation; while the emotion of fear arises in response to a specific and immediate danger, anxiety sometimes refers to some danger that is farther in the future.[43] In this usage, anxiety refers to what might happen, not to an existing danger. For example, people would be afraid when they see a snake but would be anxious if worrying that a snake might appear around the next bend of a path. However, such temporal usage is not at all uniform. For example, Freud—who coined the use of the term "anxiety neurosis" in medicine—employed the term "primary anxiety" to refer to fear that develops during actual confrontations with danger, in contrast to "signal anxiety," which is a response to the expectation of some future danger.[44] However, some thinkers have placed fear in general as a reaction anticipating the future, as in Socrates' definition of fear as "expectation of evil." In such an approach, even the fear of an immediate threat is always a fear of what is likely to happen next as a result of the threatening object, and thus is in fact a feeling about the future.[45]

A second use of "anxiety" refers to broader fearful emotions—though not entirely undirected—that are about such issues as the meaning of life, human mortality, or uncertainty about major issues or conflicts. For example, the Danish philosopher and psychologist Soren Kierkegaard developed a conception of anxiety (*Angst*) that refers to a generalized anticipation of the future.[46] Kierkegaard distinguished between fears that have specific objects and the natural emotion of *Angst* that stems from thinking about eternal dilemmas of human existence. This distinction corresponds to the notion that people *have* fears, whereas they *are* anxious.[47] Kierkegaard emphasized both the normality and the universality of anxiety: "Deep within every human being there still lives the anxiety over the possibility of being alone in the world, forgotten by God, overlooked by the millions and millions in this enormous household."[48] For Kierkegaard, anxious despair over such universal concerns as the existence of God, the inevitability of death, and the threat of meaninglessness was a natural part of the human condition. The German philosopher Martin Heidegger vividly described this sense of anxiousness when he said that the "breath" of anxiety "quivers perpetually through human existence."[49]

Another use of "anxiety"—perhaps the most common in psychology—refers to a type of bodily arousal that involves feelings of dread or fear without necessarily implying that the individual is conscious of a threat.[50] So, unlike fear, anxieties need not be, at least consciously, directed at any particular object or be about any particular thing. Instead, anxiety is a threat that emerges from internal sources and is not attached to a specific object. The feeling of anxiety is similar to the feeling one has when one is afraid of something; that is, fear simply consists of anxiety that is directed at an object. Anxiety, therefore, is just the feeling of fear but is sometimes directed at something concrete and at other times is an undirected feeling of plain anxiety that is unattached to any object.

"It will not have escaped you," Freud aptly noted, "that a certain ambiguity and indefiniteness exists in the use of the word anxiety."[51] To minimize such ambiguity, we use "fear" (and sometimes "worry" or "concern") to refer to an emotion directed at some object, and "anxiety" as a more inclusive term that refers to any experience of the feeling of anxiety either by itself (undirected at any object) or as part of an emotion of fear (directed at an object). In our usage, anxiety is a feeling that can either be free-floating, vague, and/or amorphous, or can take the form of a concrete fear directed at some immediate or future threat.

According to this usage, both fear and anxiety can be normal or disordered, and fear disorders—as in the *DSM*—are anxiety disorders. We use the term "fear disorders" to refer to disorders in which the feeling of anxiety toward some particular object or situation is misdirected or overly intense, as in phobias. "Anxiety disorders" encompass both disorders of fear, where there is an object at which the feelings are directed, and disorders of the sheer feeling of anxiety without any object at which it is directed, as in panic attacks and certain forms of generalized anxiety disorder. As shorthand, because most (but not all) normal anxiety conditions are fears rather than undirected anxiety, we sometimes distinguish the normal from the disordered by the phrases "natural fears" or "realistic worries" versus "anxiety disorders."

In sum: When we refer to a disordered condition of the fear response, like the *DSM* we generally use the term "anxiety disorder." Because most normal fear responses involve awareness of the object at which the fear is directed, when writing of normal conditions we will generally use the terms "fear" or "worry." Finally, the terms "anxiety" or "anxiousness" without a qualifier such as "disorder" refer to the general emotion that is sometimes natural and sometimes disordered.

CONCLUSION

Developing adequate distinctions between normal and disordered fears is fraught with complexity. Nevertheless, the activities of psychiatry and allied mental health fields must be based on the best possible definitions of normality and pathology. Grounding the classification of anxiety and its disorders in their evolutionary underpinnings provides a good starting point for a fruitful understanding of anxiety.

CHAPTER 2

An Evolutionary Approach to Normal and Pathological Anxiety

In this book, we attempt to understand and evaluate how psychiatry—and consequently our society at large—has reacted to and classified the multiplicity, irrationality, and vagueness of anxiety states. It is especially important to develop adequate conceptions of anxiety disorders because the diagnostic criteria that stem from them are the only tools mental health professionals have to separate natural from disordered conditions. In other areas of medicine, biological markers exist that can indicate the presence of a disease and confirm or refute a diagnosis: cardiologists use PET scans to see if a heart has tissue damage, nephrologists take x-rays to find the presence of a kidney stone, oncologists employ laboratory tests to detect cancerous cells, etc. Psychiatrists, however, have none of these tools. Instead, patient self-reports and, sometimes, clinician observation constitute their sole diagnostic resource. At present, no independent criteria exist that might verify the accuracy of a clinician's assessment of an anxiety disorder. Making the correct distinction between normal fears and anxiety disorders on the basis of a clinical picture is particularly challenging because many of the typical diagnostic indicators used to separate natural distress from disordered conditions do not work well in the case of anxiety.

We will consider psychiatry's response to anxiety through the prism of our evolutionary view of the concept of disorder, according to which a disorder is a harmful failure of fear mechanisms to perform the functions they were biologically designed to carry out. Before explaining this approach, we first review five alternative views of disorder—the biological, learning, social values, statistical, and impairment approaches—and explain why they cannot adequately separate anxiety disorders from natural fears. This initial discussion of how we do and do not understand the concept of disorder sets the stage for the discussion of anxiety and its disorders throughout the book.

DISORDERS AS DIFFERENCES IN BRAIN FUNCTIONING

At present, biological views of disorder dominate the study of anxiety in psychiatry. A common belief is that examining brain functioning and identifying biological differences that signify disorder versus normality allow us to escape from the conceptual complexities and uncertainties of distinguishing normal from disordered fear and anxiety. Despite the lack of biological markers that can aid in making diagnoses of anxiety disorders, psychiatrists often assert that anxiety (and other mental illness) is a brain disease. "People who suffer from mental illness," according to biological psychiatrist Nancy Andreasen, "suffer from a *sick or broken brain*, not from weak will, laziness, bad character, or bad upbringing."[1] More recently, the National Institute of Mental Health has launched an initiative, the Research Domain Criteria Project, which strives to classify mental disorders based on their neurobiological correlates.[2] "The power of modern computers," notes one science writer, "allows geneticists to trawl through immense heaps of data in an attempt to pinpoint the genes responsible for panic disorder."[3] Such efforts may well succeed in the long run, but they are more of a hope than a reality at this point in history. Aside from the formidable empirical and methodological challenges in such research and the repeated disappointments of such hopes in the past, examining brain functioning is not as straightforward a way as it seems to answer the conundrum of which anxieties are normal and which are disordered.

The reason is simple: both normal and disordered fear and anxiety are unquestionably associated with certain forms of brain activity. Thus, discovering a difference in biological processes between two groups does not in itself tell you whether you have discovered a difference that signifies disorder versus non-disorder as opposed to two normal variations or two disorders. One cannot leap directly from observing that there is a brain process that produces anxiety to a conclusion about what is normal versus disordered. Natural fears are equally as likely as disorders to be related to brain circuits and neurological underpinnings, so correlations of such activity with anxious states do not indicate whether the condition is a normal or a pathological one.

Think back to the panic-like symptoms that Kenneth Kendler experienced while hanging over a precipice. We can presume that a scan of Kendler's brain at that moment would show quite intense activity in his amygdala, activity that looks like the brain of a panic-disorder patient during an attack. Analogously, the brain scans of depressed patients strongly resemble the brain scans of actors asked to pretend that they feel intensely sad because both are generating intense feelings of sadness.[4] Or, imagine looking at brain scans of soldiers going out on patrol in an Afghan neighborhood in which there has been recent violence and in which hypervigilance is essential. These scans might reveal brain activity in anxiety-generating centers at the same or higher levels as among people with anxiety disorders, yet this anxiety would be an entirely normal response to extraordinarily threatening circumstances. The brain scans themselves, however, would not reveal that the condition is a natural response to an extreme environment rather than an anxiety disorder. The same configuration of neurochemicals or electrical activity that might be normal in the face of a direct threat might indicate a disorder when no danger exists.

Anxiety disorders and normal intense anxiety share a major characteristic—intense anxiety. The sheer amount of anxiety or of the underlying brain activity does not in itself indicate an anxiety disorder because extreme anxiety that arises because of a real, severe threat in the environment is normal. In such cases, heightened levels of brain activity and perhaps special brain circuitry might come into play as part of a normal, biologically designed response. Thus, looking at the intensity of amygdala activity is not a way to "see disorder" in the brain. Nor is there just one brain circuit triggering amygdala activity that represents normal anxiety; research shows that normal anxiety can flow through multiple neuronal pathways. Except in cases of gross trauma to the brain or other rare cases where we already know there is brain pathology, to search for a "broken brain" we have to know how to recognize the kind of brain state correlated with disorder. To do that, we have to go outside of the biological level and consider the context to which the intense anxiety is a response, and the likely brain design for anxiety responses, so that we can judge whether the brain-generated anxiety is normal or not.

It is quite possible that markers of brain differences between normal and disordered anxiety will emerge eventually. To identify such differences, we will have to know which contextual cues normally give rise to what levels of anxiety, as well as the normal range of abilities to inhibit anxiety. At present, however, researchers don't know which of such features cause anxiety feelings to be severed from their biologically designed contextual cues. Thus, at least for the time being, only consideration of the context in which anxiety emerges allows one to judge whether it is a normal reaction or a psychiatric disorder.

DISORDERS AS LEARNED EXPERIENCES

For much of the twentieth century, behavioral models that focused on life experiences dominated the study of anxiety, especially within the field of psychology. Behavioral psychologist John Watson (1878–1958) presented the most uncompromising view of this model. He asserted that almost any learned, conditioned cue could become a source of intense anxiety, especially if it occurred during early childhood. If a naturally frightening event occurred along with a more neutral event at about the same time and place, then the neutral event is thenceforth likely to be associated with—and in the future trigger—a fear reaction.

Watson provided perhaps the most famous example of a learned fear. Along with Rosalie Raynor, he set out to demonstrate that an 11-month-old boy initially unafraid of rats could be conditioned to fear them when they were presented to him along with the naturally frightening stimulus of a loud noise.[5] First, they allowed the boy to engage in long periods of play with a rat. Then, they created sudden, loud, and unpleasant noises whenever the boy played with the rat. After a few trials, the infant would cry in the presence of the rat without any noise. Moreover, he developed intense fears not only of rats but of a range of furry animals and objects. A large subsequent body of literature with both people and other animals indicates how learned, conditioned stimuli are cues that produce aversive responses leading animals to focus their anxiety on some particular object or event.[6]

Some intense fears undoubtedly do stem from learned experiences and their accompanying meanings. For example, studies suggest that dental phobia (i.e., fear of going to a dentist), which has little plausible rationale as an evolutionarily prepared fear, is associated with previous traumatic experiences in the dentist's chair. Aversive dental experiences among children and young adolescents cause greater dental (but not other) fears at later ages. Such studies confirm that dental fear is directly related to previous negative experiences and is presumably due to a conditioning process.[7]

Moreover, much research indicates that fear and anxiety need not stem from direct experience; they can also be learned by observing and imitating the responses of others.[8] Such learning-at-one-remove takes place constantly as a part of social interaction. For example, studies in the military show that some airmen acquired intense fears after seeing a crewmate express such fears, and that large numbers of soldiers developed intensified fears after seeing a comrade "crack up" under the stress of battle.[9] Likewise, the children of parents who display great fear when confronted with particular types of objects can develop a similarly intensified fear. The extent of children's fears during the London air raids in World War II, for example, strongly correlated with the extent of their mothers' fears.[10]

In addition to direct conditioning and vicarious learning, humans uniquely use linguistic communication and their sophisticated cognitive capacities to associate cues and responses with danger. This can lead us to react to stimuli very distant in content from anything for which we are biologically prepared to be afraid.[11] For example, people may experience anxiety when they see a newspaper headline reporting a major drop in the stock market or the discovery of excessive mercury in tuna fish, especially if they own stocks or regularly eat sushi, respectively. Similarly, for the anxious air traveler, a change in the sound of the plane's engines can trigger intense anxiety—even though that sound did not exist in past environments and has no conditioning history in the individual's life—through a series of inferences mediated by sophisticated beliefs about how airplanes stay up in the air, how engines work, and so on. Such fears arise when cognitive processes mediate the fear response in such a way that more primitively feared possibilities of, for example, death, loss of health, or loss of resources, territory, or status are linked to more abstract events.

Despite tremendous progress in research about the nature of learning, two major problems exist with the view that anxiety disorders stem from learned conditioning. First, the belief that normal processes of learning could produce fear of just about any sort of object has turned out to be simply wrong. Watson and the behaviorist tradition that followed his work emphasized how fear stimuli typically were not innate but arose from environmental conditioning; indeed, Watson thought that loud sounds and the loss of a mother's support were the only two inherited concerns that led infants to develop fear responses.[12]

Yet, despite the great differences in people's conditioning histories, most individually learned fears fit into evolutionarily designed categories of threatening objects and situations. People are pre-prepared to fear some objects more than others: the set of things to which people develop intense fears is overall quite limited and predictable, not a random assortment of objects that the conditioning theory might predict.[13] For example, children are far more likely to develop fears of the dark than of sunlight and of strange rather than familiar objects. Similarly, infant monkeys develop lifelong fear of snakes after they observe that their mothers are terrified of snakes.[14] Freud's analysis of Little Hans's phobic fear of horses provides another example. In a famous paper, psychologist Martin Seligman argued that the boy's horse fear was not simply a result of his particular unconscious or conscious learning history but also involved pre-prepared evolutionary cues.[15] Little Hans would not have been likely to become afraid of lambs, for example, regardless of his prior experiences. What people learn to fear is not so much a product of idiosyncratic learning as of our evolutionary history. The conditioning theory of phobias as an all-encompassing theory is inconsistent with the evidence.

The second major problem with the learned conditioning view is that it lacks criteria to separate normal from disordered fear and anxiety. A basic tenet of the behavioral model is that all forms of anxiety result from the same processes of conditioning. Thus, the learning model implies that disordered fears cannot be distinguished from normal ones. For example, the fear of furry objects held by the boy in Watson and Raynor's experiment was neither more nor less abnormal than any other conditioned experience. The learning model, therefore, has no criteria to distinguish natural from pathological anxiety because both types stem from similar, earlier conditioning experiences. Yet, in fact, there are clear cases of anxiety disorder versus normal fear.

There is no doubt that individual conditioning powerfully shapes the formation of intense anxiety. Indeed, the basic brain mechanisms of conditioning, which appear to be the same in humans and other animals, have recently started to be elucidated at the neuronal level.[16] Unconscious fear memories become indelibly burned into the brain and can stay with us for life. According to neuroscientist Joseph LeDoux, "We may not be able to get rid of the implicit memories that underlie anxiety disorders. If this is the case, the best we can hope for is to exercise control over them."[17] The nature of our fears depends on the interaction of learning with biologically shaped innate dispositions to fear. Learned conditioning, in itself, however, cannot account for whether what is conditioned is within normal limits or has become abnormal.

DISORDERS AS SOCIAL VALUES

One response to the lack of objective physiological indicators for defining mental illnesses is to assert that mental disorders do not exist in nature at all, but rather that their definitions reflect social values. For example, philosopher Laurie Reznek asserts, "Whether some condition is a disease depends on where we choose to draw the line of normality, and that is not a line we can discover. Rather, we invent disease status by imposing our distinction between disease and normality on the world."[18] This type of analysis, which is common among many social scientists, historians, and critics of psychiatry, argues that mental disorders are whatever a given society defines as such: no independent criteria exist that could define disorder apart from cultural norms and definitions. From this point of view, mental disorders reflect violations of certain kinds of social values.[19] British sociologist Peter Sedgwick stated this doctrine in an extreme and clear form:

> Outside the significances that man voluntarily attaches to certain conditions, *there are no illnesses or diseases in nature.* . . . Are there not infectious and contagious bacilli? Are there not definite and objective lesions in the cellular structures of the human body? Are there not fractures of bones, the fatal ruptures of tissues, the malignant multiplications

of tumorous growths? . . . Yet these, as natural events, do not *prior to the human social meanings we attach to them* constitute illnesses, sicknesses, or diseases. The fracture of a septuagenarian's femur has, within the world of nature, no more significance than the snapping of an autumn leaf from its twig. . . . Out of his anthropocentric self-interest, man has chosen to consider as "illnesses" or "diseases" those natural circumstances which precipitate the death (or the failure to function according to certain values) of a limited number of biological species: man himself, his pets and other cherished livestock, and the plant-varieties he cultivates for gain or pleasure. . . . Children and cattle may fall ill, have diseases, and seem as sick; but who has ever imagined that spiders and lizards can be sick or diseased?[20]

In such views, concepts of disorder are human-made inventions that are unconstrained by any broader conceptual unity.

In contrast to Sedgwick's dramatic statement, in fact, lizards and spiders can become diseased. But a more important point in response to this sort of values-based view is that there is a scientific reason, quite aside from human values, as to why the snapping of a septuagenarian's femur is considered a disorder whereas the snapping of an autumn leaf from its twig is not: leaves are biologically designed to separate from twigs in autumn, whereas femurs are biologically designed to support movement, not to snap. Grounding the concept of mental disorder in biological dysfunction resolves the relativity inherent in the view that mental disorders are solely social constructions.

Another problem with the values-based position is that just because a condition is disvalued does not imply that it is a disorder. The values view fails to address a major challenge in analyzing the concept of disorder: what criterion distinguishes those disvalued conditions that are considered disorders from those that are not? We do not consider many undesirable conditions, ranging from shyness and modest IQ to shortness and rudeness, to be disorders. The values approach cannot distinguish violations of social norms arising due to mental illnesses from many other disvalued traits such as deviance, bad manners, ignorance, lack of skill, or malice. It therefore becomes amenable to defining a vast range of behaviors as mental disorders. Any criterion that separates mental disorders from other disvalued traits must go beyond the disvalued nature of the condition.

A further difficulty with the values view is that if definitions of mental illness are relative to specific times and places, it becomes impossible to compare them across cultures. For instance, a scholar of obsessive-compulsive conditions notes, "We have to posit a specific time and place where 'obsession,' as a shifting term, is understood one way, and then another specific time and place when it is under-stood another way."[21] Yet, if we endorse this view, there is no standpoint that allows us to say that two different conceptions of, in this case, "obsessions" are actually instances of the same phenomenon. The only possible way of making comparisons is by positing some conception that shows how varying expressions are different manifestations of some comparable underlying entity.

Finally, the values conception cannot separate correct from incorrect definitions of disorder. According to it, if a definition accords with current social values, it cannot simply be *wrong*. Yet surely their values often mislead people into mistakenly thinking that a normal condition is a disorder. For example, nineteenth-century psychiatrists, reflecting the cultural values of the Victorian era, thought masturbation was a sign of a serious mental illness.[22] It turned out that Victorian definitions of masturbation as a mental disorder were erroneous, just as antebellum Southern doctors incorrectly believed that runaway slaves suffered from a psychiatric disorder and Soviet psychiatrists misclassified political dissidents as disordered. Judgments that some conceptions of mental disorder are more valid than others require a standard that goes beyond local values and can accurately separate truly pathological conditions from those that reflect socially disapproved behaviors.

STATISTICAL CONCEPTIONS OF DISORDER

A fourth common response to the absence of objective indicators in psychiatry is to use statistical rarity rather than social values as a standard to help define disordered conditions in a more scientifically objective way.[23] From the statistical point of view, mental disorders are defined by being at the extreme tail of a statistical distribution. Normality and disorder are not discontinuous; they lie on different points of a shared spectrum, with disorders varying only in degree but not in kind from normal emotions. Psychological traits such as fear are seen as lying on a bell-shaped curve featuring low, average, and high levels. This approach has a certain moral appeal, since it appears to break down the barriers between people with mental illnesses and normal individuals. In addition, a verbal ambiguity encourages this approach: "abnormal" can describe unusual as well as pathological conditions.

The statistical approach to anxiety disorder is seriously flawed. Rarity and disorder are simply different ideas; there are rare normal conditions and common disorders. A rare reaction might be quite normal (as in any odd but normal variation, from green eyes to dislike of sports), and a very common reaction could be a mass disorder (as in conditions such as atherosclerosis or gum disease). Severely threatening circumstances can lead huge proportions of given populations to develop disorders. For example, a majority of fighter pilots who flew numerous combat missions in World War II developed anxiety disorders.[24] Such disorders can also be rampant and prolonged in populations that face intense stressors such as civil wars, involuntary migrations from homes, or refugee status in an alien country. Having symptoms that lie on the high end of a continuum of anxiety cannot in itself indicate the presence of a disorder.

Moreover, the intensity of one's anxiety does not validly indicate whether the feelings are disordered or not. Severe yet normal anxiety feelings often arise in response to severe actual or imagined threats. Consider, for example, the emotions of the author J. K. Rowling, who confessed her trepidations before addressing a convocation at Harvard: "The weeks of fear and nausea I've experienced at the thought of giving this commencement address have made me lose weight."[25] Yet, once the speech was over, Rowling's symptoms disappeared, indicating that they were an intense response to a given context that vanished as soon as the occasion was over. Unmarried women deciding whether to have a child or an abortion, parents confronted with the life-threatening illness of a child, students facing decisions to drop out of college because of mounting debts, or children pondering their first day at a new school often experience high levels of anxiety because they have something serious to worry about.

When threats are enduring they can lead to persistent, extreme levels of non-disordered anxiety. For example, one Iraqi psychiatrist describes the typical psyche of his countrymen during the period of civil war and American occupation: "Anything can happen at any moment. You can't plan for the next day or the next hour. You are always afraid, in every waking hour and in your sleep."[26] In addition to intense normal reactions to specific circumstances, there is also natural variation in human temperament and in the tendency to respond more or less intensely to stress. Consequently, elevating statistically high intensity into a criterion for anxiety disorders would pathologize the upper end of the normal distribution in emotionality. The statistical view's implication that anxiety disorders must be infrequent is simply incorrect.

DISORDER AS IMPAIRMENT

A final criterion sometimes used to define disorder lies in the distressing, disabling, impairing, and otherwise harmful consequences of a condition.[27] For example, the *DSM* embraces this approach as one part of its definition of disorder through its "clinical significance criterion," which requires that symptoms must entail distress or role impairment to be considered a disorder. Certainly conditions are only properly classified as medical disorders if they also are considered harmful or undesirable in one way or another; a harmless or beneficial condition is not a disorder. However, this perspective goes further and sometimes uses harmfulness as a sufficient criterion for the presence of an anxiety disorder even when the condition is a normal one.

Distress and suffering in themselves are obviously part of our natural range of responses to difficult circumstances. However, it is easy to think that anxiety is disordered when it goes beyond misery to entail harms such as significant financial costs, increased physical health problems, marital instability, and impaired familial, educational, and occupational functioning.[28] For example, psychiatrists distinguish the mental disorder of social phobia from normal shyness because social phobics are more likely to drop out of school, quit their jobs, drink heavily, and suffer from other impairments.[29] Because people who meet the symptom criteria for some anxiety diagnoses face more personal, social, and health disabilities than those who don't, their handicaps are presumed to validate that their conditions are genuine anxiety disorders.

One problem with using impairment as the criterion to distinguish disorders from normal negative emotions is that individuals who *naturally* become anxious in the face of highly threatening situations also often suffer from social, occupational, and health disabilities. Shy people, for instance, as well as those with social anxiety disorders, can face social disadvantages. Likewise, people who have anxious concerns about a sick relative for whom they are caring often display absenteeism from work, lower social functioning, and worsened health outcomes. Short stature, divorce, bereavement, and taking up running are all associated with elevated risks of myocardial infarction, yet the risk of negative effects does not mean that any of those conditions are disorders.[30] The same is true of anxiety reactions and their negative sequelae. Problematic consequences, however undesirable or ultimately impairing they might be, do not necessarily indicate the presence of a disorder because many non-disordered conditions are harmful, and there is nothing wrong with people who become anxious when they face threatening situations, even if such anxiety might at times be harmful. While it is true that conditions that entail no harm should not be considered disorders, harm in itself is not a sufficient criterion for a disorder.

Moreover, the impairment criterion can turn social and occupational challenges into criteria for mental disorders. Normal levels of aversion to enclosed spaces might be disqualifying for a tunnel digger, just as normal levels of height fear might be crippling for workers who build skyscrapers.[31] Likewise, being anxious to a higher degree than others about speaking to strangers can be impairing to a salesperson but not to a mechanic. Surely the job one holds cannot determine whether one has a disorder. Nor can the society's general occupational requirements in and of themselves determine whether there is a biological dysfunction.

This is not to say that impairment is never indicative of disorder—obviously sometimes gross or basic impairment can strongly suggest disorder. But it all depends on the kind of impairment. Some role capacities are biologically shaped in such a way that role impairment implies biological dysfunction. For example, if social phobia when interacting with family members impairs basic role functions such as parenting and sexual interaction, this role impairment is also biological dysfunction. But as a general criterion, impairment and related forms of harm do not offer a valid way to distinguish disordered anxiety from all the normal anxieties that may also impair performance.

THE EVOLUTIONARY FOUNDATION OF ANXIETY

We have examined and found wanting five common ideas about how to tell the difference between anxiety that is normal and anxiety that represents a disorder. One thing that all these views of disorder have in common is that they ignore the distinction between conditions that are natural—that is, biologically designed—and those where something has gone wrong with the way the individual's anxiety mechanisms are functioning. Yet these notions of how the organism is biologically designed to function and whether something has gone wrong with such functioning are at the heart of the concept of disorder.

Indeed, the most fundamental distinction in medicine is between the normal and the pathological. Adequate conceptions of normality are foundational for accurate knowledge about what is pathological.[32] Psychiatrists, however, rarely consider what appropriate psychological functioning involves. "It is indeed astonishing," exclaims neurologist Antonio Damasio, "to realize that (medical) students learn about psychopathology without ever being taught normal psychology."[33] The idea that mental disorders exist when some aspect of mental processes are not functioning properly requires consideration of what constitutes normal functioning of psychological mechanisms. This means that pathology cannot be equated with the sheer presence of negative emotions, since bad feelings can often exist for good reasons and be normal.[34]

A disorder indicates that something is *wrong* with some (possibly inferred and as yet unknown) internal mechanism that is biologically designed to do something but is failing to do it—or is designed *not* to do something that it is doing, as in panic attacks when no threat is present. This view contrasts with anchoring disordered conditions in brain physiology, learned experience, social values, statistical rarity, or impairment—for both normal and disordered anxiety can have each of these features. A crucial corollary of the evolutionary view, to which we now turn, is that knowing when something is wrong with a psychological mechanism requires knowing not just emotional symptoms and their severity and duration but also the context—both social and biological—in which natural selection designed that type of emotion to arise.

NATURAL FUNCTIONING

An understanding of the natural functioning of any feature, whether physical or psychological, must consider both the function of the feature—that is, the effect it had that enhanced fitness in the environment when the human genome was formed—and the sort of environment for which the trait proved adaptive. It is generally easy to define in a rough way the normal and pathological functioning of most physical organs. Evolution biologically designed the eyes to see, the heart to pump blood, the kidneys to eliminate waste, and the lungs to enable us to breathe. These structures are healthy when they are carrying out the functions that evolution designed them to perform. Conversely, they are diseased when they are unable to accomplish their biologically designed functions.

Likewise, mental illnesses are failures of minds to function as natural selection designed them to function. Those internal processes that can be disturbed include emotion, thought, perception, motivation, language, and intentional action. The mind—and the brain, which is the organ in which most mental processes occur—has many special features, such as learning, cultural shaping, plasticity in taking on new tasks, and interpreting the meanings of contextual events, which makes the health/disorder distinction more complex than in physical medicine. Nevertheless, the ultimate benchmark for health and disorder is the same in psychiatry as it is in physical medicine, namely, whether the individual's internal processes are performing the functions they were biologically designed to perform. Thus, the definition of mental dysfunction is conceptually analogous to the definition of physical dysfunctions: mental disorders exist when a psychological mechanism is unable to perform its evolutionarily designed function.

Despite the conceptual similarity in defining mental and physical disorders, it is far trickier to make decisions about whether psychological mechanisms such as those that generate anxiety are accomplishing their designed function than whether physical organs are functioning appropriately. Two intrinsic difficulties make definitions of normal and pathological psychological functioning much harder to develop than comparable definitions of physical functioning. First, most bodily systems function constantly and do not turn on and off. A heart that stopped pumping blood, a lung that cannot breathe, or a kidney that does not process wastes indicates a serious and often deadly pathology. For the most part, therefore, physicians don't need to understand the context in which a bodily disturbance occurs; they need only to assess the performance of the system in question.

Unlike the bodily systems that medicine treats, psychological mechanisms are *contextual*. The brain is an intensely social organ that inherently responds to its environment. "Our inner faculties," psychologist William James observed, "are adapted in advance to the features of the world in which we dwell."[35] Because mental structures are generally sensitive to context, definitions of both normal fear and anxiety disorders must take into account situational factors. Fears, worries, and concerns that arise in the kinds of threatening circumstances they were designed to respond to are natural and not disordered.

Second, for the most part, the aspects of the environments in which physical organs currently function are similar to those that existed during the evolutionary period in which they developed.[36] The natural functions of, say, the heart, lungs, or kidneys are performed in much the same way now as they were when the human genome developed. In contrast, psychological traits were selected into the human genome to deal with circumstances that might have little or no relationship to present-day contexts because of rapid changes in the social environment. Emotional algorithms, according to evolutionary psychologists John Tooby and Leida Cosmides, "lead organisms to act as if certain things were true about their present circumstances, whether or not they are, because they were true of past circumstances."[37] Psychological functions arose to respond to prehistoric, not contemporary, conditions.

The Environment of Evolutionary Adaptation (EEA)—that is, the environment with its distinctive challenges to which human beings were responding when natural selection shaped their mental features—is the starting point for the study of how evolution designed emotions such as fear and anxiety to function and why they are—or were—adaptive.[38] The EEA generally corresponds to the time when humans lived in hunter-gatherer societies, first on the African plains and then in dispersed locales, between two million and ten thousand years ago. Generally, people react to cues that lead to responses that had evolutionary payoff in the EEA. Psychological traits that were adaptive during the EEA are currently adaptive only to the extent that the problems that these traits evolved to solve resemble those that humans presently face. "The world in which we dwell" is changing rapidly, and many situations no longer hold the dangers that they did when an emotional system was being naturally selected.

The human taste for fats, sugars, and salt provides a good example of a trait that was adaptive in the past but is currently maladaptive.[39] Maximizing caloric intake was a good strategy to enhance survival and reproduction when calories were scarce in prehistoric times. Tastes that led people to ingest as many calories as possible were useful in such environments. In the modern world, where calories are all too readily available, these ancestral tastes can lead to obesity and associated elevated risk for many diseases. Although these traits are no longer adaptive, they remain part of our ancestral inheritance. Tastes for fatty, sugary, and salty foods are not disordered, however harmful their consequences might presently be.

Like our taste for unhealthy calorie-laden foods, emotional responses that evolution engineered for recurrent problems in the ancestral world are often not well designed for the modern world.[40] Humans now face very different circumstances than those when emotions developed, such that *appropriately* functioning psychological mechanisms might not produce emotions that are adaptive in present-day conditions. The kinds of dangers that were common in prehistory—wild animals, strangers, rejection by one's social group, and the like—continue to be common sources of anxiety in the modern world despite posing threats less often now than they did back then. Fears of snakes, spiders, darkness, or heights that made a great deal of sense in ancient environments are usually unreasonable now. Our stone-age emotional systems might be working appropriately, but in environments where they were not designed to function.

This leads to the question of whether psychological mechanisms that are functioning as they were designed to function but that are maladaptive in current circumstances are disorders or not. An analogy is the situations of people who are under water or in outer space without breathing aids. In the absence of mechanical forms of assistance, human lungs cannot perform their natural function of taking in oxygen, and therefore certain death will result within a few minutes. Nevertheless, individuals who find themselves in these situations without an air supply do not suffer from a lung disorder: it is just that perfectly normal lungs cannot function in environments that lack oxygen. A mismatch between some mechanism and its current environment does not indicate a disorder when the mechanism remains capable of functioning appropriately within the range of environments for which it was designed to function.

However, conditions in novel environments can sometimes cause disorders. Therefore, formulators of diagnostic criteria must not only consider whether anxiety arising as a response to prehistoric dangers that are not currently dangerous is disordered. In addition, they must ask if such mismatches with contemporary circumstances have caused a failure of fear mechanisms to be able to perform their designed functions and, therefore, have led to an anxiety disorder. The lungs, for example, were not designed to ingest pollutants from toxic environments. Inhaling such poisons in large amounts or over long periods of time can lead the lungs to be unable to perform their natural functions. For example, rescue workers who were exposed to thick dust clouds after the September 11 attack on the World Trade Center still had abnormal lung functioning seven years after the attack.[41]

Likewise, evolution did not design people to respond effectively to some conditions they confront in current environments, such as modern warfare. The traumas of combat can alter designed brain functioning and create enduring pathological effects on memory, cognition, and mood. In such cases, environmental circumstances render some natural emotion unable to perform its designed function.

Modernity can not only lead to a mismatch between natural emotions and situations, it can also cause emotional mechanisms to break down partially or completely. Naturally functioning emotions that are mismatched with current conditions need to be distinguished from disordered emotions that may result from the impact of novel environments. Needless to say, it is not always easy to make the distinction between mismatched and disordered emotions.

THE FUNCTIONS OF FEAR AND ANXIETY

The best way to understand an emotion is to describe its functions—the specific adaptive problem that natural selection designed it to solve.[42] A natural function of a mechanism is part of the explanation for why the underlying mechanism exists and is structured the way that it is. Different emotions have diverse functions that deal with distinct kinds of problem situations and therefore have separate brain systems devoted to them. These functions adjust physiological, psychological, and behavioral processes to respond to the particular characteristics of challenging social and other environmental situations.

Arguably, the natural functions of anxiety are better understood than those of any other emotion, forming a solid basis for *prima facie* inferences regarding normality and disorder (which the next chapter considers in more detail). Unlike the puzzlement that exists about the reasons why many other emotions (e.g., grief, joy) are present in the human genome, it is easy to broadly understand the evolutionary functions of anxiety. Any situation that creates harm sufficient to impair a life form's chances of survival and reproduction will potentially influence selective pressures. At the most basic level, defenses against immediately life-threatening dangers must be any organism's highest priority, whether those dangers stem from predators and other organisms, natural forces, or social factors.[43] Organisms whose fear motivates them to recognize and to avoid situations that threaten harm or death are more likely to survive and reproduce than ones that are not able to escape from dangerous circumstances.

Natural selection is responsible for genetically transmitted fear mechanisms. Evolution generally proceeds through preserving and building upon older mechanisms rather than replacing them wholesale with new mechanisms.[44] The ability to take defensive actions that allow organisms to avoid danger has ancient origins that long precede the evolution of humans. All living creatures, even the most elementary bacteria, have some innate mechanism that allows them to react defensively in response to threats. For example, one-celled stentors, tiny creatures that live in ponds, make graded responses to threats depending on their severity.[45] In the case of anxiety, evolution has maintained a core of ancient emotional behaviors.

Anxiety was designed to respond to environmental threats through focusing attention on perceived risks, preparing the body for flight, and maximizing opportunities to escape from dangerous situations.[46] Even at present, people with high levels of anxiety are less likely to die from accidents, most likely because they are more likely than others to avoid risky behaviors and situations.[47] If anxiety has such a basic function to play in responding to environmental dangers, the implication is both that it is transmitted as part of the human genome and therefore is found among virtually all normal humans, and that it is found in all cultures. Considerable evidence indicates that anxiety is indeed a universal emotion.

THE UNIVERSALITY OF FEAR AND ANXIETY

Just because an emotion is found in all cultures does not necessarily mean that it is also biologically rooted.[48] For example, certain sorts of fears might inhere in the human condition rather than in human biology. Thomas Hobbes, for example, famously considered that humanity's natural state was to be overwhelmed with fear: "his heart all the day long gnawed on by fear of death, poverty, or other calamity. . . (he) has no repose, nor pause of his anxiety, but in sleep."[49] Likewise, Soren Kierkegaard emphasized how choices between various courses of action are an inherent part of human existence that inevitably leads to anxiety over what people decide to do or not do.[50] Such fears are at the same time cultural products and human universals.

Fear response mechanisms, however, seem to be grounded in genetically transmitted brain circuitry and thus are not only cultural universals but also common to all humans who have normally functioning brains. One powerful reason for thinking that anxiety is a universal emotion lies in the commonalities across species in basic fear response mechanisms. "Most living creatures," notes psychophysiologist Arne Ohman, "risk ending up on a predator's menu."[51] Consequently, normal brains need to have mechanisms that detect danger and respond appropriately and quickly to it. All organisms must have some way to escape from danger if they are going to be able to survive.

Some types of cues that evoke fearful responses are common across species, such as loud noises or expectations of pain.[52] Abrupt, intense, irregular, and rapidly increasing stimuli also produce fear responses. Likewise, unusual objects, strange foods, or novel situations are widely associated with fear. Land-dwelling species fear heights and withdraw from edges of cliffs. Most organisms become afraid if there is too much or too little space or light around them.[53]

Every species has a genetic heritage that preprograms it to recognize some predators the first time they see them. For example, rats that are born and reared in laboratories freeze or try to escape when they confront a cat for the first time.[54] Baby birds show inhibited physiological and motor responses whenever large objects fly over their nests. Likewise, numerous mammals, including humans, are alarmed by snake-like cues despite never having experienced traumatic encounters with snakes.[55] It is far easier to condition fears to objects or situations that posed threats in prehistoric times than to dangers that are of modern origin.[56] Thus, laboratory-reared monkeys who have never seen snakes are easily conditioned to fear them after viewing films of older monkeys demonstrating intense snake fear.[57] They do not, however, develop fears of stimuli such as flowers or mushrooms when they observe older monkeys responding fearfully to these innocuous stimuli.[58]

Humans inherit proneness to many fears and responses to threatening situations from their evolutionary ancestors. Darwin noted that fear was probably the evolutionarily oldest emotion and was expressed in almost the same way among humans and their remote ancestors alike.

> Fear was expressed from an extremely remote period, in almost the same manner as it is now by man; namely, by trembling, the erection of the hair, cold perspiration, pallor, widely opened eyes, the relaxation of most of the muscles, and the whole body cowering downwards or held motionless.[59]

Darwin also explained why these expressions still arise:

> Men, during numberless generations, have endeavoured to escape from their enemies or danger by headlong flight . . . And such great exertions will have caused the heart to beat rapidly, the breathing to be hurried, the chest to heave, and the nostrils to be dilated . . . And now, whenever the emotion of fear is strongly felt, though it may not lead to any exertion, the same results tend to reappear, through the force of inheritance and association.[60]

In addition, he observed that fear can be literally "hair-raising," a now useless retention through inheritance of a relic of animal fear response.[61]

Current research following in the Darwinian tradition indicates, according to neuroscientist Richard Davidson, "a remarkable convergence between findings at the animal and human levels."[62] Among both human and non-human primates, fear expressions involve open eyes with tense lower lids, whites of the eyes that show above but not below the iris, forehead and brows raised and drawn together, and lips slightly retracted horizontally.[63] Expressions such as widened eyes and rising eyebrows allow animals to see and hear better so they can respond to danger more quickly and effectively. A genetically inherited biological base produces a universal grammar that constrains (but does not determine) the surface expressions of fear.

A second line of research regarding the universality of fear relies on research among infants who are too young to be influenced by cultural systems of learning. Here, too, Darwin was a pioneer. He noted that fear was among the earliest feelings infants experienced, "as shown by their startling at any sudden sound when only a few weeks old, followed by crying."[64] Their bodies become momentarily rigid, their eyes tend to close somewhat, their heads bend awkwardly, and their mouths contort into a cry and crying ensues. More recent research confirms that specific childhood fears are natural results of preprogrammed dispositions so that children develop fears in certain situations at certain ages. Psychiatrist Isaac Marks showed how children develop a predictable sequence of fears over the course of normal development: fear of separation and strange adults develops at 4–9 months and persists to about the age of 2 years, followed by fears of animals from ages 2–4 and of the dark at ages 4–6.[65] Night terrors and fear of darkness typically arise among children around ages 1 and 2.[66] Marks also noted how his own 2-year-old son was terrified at his first sight of strands of seaweed that looked as if they were snakes.[67] As Sigmund Freud and John Bowlby emphasized, actual or anticipated separations from mothers and mother-figures are especially important sources of anxiousness.[68] Such separations might be related to the universal fear of getting lost.[69] Comparable fears, especially fears of certain animals and of darkness, are found all over the world and often among young primates as well.

The hallmark signs of normal fears are that they arise around the age when they would have been adaptive during prehistory. Fears of strangers and of animals universally arise just when babies start to crawl away from mothers at about six months of age and so would have been easier victims for predators. Fear of heights likewise develops when the very young start to become mobile.[70] Notably, virtually all of the things that children fear have ancestral roots. Young children are easily conditioned to fear crawling animals but not, for example, opera glasses.[71] Conversely, children rarely fear things that were harmless in the past but are harmful at present. Parents, for example, must make extensive efforts to get children to refrain from crossing busy streets, handling sharp objects, or investigating electric outlets, but not to have them avoid snakes, spiders, and crawling insects.

A third source of evidence for the universality of fear stems from cross-cultural similarities in this emotion. Again, Darwin relied on this method, using a far-flung network of personal informants to confirm his judgment that expressions of fear would be normal:

> With respect to fear, as exhibited by the various races of man, my informants agree that the signs are the same as with Europeans. They are displayed in an exaggerated degree with the Hindoos and natives of Ceylon. Mr. Geach has seen Malays when terrified turn pale and shake.[72]

Darwin noted that 20 of 24 persons shown a photograph of a fearful man identified "intense fright" or "horror" as the correct expression. More recently, the psychologist Paul Ekman used less obviously culturally biased research to show agreement across cultures about facial expressions of fear. Ekman found agreement in judgments of pictures of fear in Japan, Brazil, Chile, Argentina, and the U.S. ranging from 71% to 77%, 78%, 68%, and 88% respectively.[73] The overwhelming majority of the Fore of New Guinea, who had no previous contact with Western culture, could discriminate expressions of fear from those of anger, disgust, or sadness (although less than half accurately distinguished fear from surprise). Because Ekman's method uses photographs and is not dependent on linguistic terms, it is not subject to charges of imposing unsuitable culture-bound categories of expression.

Even many cultural anthropologists, who rarely find evidence of universality of emotions in the groups they study, view fear as an exception. For example, anthropologists Richard Shweder and Jonathan Haidt closely analyzed the Rasadhyaya, a third-century CE. Sanskrit text in India.[74] They found very few emotions that contemporary Westerners would identify. Fear, however, was an easily recognizable exception, along with anger and sorrow. Many biblical descriptions, as well, clearly describe emotions of fear that resemble Darwin's descriptions to a remarkable extent. Job's experience is illustrative: "In thoughts from the visions of the night, when deep sleep falleth on men, fear came upon me, and trembling, which made all my bones to shake. Then a spirit passed before my face; the hair of my flesh stood up."[75] A wide range of evidence from other species, pre-socialized children, and other cultures, therefore, indicates the universality of anxious emotions.

INNATE FEARS: THE EXAMPLE OF FEAR OF HEIGHTS

As early as 1877, Charles Darwin proposed that innate fears might arise from natural selection. After observing his 2-year-old son's fear of large zoo animals, Darwin asked, "May we not suspect that . . . fears of children, which are quite independent of experience, are the inherited effects of real dangers . . . during savage times."[76] Fear of heights provides a good example of such an innate fear. Indeed, fear of heights might be called a "prototypical" evolutionarily relevant fear because of the obvious threat from falling to all humans, but especially to children. As a result, the fear of heights seems both innate and universal.

Research with babies demonstrates how the fear of falling is hard-wired and precognitive. The classic "visual cliff" experiments of psychologists Eleanor Gibson and Richard Walk provide a particularly good illustration of the instinctive nature of fear of heights. The visual cliff is an apparatus that is half board with a pattern and

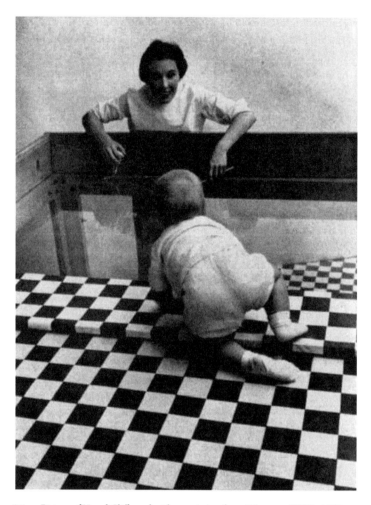

Figure 2.1: Picture of Visual Cliff, used with permission from Gibson and Walk, 1960.

half glass supported several feet above the floor, with a continuation of the board's pattern on the floor several feet under the glass. At the end of the board there is what appears to be a sudden drop to the floor, although in fact there is a continued solidity of the glass.

Gibson and Walk placed 36 infants ranging in age from 6 months to 14 months on the center board.[77] The child's mother would then call from the deep side and the shallow side alternately. Even when its mother beckoned from the other side, a baby would not crawl out onto a clear glass plate, no matter how many times it was shown by placing its hand or body on the glass that there was a solid object there upon which to crawl. All of the 27 infants who moved off the center board crawled onto the shallow side at least once; only 3 of them ever crawled onto the deep "cliff" side, illustrating some small degree of normal variation in such fears or in the ability to overcome them even when very young. Many infants crawled away from their mother when she called to them from the deep side. Others would pat the glass but, despite the tactile evidence that the "cliff" was in fact a solid surface, would refuse to cross it. Still others would peer down through the glass on the deep side and then back away. Some simply cried. Even though babies can touch the glass and feel its solidity all they like, most will not crawl onto the solid glass surface. These hard-wired fears provide an evolved protection from injuries due to falling—a major cause of injury and death even into adulthood. We seem to be naturally selected to visually recognize sudden drops in elevation of the ground and to possess an innate, biologically designed fear of such drops that develops around the time of self-loco-motion even without any previous experience or conditioning.[78]

A more recent study confirms that fear of heights is innate and not developed through learning or as a result of earlier traumatic experiences. This study finds that falls are the most common accident occurring to children up to 9 years. Yet, it is not children who have suffered injury from serious falls who are more likely to subsequently develop fears of heights. Instead, "falls resulting in serious injury between 5 and 9 years occurred with greater frequency in those *without* a fear at age 18. Of greatest importance, *no* individual who had a height phobia at age 18 had a history of a serious fall before the age of nine."[79] Height fears did not result from conditioning experiences, but from inborn tendencies that are protective.

Fear of heights is not limited to humans. Findings from other terrestrial species are largely consistent and equally dramatic. Due to their early self-produced loco-motion, chicks, kids, and lambs could be tested on the first day of life as soon as they could stand. *No* chick, kid, or lamb tested with the visual cliff ever stepped onto the glass on the deep side, even at one day of age.[80] When lowered onto the deep side, kids and lambs would initially refuse to put their feet down. They then adopted a defensive posture and their front legs became rigid and their hind legs limp. From this immobile state they would often leap in the air to the apparent safety of the center board, rather than walk on the glass. Few fears appear more consistently in terrestrial animals: researchers have noted similar findings with cats, land turtles, dogs, pigs, and neonatal monkeys, to name but a few.[81] Unlike land-dwelling ani-mals, aquatic species such as ducks and water-dwelling turtles, which have little reason to fear a perceived drop, readily cross onto the deep side.[82]

Findings about the fear of heights have a number of important implications. A variety of species possess innate fears of heights that appear by the time babies are locomotive. Such fears are present in pre-socialized infants who have no language skills, so this fear has a precognitive, instinctual basis. Moreover, these fears are common to all land-dwelling species and therefore must have been inherited through processes of natural selection. Finally, height fears among older age groups are not related to previous experiences of falls and thus are not products of learned conditioning. There is little doubt that humans, like many other species, are naturally designed to fear high places.

CULTURE AND UNIVERSALITY

Despite the varying array of evidence for certain kinds of universal fears, many social scientists deny the existence of worldwide, biologically grounded emotions.[83] Social constructionists, for example, often sharply distinguish between factors having to do with the mind, which language and culture profoundly influence, and those dealing with the body, which nature primarily shapes. Instead of assuming the existence of objective disease processes, constructionists often emphasize that cultural "display rules" dictate how emotions of anxiety should be evoked, felt, and expressed. "The attitudes that entered into the ideological construction of the emotions in ancient Greece," asserts historian David Konstan, "are not the same as ours."[84] According to this view, because these rules differ so drastically both across different societies and across different social statuses in the same society, fear and anxiety must in essence be culturally relative emotions.

Many strands of social constructivist accounts of how culture shapes emotions are helpful in illuminating fear's enormous cultural variability. There is no doubt that, while the roots of anxiety are found in shared human biology, culture also has profound influences on this emotion. For one thing, constructionists rightly emphasize how culture shapes norms for the appropriate expression of anxiety. For example, symptoms of social phobia among Japanese commonly take the form of a fear of offending others; analogous symptoms among Americans are expressed through intense fear of personal embarrassment.[85] Cultures also provide people with the tools to exert control over emotions and the thresholds when they are triggered. The ancient Greeks, for example, both recognized the power of emotions of anxiety and the necessity to train soldiers to resist these emotions while in combat.[86]

It is also the case that different cultures socialize their members not only to certain styles of expressing and controlling fear and anxiety but also to the particular groups, objects, conditions, and situations that are appropriate to fear. These anxiety-producing stimuli are neither inherited nor results of idiosyncratic learning, but emerge from socially shared foundations. It is reasonable to fear whatever cultures emphasize as sources of danger, regardless of the objective environmental grounding of such fears. Unlike natural fears, which are inherited and pretty much universal within the parameters of enormous individual variability, standards of reasonableness vary from culture to culture. A person in medieval times would have reasonably feared demons. Likewise, residents of sixteenth-century English villages had a reasonable fear of witchcraft, magic, and ghosts. Cultural norms in Western societies in the nineteenth century led the consequences of masturbation to be a particularly powerful source of anxiety.[87] In the absence of participation in some unusual subculture, fears of demons, witchcraft, ghosts, or masturbation are not reasonable at present, at least, in modern, developed societies. In contrast, such prevalent fears in the twenty-first century as germs and food allergies might seem laughable in other cultures.

Moreover, cultures not only provide particular objects of fear but also influence the quantity of fearfulness that is found in given groups. While some cultures, such as the Dobuans of Melanesia, fear a wide variety of objects and situations, others, such as the Tasaday who live in the highlands of the Philippines, have few fears.[88] Indeed, omnipresent fears can mark whole historical periods, such as the late Middle Ages in Europe.[89] Groups with communal norms that emphasize cooperation foster less anxiety than those that promote competitiveness among their members.[90] As well, cultures that feature consistent and stable meaning systems that offer socially shared interpretations of threatening situations should have fewer fearful members than those that lack these qualities. Likewise, cultures can provide ritualistic systems consisting of rules that, when followed, offer reassurance in the face of threatening situations. Their cultures thus to some extent provide people with the particular objects that are appropriate to fear, the proper ways to express their fears, and the conventions, norms, and habits that they use to manage their concerns and worries.

Nevertheless, despite these culturally induced variations, the fact remains that across cultures, there is a remarkable agreement over many objects and types of fear, and most culturally feared objects fall into evolutionarily pre-prepared categories. Moreover, the very fact that fear exists across cultures in a fully recognizable form similar to that in other species cannot be explained by the constructivist account and must be due to biological design. Aside from standard fears of such things as snakes and heights, as Chapter 3 discusses in more detail, these universal threats include, for example, uncertain and novel situations, encounters with social superiors, and strangers. Throughout history people have been far more likely to project their fears onto out-groups than in-groups; more socially distant populations are universally the object of heightened levels of fear. Socially marginal people are more often feared than the socially respectable, strangers more than intimates, and members of more distant cultures more than fellow group members. Such cultural processes reflect evolutionarily grounded fears of unfamiliar persons, although cultural learning buttresses the universal template to fear distant social groups. Ultimately, different expressions of anxiousness are culturally influenced variants of common underlying emotions with parameters waiting to be filled by cultural meanings. Cultural construction is not antithetical to, but is coordinated with, biological design.

STRANGER ANXIETY AS BIOLOGICALLY AND CULTURALLY INFLUENCED

Cultural shaping and naturally evolved fears are typically not two distinct dimensions; rather, they usually interact with each other. For example, fear of strangers among young children seems to be universal. Consider children's crying with distress when a stranger approaches them, long recognized as a basic emotion. Freud, for one, says, "Only a few of the manifestations of anxiety in children are comprehensible to us, and we must confine our attention to them. They occur, for instance ... when [a child] finds itself alone with an unknown person instead of one to whom it is used—such as its mother. . . . Here, I think, we have the key to an understanding of anxiety. . . . anxiety appears as a reaction to the felt loss of the object."[91]

Figure 2.2 shows how both the underlying pattern and innate triggers of stranger fear are similar across cultures; in all cultures this fear reaches a peak at about the same age, with children younger and older showing less frequent fear responses.[92]

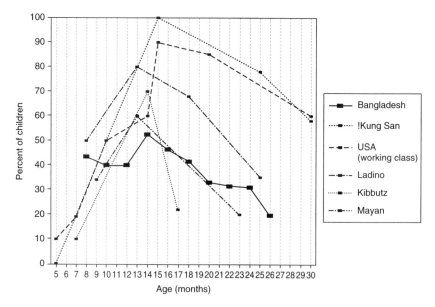

Figure 2.2: Crying at Mother's Departure, used with permission from Super and Harkness, 2008.

Presumably, the period around one year of age is when strangers posed a particularly great threat to a developing child not yet old enough to run away or seek help.

Yet, innate triggers of fear and cultural variation both influence stranger anxiety. These data also show that culture strongly influences the frequency of children who respond to the trigger with fearful crying and the persistence of stranger fear. Infants in all sampled cultures rarely cry at maternal departure until around 7 or 8 months, followed by a peak shortly after the first birthday, with a subsequent decline.[93] In contrast to the similarity in timing for the rise of distress, these cultures vary dramatically in not only the overall rate of crying but also the rate of disappearance of the fear with age. This response largely dissipates among Mayan and Israeli infants by 24 months, while nearly half the !Kung San and U.S. infants still become distressed at this time. The nearly exclusive maternal care practices of the !Kung San and U.S. groups appear to extend the reaction to maternal departure, while distress quickly dissipates among Guatemalans and members of Israeli kibbutzim who have customs of shared infant care. Neither nature nor culture alone can explain these patterns: both are necessary to account for the universal emergence of stranger fears among small children and the variation in rates and endurance of these fears across cultures.

A major task of the social sciences is to reconcile biological universals and cultural variability.[94] When it comes to fear and anxiety, nature and culture are neither mutually exclusive nor distinct, but rather two complementary aspects of how anxious emotions are generated and expressed. On the one hand, because brain-based mechanisms are common across cultures and individuals, the study of psychological processes must have a strong universalistic component. The biological underpinnings of emotion do not depend on language or even on awareness. Fear and anxiety might be social constructions, but they are built upon thousands of generations of evolutionary experience.

On the other hand, the cultural and historical variation in the expressions and classifications of anxiety disorders shows that even universal phenomena require cultural understandings. Different cultures so powerfully shape biologically grounded experiences that there is no one-to-one correspondence between biological indicators and experienced or expressed emotions. Both biological and cultural explanations are needed to fully comprehend the range of anxious emotions and why a normal fear in one setting can be considered an anxiety disorder in another.

INDIVIDUAL VARIATION

Reconciling universality with differing cultural expressions is one job of an adequate evolutionary concept of anxiety. Another task is to explain how a universal emotion such as anxiety can also display a huge range in the tendencies of different individuals to feel, and manifest, fear. For example, while we have seen that height fear is universal, its extent varies substantially among individuals. Many people are terrified by experiences such as standing at the top of the Willis (formerly Sears) Tower, skydiving, or mountain climbing, yet many others crave and seek out these activities. How can a genetically rooted emotion be compatible with such a broad diversity of individual expression?

There are several reasons for why people's inclination to feel fear or anxiety might naturally vary. For one thing, most human traits—whether height, intelligence, physical strength, or beauty—are distributed along a spectrum due to genetic variation. For another, people's feelings and behavior are a result not just of their genes but also of their life histories. Some people adjust to common fears, as when many childhood concerns (e.g., fears of darkness or wild animals) wane and gradually extinguish or are overcome with aging. But for others, early life experiences maintain or intensify these fears. Consider the experience of the film director Alfred Hitchcock, whose father sent him to a police station when he was a young child with a note asking the constable to lock the boy in a cell.[95] The five minutes that Hitchcock spent in the cell had a lasting impact on him—recurring themes of arrest and a fear of confinement in small enclosed places appear in his films. Even many fears that seem to be wholly inexplicable might have a reasonable explanation in terms of normal fear conditioning when an individual's meaning system is taken into account. Psychiatrist John Bowlby relates the case of a woman who had a seemingly senseless fear that her healthy 4-year-old child was in danger of dying.[96] It turned out that the woman had a brother who died at this age, rendering her own fear comprehensible in light of her experience.

In addition, feelings result from not just one trait but from an individual's entire array of traits interacting with the situation. Thus, some people are lucky enough to have experiences that allow them to feel in control and less vulnerable and may have experienced few traumas that create salient memories that come back to trigger fear, and they thus experience less fear. Others may be better at overcoming or inhibiting or ignoring their fear, or suppressing it when initially aroused, either because of what they learned while growing up, their innate talent at doing so, or the lack of other stressors that weaken their ability to handle the fears they have. But as many thinkers from early Greek philosophers to contemporary psychologists have pointed out, courage is not a matter of feeling no fear; it is a matter of being capable of acting in accordance with what one rationally knows to be the best path irrespective of one's fear.[97] Some people may be better than others at overriding their fears with rational considerations.

Variation is also likely more than just random variation. Genetic endowment leads anxious temperaments to vary from the time of birth. Just as natural selection led to different sexes and varied eye colors, it appears to have led to equally adaptive but different levels of fearfulness. Different strategies in addressing specific threats might have been equally effective in our prehistory, and variations in fear were selected accordingly. For example, risk and reward might have covaried in such a way that there were different solutions to the equation of optimal fear. For some, high self-confidence and bravado often led to disaster but occasionally to a very high payoff with great power and high reproductive value; for others, fearful cautiousness led to safety and more modest but more frequent positive outcomes. Thus, within a certain range, many different levels of fear and biological strategies of emotional arousal—each offering its own benefits and costs—could have about equal net reproductive implications. Natural selection would favor various trade-offs of traits and turn a blind eye to the precise level of fear within this range. Variation is so common and pronounced because it turns out that, given a set of environmental challenges, there are often multiple different adaptive strategies for addressing that set of challenges.[98]

Moreover, individuals vary in ways that allow them to take advantage of different social niches, whether as trapeze artists or forest rangers, where decreased or increased anxiety is beneficial. Indeed, the very fact that some people embrace one strategy may enhance the value of other strategies for exploiting social niches, thus leading to a balance between different types in the population. In addition, when environments vary in the level of a trait that would be adaptive, as is likely the case with fear in primitive circumstances, the population tends to retain a large amount of genetic variation where different types cope better with different particular scenarios.[99] For example, those higher in vigilance and anxiety might fare better in times of generally increased danger, whereas those with calmer temperaments might be at an advantage in relatively safe and secure periods. For all of these reasons, a wide range of individual variation will always surround every innate fear.

CONCLUSION

The attempt to understand normal and disordered fear and anxiety led in this chapter to an investigation of concepts of normality and pathology themselves. Fear is perhaps the best single emotion for providing a lens to view how both brain-based and culture-based processes underlie definitions of health and disease. Both normal fear and anxiety disorders are grounded in biology: one in the normal, contextually wired brain and the other in disorders of brain-based mechanisms. Common criticisms of the supposed evolutionary groundings of processes such as cheater detection, male propensity to rape, or sexual attractiveness as fanciful "just-so" stories do not hold for fear.[100] In distinction from many other emotions, it is easy to understand the evolutionary functions of fear and why organisms that became afraid in dangerous situations were better able to survive and reproduce than organisms that didn't have these mechanisms.

While fear and anxiety are rooted in evolutionarily shaped brain circuitry, it is anything but obvious what represents the natural as opposed to the pathological functioning of this organ. The amygdala and other fear-related brain regions are designed to respond to the kinds of dangers that imposed selective pressures on organisms in the distant past but that in many cases might not pose any threats in the present. Indeed, humans tend to be naturally afraid of a small number of objects and situations, including crawling insects, snakes, carnivorous animals, thunder, darkness, strangers, closed-in spaces, heights, deep water, social scrutiny, and leaving home alone.[101] It is striking that these are the sorts of threats that plagued prehistoric people but are ones that are rarely dangerous in the modern world. Therefore, *normal* brains often react to cues that no longer indicate danger. And, reacting by way of the amygdala, these responses to some extent initially bypass higher cognitive processing. These intrinsic qualities of fear responses raise fundamental questions about the "adaptive" aspect of natural fears, since the sorts of contexts that made fear adaptive during prehistory are often no longer relevant in the contemporary world. The next chapter delves more deeply into the circumstances that make some anxiety responses natural and others pathological.

CHAPTER 3

Normal, Pathological, and Mismatched Anxiousness

The previous chapter presented an evolutionary view that we argued to be superior to the major alternatives for distinguishing natural from disordered anxiety. According to this view, pathological anxiety requires a defect in an internal cognitive or biological mechanism that regulates anxious emotions, causing anxiety that falls outside of the biologically designed range of variation of emotion. An evolutionary perspective is especially powerful because it provides a universal framework that nevertheless incorporates cultural and individual variation. This chapter considers in more detail the question of what distinguishes anxiety-producing mechanisms that are functioning naturally—that is, as they are biologically designed to function—and those that are dysfunctions of these mechanisms.

SETTING BOUNDARIES BETWEEN NATURAL AND DISORDERED FEAR AND ANXIETY

From the fact that evolution shaped fear mechanisms to be activated within specific contexts that cue anxiety arousal in a way that prepares us to deal with potential danger, we can derive some guidelines concerning the ways in which these mechanisms can go wrong and yield anxiety disorders as well as the conditions under which anxiety reactions, though intense and uncomfortable, might still be normal. One such implication is that, contrary to the tendency among psychiatrists to equate anxiety severity with pathology, pathological anxiety does not consist simply of intense anxiety.

Disordered anxiety does not lie at one end of a continuum of severity with mild fears on the other end. Intensity and disorder are two somewhat related but conceptually independent dimensions. This is because extremely threatening situations—or situations that were once extremely threatening—often produce correspondingly intense but natural amounts of non-disordered fear. Conversely, chronic mild anxiety that has no relationship to any external threat can represent a disorder of minimal severity, not a normal level of fear. Thus, although anxiety disorders tend on average to be characterized by severe anxiety, intensity and dysfunction in principle constitute two different dimensions; both normal and disordered anxiety responses can range from mild to severe. The "mild" versus "severe" distinction is not the same as the "normal" versus "disordered" distinction because the latter has to do with whether something has gone wrong with the biologically designed functioning of anxiety mechanisms, irrespective of severity level.[1]

Another implication of the evolutionary perspective is that many anxiety-provoking situations are typical of ancient situations of real danger that, through natural selection, became naturally anxiety-provoking, and they remain so whether or not they conform to what is presently dangerous. This means that fears that are unreasonable within current contexts might nevertheless emerge from naturally functioning anxiety-producing mechanisms. It is very easy to mistake such natural fears for anxiety disorders because of the lack of real danger. The importance of context and the difficulties posed by the mismatch between natural fears and current environments, as well as normal individual and cultural variation, ensure a high degree of uncertainty and indeterminacy about the borders placed around disorder.

These ambiguities explain the difficulty of making distinctions between anxiety disorders and extreme but normal-range levels of fear. While some clear cases of disordered and non-disordered forms of anxiety can be confidently recognized, the boundaries between normal fears and pathological anxiety disorders—especially when it comes to fear triggered by situations that in our environment do not involve obvious dangers—are often unclear and vague. Some of these ambiguities are not resolvable given our current knowledge of mental functioning, and some may involve inherent fuzziness that can never be fully resolved.

There need not be a precise boundary between disorder and non-disorder for the distinction to be usable and indeed crucial within psychiatry. The adequacy of a concept of mental disorder has nothing to do with whether it neatly separates conditions sharply into normal emotions and disorders. Indeed, if a large zone of indeterminacy between normal and disordered conditions exists in nature, then the most accurate concept of disorder will *not* have precise boundaries. If disorders are harmful dysfunctions, then the fact that concepts of harm and of dysfunction both come in degrees and are fuzzy concepts with lots of ambiguous boundary cases means that the concept of disorder will also be fuzzy with lots of ambiguous boundary cases. What is essential is that the concepts of normality and pathology can be clearly applied to a range of important cases. Clarity about such concepts becomes particularly important when clear cases of normality or disorder are misclassified due to conceptual confusion or poorly framed diagnostic criteria—a problem that we will argue exists in the current psychiatric diagnostic criteria for many anxiety disorders.

When vagueness does exist in an otherwise objective distinction, boundary-setting can become an intensely social process. Consider, for example, the distinction between "child" and "adult." Surely there is a real distinction between children and adults, based on an array of natural facts. The distinction is not overall an arbitrary one; it has clear cases on both sides and is important to make. At the same time, given the continuous nature of the developmental process from child to adult, there are bound to be fuzzy and ambiguous areas along the child–adult dimension. However, a sharp and enforceable boundary is often necessary for social purposes. Thus, considerations other than the concept itself, such as social values and the specific social function of the distinction in a particular setting, enter into the way the boundary is drawn. Setting the boundary may be done differently in establishing who can drink alcoholic beverages, join the military, enter into a legal contract, obtain a driver's license, engage in consensual sexual relations, or marry. Consequently, there are many distinctions between children and adults that depend on the context. As we will see in future chapters, because the boundaries between natural and pathological anxiety are so fuzzy, social processes and interests have critical impacts on where the actual dividing lines are set.

THE CHARACTERISTICS OF FEAR AND ANXIETY

Anxiety, both normal and disordered, can become manifest in a chameleon-like variety of ways. These include psychological manifestations such as nervousness, apprehension, worry, and fear; physiological symptoms including breathing difficulties, heart palpitations, trembling hands, intense sweating, and dizziness; and behaviors such as avoidance and withdrawal. Sometimes anxiety is tied to particular phobic objects or situations; other times it is objectless, as in generalized anxiety or panic disorders. The many particular expressions of anxiety notwithstanding, some general features characterize all or most of its forms.

Instantaneous activation. Because evolution originally designed fearful emotions to respond to dangers that might pose imminent threats, a central feature of natural fear mechanisms is their immediate activation in response to cues of danger. Once organisms sense danger, they must have the capacity to react more or less instantly. Yet, the biology of fear is anchored not only in the level of neurons, synapses, and neurochemicals but also in complexly organized brain-based neural circuits and cognitive processes. Fear circuitry must include mechanisms for monitoring inputs regarding potentially dangerous situations, mechanisms for appraising the degree and nature of danger when it is detected, and mechanisms that, in response to the assessment that the situation is indeed dangerous, produce the physiological, psychological, and behavioral outputs related to fear.[2] Whether implicit (outside of consciousness) via relatively automatic processes, or arising after considered judgments, consciousness of fear occurs only after some object or situation is *judged* to appear dangerous.[3]

Thinking, however, is one process that can considerably slow reaction time. Conscious appraisals inherently proceed more slowly than unconscious reactions, so initial fear responses are designed to bypass mindful thought. The Roman Stoic philosopher Epictetus recognized this aspect of fear mechanisms when he said, in the early second century CE:

> Mental impressions, through which a person's mind is struck by the initial aspect of some circumstance impinging on the mind, are not voluntary or a matter of choice, but force themselves upon one's awareness by a kind of power of their own . . . That is why, when some terrifying sound occurs, either from the sky or from the collapse of a building or as the sudden herald of some danger, even the wise person's mind necessarily responds and is contracted and grows pale for a little while, not because he opines that something evil is at hand, but by certain rapid and unplanned movements antecedent to the office of intellect and reason. Shortly, however, the wise person in that situation withholds assent from those terrifying impressions; he spurns and rejects them and does not think that there is anything in them which he should fear.[4]

Epictetus' observation anticipated biological findings that demonstrate how the necessity to act quickly in the face of sudden danger leads fear mechanisms to bypass slower thalamocortical pathways and respond without conscious appraisal and thought.[5] The primary appraisal processes regarding danger are involuntary and take place before the brain has a chance to think about what to do.

Fear responses originate in the most ancient part of the brain, the amygdala.[6] This part of the brain is found in all species that have a brain, and in all these species the amygdala, among its other functions, takes care of fear responses. This means that fearful reactions are grounded in an organ that humans have inherited from our distant evolutionary ancestors. Amygdala cells activate when they receive stimuli that signal dangers that are either innate, such as the smell or sound of a predator, or learned from past experiences.

The role of the amygdala in fear responses has remained constant over millions of years of evolution because of the efficient pathways of information transmission that exist between the thalamus (the part of the brain that processes and relays sensory information) and the amygdala.[7] These thalamo-amygdala pathways are extraordinarily fast at conveying signals of danger. Like many ancient brain processes, they are not voluntarily controlled; instead, they respond automatically to particular stimuli. The connections from cortical areas to the amygdala are far weaker than those that run in the opposite direction, which might explain why it is easier for emotional information to invade our conscious thoughts than for us to gain conscious control over our emotions. While different organisms fear different things, their neural responses to what they fear are similar.

Darwin anticipated the modern neurobiological findings demonstrating the largely unconscious nature of the fear detection system in his speculations that neural signals passing from the brain to the body bypass consciousness.[8] He thought that while willpower can sometimes mute the expression of fear, fear usually arises involuntarily. Well before Darwin, philosophers such as Plato, Aquinas, and Hume noted that reason is a slave to the emotions.[9] Modern biology indicates why this should be the case: the amygdala is wired to preempt thought in dangerous situations.[10] As the psychologist William James famously proposed in 1884, the conscious control over fear occurs only after these emotions themselves have arisen.[11]

Initial responses to danger are thus not deliberate choices but unconscious programs that emerge and function in evolutionarily old brain structures, without restraint by conscious thought. Psychological experiments indicate that subliminal exposure to evolutionarily relevant fear cues such as spiders and snakes, but not to unthreatening stimuli such as flowers or mushrooms, activates physiological fear responses.[12] Likewise, experimental subjects who are exposed to angry faces demonstrate far more neural activity in their amygdalae than those exposed to neutral faces, even though their exposure to both types of faces is too brief to be consciously perceived. The normal biology of fear bypasses conscious and rational systems of control in initial stages of response and activates very rapidly when evolutionarily relevant cues are aroused. Consequently, while fear can be cognitively and culturally controlled, it is extremely difficult to suppress completely.

Low threshold. The second characteristic of fear-generating danger detection mechanisms is that they are biased toward perceiving threats. Normal fear responses are preprogrammed to more easily mistake safe situations for dangerous ones than to make the opposite error of assuming safety when danger in fact exists. From an evolutionary perspective of surviving to reproduce, it seems that it is indeed better to be safe than sorry. For example, people who overestimate the chances that the smell of rotten eggs indicates a natural gas leak are likely better off in the long run than those who erroneously think the smell of leaking gas likely stems from foul eggs. The reason for this is obvious: while in the short term such overestimation of danger may cause some wasted time and energy through incorrectly reacting fearfully in safe situations, these minimal costs are far outweighed in the long run by the survival advantages of more effective responses to true emergencies, when a defensive response may save one from an actual threat that is life-threatening.

Evolutionary psychiatrist Randolph Nesse calls the bias of fear mechanisms toward interpreting danger the "smoke detector principle."[13] Smoke detectors are often deliberately set sensitively, and as a consequence they often will sound an alarm when smoke harmlessly arises from cooking or a cigarette; though they unfortunately react to many false threats, they are also more likely to react to even a modest real one. The alternative, an alarm with a higher triggering threshold that rarely responds in the absence of a real fire but also has a substantial probability of missing an actual fire, would be much less desirable because false alarms are annoying but not terribly damaging, whereas it takes just one missed fire to harm you or your possessions.[14]

Many warning mechanisms in nature are biologically designed on the smoke detector principle to yield many false warnings for every rare occasion when there is a real danger.[15] "From my own recollection," noted Darwin's cousin Francis Galton, "I believe that every antelope in South Africa has to run for its life every one or two days on average, and that he starts or gallops under the influence of a false alarm many times a day."[16] Similarly, beavers tend to beat their tails upon the ground and make thumping sounds to warn of danger. However, the various signals that trigger this response are only occasionally linked to a real predator, so most of the time the signal responds to some sound or other cue that turns out to be innocuous. Such false alarms are costly in terms of lost time and expended energy, but are still a net gain for the organism due to the occasional success. Comparably, fear mechanisms can be biologically useful on balance even if they often are "wrong" when they trigger fear—as when one reacts with a startle response to some innocuous sound.

In addition to an inherent tendency to overstate the degree of threat in response to evolutionarily relevant fear stimuli, the evolutionary perspective suggests that organisms should have natural biases to retain and remember rather than to forget fearful situations.[17] For example, many cases of post-traumatic stress disorder are products of evolutionary tendencies to heighten fear sensitivities so that similar situations might be avoided in the future. The grossly exaggerated senses of danger that people with anxiety disorders display extend natural tendencies to amplify the dangers posed in any given situation.

Responsiveness to unusual and uncertain situations. A third quality of fear responses is that the inherent bias toward perceiving danger is particularly apparent in the processing of novel, surprising, and ambiguous stimuli.[18] The strangeness and consequent uncertainty of a new or unusual situation is a principle source of fear. Even the simplest one-celled animals are sensitive to unexpected and unfamiliar events.[19] Because organisms have no experience of—and thus no conditioned cues to—such stimuli, and because novel situations are occasionally highly dangerous, such situations are more likely to be treated as potential sources of danger than of safety. People are preprogrammed to fear the unexpected, the strange, and the indefinite, whatever particular forms these take in a given context or social group.

Future orientation. A final characteristic of fear lies in its forward-looking nature.[20] Fear about the past would activate the organism to deal with a challenge that no longer exists, wasting resources. Fear is an anticipatory emotion: we fear what might happen to us, not what has already occurred. People are fearful when they anticipate entering combat, giving a speech, having a medical operation, reacting to an impending traffic accident, taking an examination, or getting punished.[21] Likewise, they become anxious regarding general uncertainties about the future. For example, young people in seventeenth-century England complained "about the anxieties of courtship and marriage and the uncertainties of getting a living and bearing children, problems that accompanied the transition from youthful dependence on parents and masters to full independence as married adults."[22] The future orientation of anxiety enhances our ability to anticipate and plan for upcoming challenges and enables us to prevent potential harm to ourselves.

The forward-looking thrust of anxiousness contrasts with most other emotions, such as sadness, hatred, or jealousy, which are more oriented to reviewing past experiences. For example, events that pose dangers to future welfare predict anxiety, while events that entail some loss that has already occurred are more likely to lead to depression.[23] Once a feared event is over, other emotions—whether depression, anger, relief, or joy—come into play.

The biology of fear, then, entails many unpleasant features. It emerges quickly, is difficult to consciously control, arises at low thresholds, motivates us to avoid novel and uncertain situations, and is oriented to anticipating future dangers. Its hallmark symptoms—highly uncomfortable subjective feelings of anxiousness accompanied by such physiological indicators as sweating, rapid heartbeat, and/or muscle tension as well as the narrow focusing of attention on a potential threat—are all naturally selected responses to threatening situations. The way intense fear transforms perception and attention is part of how it enables the organism to deal with the immediately pressing situational challenge. Information-gathering and memory become narrowly focused on the particular danger. Safety becomes a prioritized goal as the organism, with heightened cognitive vigilance and apprehensive expectation, scrutinizes methods of avoidance.[24]

We can, of course, make deliberate attempts to override our unconsciously generated anxiety reactions with subsequent reasoned actions. We are stuck, though, with being biologically designed in such a way that it is easier for our anxious emotions to influence our thoughts than it is for our thoughts to gain control over these emotions. We have no choice about the fact that our brains are designed with mechanisms that activate strong emotional responses quickly and unthinkingly to perceived threat as a priority. Moreover, these emotions automatically respond to situations that, because they were evocative of danger in ancient times as well as realistic dangers in the present, have become innate triggers of fear responses. We also are designed to recollect traumatic occurrences, however painful such memories might be and however strongly we might wish to forget them. These features of fear response mechanisms help explain why anxiety so often seems irrational to both anxious people and those around them. These qualities are not just the burden of people with anxiety disorders but, to a greater or lesser degree, of all of us. "We are," observes neurobiologist Joseph LeDoux about human emotions of fear, "emotional lizards."[25]

Normal Anxiety

Evolution designed anxiety to arise quickly, automatically, and at low thresholds in response to a variety of dangerous and uncertain situations. This means that, as philosophers and theologians, not to mention psychiatrists, have long recognized, levels of normal anxiety will tend to be high. The commonness of the sorts of experiences that naturally lead to anxiousness ensure that fear and anxiety are ubiquitous phenomena.

Immediate threats of harm produce anxiety among virtually all people who experience them. Combat provides a classic example of an imminently dangerous situation. Systematic observations of soldiers anticipating combat reveal that the vast majority experience at least some fear. Only 7% of infantrymen who participated in a study during World War II reported never feeling afraid. About 90% had trouble getting to sleep, 87% experienced violent pounding of the heart, and 85% were troubled by sweating palms.[26] "A state of tension and anxiety is so prevalent in the front lines," noted military psychiatrist Herbert Spiegel in 1943, "that it must be regarded as a normal reaction in this grossly abnormal situation."[27] Well before this, the Roman philosopher Seneca noted, "Even the man who is generally very brave grows pale when putting on his armor; the fiercest of soldiers is weak at the knees when the signal to engage is given; a great general's heart pounds before the lines of battle meet."[28] Any situation that leads to perceptions of urgent, mortal danger induces intense and immediate anxiety among normal people.[29]

Fears naturally develop not just during the expectation of imminent harm but also from anticipated threats. Uncertainty about the nature of future dangers is particularly conducive to anxiety. Most people are fearful before learning the results of a medical test for a serious illness, giving an important talk, taking a consequential exam, starting a new school or job, entering an athletic contest, or hearing a judge's sentencing about punishment.[30] Periods of economic insecurity and recession are especially likely to lead to worries and concerns among a large proportion of the affected population. Likewise, even after the immediate dangers from extremely stressful events such as natural disasters have passed, many people experience very high levels of anxiety because of persistent insecurity about the future they create.[31]

Because it is tied to particular contexts, normal anxiety dissipates once the uncertainty of a threatening situation has been resolved. For example, in the movie *Cleo from 5 to 7*, Cleo becomes extremely anxious when she learns she might have a fatal form of cancer. When her biopsy reveals that several months of chemotherapy should cure the cancer, hope for her future immediately replaces her anxiety. The normality of her initial anxiousness is tied to its context of a life-threatening situation; once the uncertainty of this situation is resolved, her distressing emotions disappear.

There are, then, numerous sources of normal anxiety. Some stem from life events that threaten individuals, such as the prospect of a home foreclosure, a serious illness in oneself or an intimate, the loss of a valued job, or fear that a romantic partner will leave a relationship. Daily living also entails routine threats such as being late for a meeting because of a traffic jam, missing work because of a sick child, or wearing the wrong clothes to a dinner party. Others characterize entire communities that undergo the loss of a major employer or a natural disaster, or whole countries that are in the midst of wars, revolutions, and foreign occupations. Social life is full of things—ranging from the mundane to the cataclysmic—that normal people worry about. We now consider the ways in which our anxiety-generating mechanisms can go wrong, leading to worries that constitute psychiatric disorders.

Anxiety Disorders

Current classifications of anxiety disorders, which Chapter 5 considers in detail, focus on specifying the particular symptoms of a variety of anxiety disorders including phobias, panic, obsessive-compulsive behavior, generalized anxiety, and a few other conditions. Here, instead, we focus on the more basic question of what makes any specific anxiety condition a disorder. In particular, we consider three general indicators of disordered anxiety mechanisms, all of which involve a divergence between a context and the resulting level of anxiety. First, anxiety arises in the absence of appropriate evolutionary or cultural contexts. Second, anxiety might emerge after appropriate cues but then come to involve symptoms of excessive severity or duration that are disengaged from the initial threatening context. Finally, the inability to become anxious when a dangerous context arises can indicate an anxiety disorder.

Anxiety without Appropriate Cause

Anxiety disorders typically involve people who become extremely anxious in the absence of appropriate indications of danger. In one type of situation, anxiety develops and persists when no fear cues are present, indicating that the natural danger-signaling functions of fear mechanisms are not working properly.[32] Sometimes, as in cases of generalized anxiety disorder, people can feel omnipresent anxiety without any signs of threat. Such a constantly fearful person cannot adapt to changing circumstances and presumably has an anxiety disorder.[33]

Panic provides an example of a condition that naturally arises after cues that correspond to increased risk of attack and therefore would be useful in life-threatening situations. It alters cognition, behavior, and physiology so that people can react with heightened alertness, focus, speed, and effectiveness. Sudden panic episodes that arise in the absence of severely threatening situations (for example, in a grocery store) appear to be misfirings of whatever mechanism is responsible for generating panic-type feelings in response to acute threats.[34] Similarly, the fear of leaving one's home (agoraphobia) can be adaptive in dangerous environments but is not otherwise understandable as a biologically designed response. Social anxiety that arises in situations that do not involve social threats, humiliation, or scrutiny can also indicate a disordered state. For example, the social anxiety of someone who is sitting in a large lecture hall with little interaction between students and an instructor might be a sign of a disorder in which something has gone wrong with the functioning of social anxiety mechanisms.

Obsessive-compulsive behaviors are disorders because they have no triggers but must be performed regardless of their context. Thoughts and behaviors become preoccupations that require elaborate rituals to allay anxiety. Media personality Howard Stern describes an array of such activities, including having to read sentences exactly three times, performing elaborate rituals involving changing television channels in certain ways before he could go to sleep, or conducting a variety of activities when a clock read even and not odd numbers because he perceived odd numbers were luckier than even ones.[35] "It got so bad," Stern notes, "that if I was studying in the library and I had finished and wanted to take a break, I would look up at the clock. If the clock read 3:06, I would have to sit in my chair and wait until it turned 3:07 because I had somehow convinced myself that odd numbers were luckier than even ones."[36] The context in which these behaviors were performed was irrelevant: Stern had to perform them regardless of any other consideration. Such compulsive thinking and behavior can vary in severity from very mild to extremely disabling.

Stern's condition can be considered a disorder because it both involved a substantial amount of impairment and is neither directed at current or evolutionary dangers nor responsive to contextual changes. Often, however, obsessive tendencies can be channeled into socially acceptable modes such as housecleaning, stamp collecting, or compiling baseball statistics. Such cases might meet the criteria for a dysfunction but would not be disorders unless they are also impairing.

Not just the absence of appropriate cues but also the presence of the wrong cues can signify an anxiety disorder. In such cases, fear becomes attached to objects or situations that do not seem to be either natural or culturally reasonable sources of fear. Fears of objects or situations that generally are not sources of fear indicate that something has gone wrong with anxiety-generating mechanisms. For example, intense fears of being observed while eating, drinking, or writing have no plausible rational, evolutionary, or cultural basis and most likely are anxiety disorders.[37]

Anxiety disorders arise when people are constantly anxious when they have nothing to fear, become anxious about objects that pose neither evolutionary nor current threats, or must perform elaborate rituals that are not culturally appropriate to ward off anxiety. Such cases of groundless anxiety without any appropriate cause seem to be relatively rare. Most fears are related to actually threatening contexts or evolutionarily or culturally proper stimuli.

Excessiveness of Anxiety Responses

A second type of anxiety disorder stems from the consequences of threatening situations. Normal fear is triggered by danger and dissipates as the danger wanes, returning transiently as emotional memories when circumstances resemble the original threatening situation. Heightened states of arousal that lead to sleep difficulties, enhanced alertness, or increased heart rate are adaptive in the presence of actual danger, and perhaps briefly when new situations seem to resemble the ones in which the earlier danger occurred. These fear mechanisms were designed to respond to immediate threats and then to gradually subside except when emotional memory might warn of a return of the threat.[38]

Disorders can thus arise when anxiety that initially emerges as a prepared response to a dangerous situation becomes detached from the dangerous context and endures well beyond the persistence of the threat, not as a transient emotional memory limited to very similar circumstances but in a more general way that reshapes a life to the demands of grappling with endless anxiety. For example, post-traumatic stress disorders are conditions in which anxiety evoked by an environmental precipitant causes a subsequent breakdown in the ability of fear mechanisms to perform their designed functions due to an overly generalized continuing intense fear. Likewise, sustained anxiety states that are unrestricted by an immediate threat, such as continuous phobic arousal when no dangerous object is present, are often disordered. An individual who becomes hypervigilant and has trouble sleeping or attending to other tasks immediately after hearing a strange sound in the basement is responding adaptively, but if the individual maintains this state for several months without hearing similar sounds and without good reasons for believing the sounds represented a threat, then the initial vigilance may have become a disorder. In such cases, one would expect that neither the cessation of the fear-arousing stimuli nor withdrawal from the threatening situation reduces the anxiety.

It is very difficult to separate responses that display disproportionate duration and severity to an initial threat from high-range but normal personality dispositions. People who score high on scales indicating "neurotic" personality dispositions respond to stressful situations with high amounts of anxiety that can reflect an anxious temperament rather than an anxiety disorder. No means are currently available that can separate disproportionately high levels of anxiousness that are related to personality dimensions from those that are disordered. The resulting vagueness of boundaries means that the demarcation of "excessive" from "proportionate" anxiety can be set at many points along a wide range. Whatever particular point is chosen will inevitably have a large degree of arbitrariness.

Deficient Amounts of Fear

Human beings as well as cultures vary in anxiety intensity and its expression, and individuals vary in general resilience to stress as well as the degree to which they have cultivated methods of controlling or suppressing anxiety, sometimes to the point of great courage. Moreover, much of our anxiety is unnecessary given the relatively safe environments in which we live and the ancient and no-longer-threatening sources of some of our anxieties, so that lacking such anxieties would not be harmful and thus not a disorder. One certainly would not want to confuse a naturally calm temperament, a lucky lack of needless distress, or virtues like resilience or courage with disorder.

Nevertheless, in rare cases an extreme lack of capacity to generate anxiety even in the face of substantial immediate threat can indicate a disorder. The lack of ability to respond with anxiety to genuine threat can deprive the individual of crucial means for responding effectively, resulting in foolish or even reckless action that leads to outcomes such as injury, imprisonment, or death. Recklessness can of course be a normal variation of judgment up to a point, but when actions are not sensitive to risks because they are not guided by anxious emotional responses to threat, that could reflect a disorder. Analogously, even though it is sometimes a helpful virtue to be stoic and ignore physical pain, and sometimes it is reckless though not disordered to do so as one aggravates or prevents the healing of a painful injury, the inability to feel physical pain is a disorder of pain-sensing mechanisms that generally leads to early death from injuries and infections due to failure to respond effectively to physical insults to the body.

Consequently, organisms unable to be fearful even at a minimal level in species-typical ways when real threats are present must be considered disordered.[39] Creatures that can't detect and respond to danger—and thus are fearless and even reckless in the face of threatening situations—are likely to perish. This was the fate of the dodo bird, which evolved on an island with no predators and hence developed no instinctual fears. Once predators—namely, human beings—were introduced into its environment, the defenseless dodo was quickly exterminated. The dodos were just unlucky, not disordered, because nothing in their genetic heritage or personal experience had prepared them for the danger from humans when their island was colonized. However, the failure of species-typical fears to appear in the face of the real danger to which they are a biologically designed response can indicate a disorder.

Damaged brains, which many writers recognize as the only cause of genuine mental disorders, occasionally underlie anxiety disorders that involve lack of capacity for biologically designed anxiety responses.[40] Notably, when certain lesions in the amygdala occur, they lead to *incapacities* in expressing anxiety, not to excessive amounts of anxiety. For example, the neurologist Antonio Damasio found one rare patient with a damaged amygdala.[41] This patient showed little capability to respond to attempts at fear conditioning. Indeed, although she was able to identify most types of facial expressions, she was unable to identify faces that showed fear. Another type of brain lesion occurs when prefrontal lobotomies sever the connections in the deep white matter of both frontal lobes. These operations leave intellectual capacities undisturbed but almost immediately abolish anxiety and agitation; after undergoing these procedures, patients become extremely calm and unable to suffer. The implication is that *normal* brains are marked by the capacity to have high levels of arousal and vigilance; demonstrable brain lesions impair the natural ability of the brain to become anxious.

Too little anxiety is harmful and likely was naturally selected against. For example, children with little or no fear of heights are likely to suffer more falls than those with higher levels of fear. Likewise, adults who report an absence of height fear have elevated histories of serious falls in childhood.[42] Because evolution designed normal fear responses to arise quickly and easily, disorders that involve the absence of fear are unusual. People with little capacity to be anxious rarely visit psychiatrists but are often found in jails, hospitals, and cemeteries.[43] Under the right circumstances, especially in emergencies or combat, people with slight or no anxiety are highly valued, reaping praise, awards, and medals for heroic responses that disregard their own safety, yet the same individuals may get themselves in great trouble in other contexts where their lack of anxiety fails to guide them into prudent behaviors. Philosophers throughout the centuries have been at pains to distinguish such reckless behavior, no matter how occasionally accidentally useful, from true courage where potential fear is set aside or overcome in the service of a culturally or personally valued goal.

No category of anxiety disorder currently in the *Diagnostic and Statistical Manual* refers to any condition that features insufficient amounts of anxiety. Perhaps this is a rare condition, and perhaps as long as an individual is in a relatively safe environment, the lack of anxiety might be construed as a lucky, harmless break and not a disorder. Also, such individuals may perform dangerous tasks that others would avoid. Such social factors can determine whether there is harm and thus whether a dysfunctional psychological mechanism constitutes a disorder or just a benign anomaly.

MISMATCHES OF FEAR TO OBJECTS AND SITUATIONS

It is intrinsically difficult to separate mental disorders from distressing but natural emotions. This distinction is even harder to make for anxiety disorders than other conditions. Evolution designed anxiety to emerge not just from imminent dangers and uncertainties but also from cues that signaled danger in ancient environments but that are not necessarily currently dangerous. The huge prevalence of putative anxiety disorders is largely due to the widespread existence of evolutionarily normal fears that were reasonable during prehistory but that no longer have any rational basis.

Consider the eminent American psychologist G. Stanley Hall's (1844–1924) musings on the most common fears of late nineteenth-century Americans:

> Night is now the safest time, serpents are no longer among our most fatal foes, and most
> of the animal fears do not fit the present conditions of civilised life; strangers are not

usually dangerous, nor are big eyes and teeth; celestial fears fit the heavens of ancient superstition and not the heavens of modern science.[44]

Hall realized that such fears were genetically transmitted relics of the sorts of dangers that humans faced in prehistoric, not in current, environments.

In most modern environments, animals rarely pose dangers to humans, groups are culturally heterogeneous, and technology helps us control many external threats. Nevertheless, normal brains are programmed to respond to danger and to produce fear responses that worked effectively during the period when our fear responses were selected, and so people are often afraid of things that often pose no present danger. For instance, as Hall noted, objectively speaking, darkness is the safest time of day. With rare exceptions, such as sudden infant death syndrome, harms rarely happen during the night and people are generally exposed to far more dangers during daylight. Yet, we—especially children—often retain intense fears of the dark that are evolutionary vestiges of a formerly rational fear.

Indeed, many, or even most, conditions that are currently classified as phobias (by far the most common form of anxiety disorder) result from species-typical fear mechanisms of situations that posed genuine threats in prehistory but that are quite distinct from those facing present-day humans. Consider that the most prevalent sorts of specific fears among modern Americans are still of snakes, spiders, heights, and darkness.[45] Fears when being alone at night, unexpectedly confronting a stranger in an open space, or seeing a snake would be cues that long ago indicated possible danger from a predator. The common thread among these fears is that they would have been sources of danger during prehistory but rarely pose threats at present. Or, think about the intense fears that many children have of darkness or of animals that they have never seen and are not likely to ever confront. Such fears are not proportionately related to any actual environmental threat and might seem to indicate anxiety disorders when they reach a certain level of intensity. Yet, despite their current unreasonableness, they stem from naturally transmitted brain circuitry that arose millennia ago to respond to realistic threats in ancient environments.

Only minimal cues are necessary to generate ancestral fears. For example, children still report intense fears of snakes, especially between the ages of 4 and 6. Indeed, surveys show that snakes are the single most disliked animal of any.[46] Small children also often demonstrate extreme fears of darkness, being alone, separation from mothers or other intimate caretakers, getting lost, strangers, or animals such as lions or wolves that they are unlikely to actually encounter.[47] The commonality among these childhood fears is that they represented genuine fears in human prehistory, although they are rarely threatening in modern environments. Children who have powerful fears of darkness, strangers, or animals that pose no actual danger to them usually are responding to innate predispositions, perhaps triggered by minimal cues, not to idiosyncratic learned experiences. Conversely, children are unlikely to naturally fear current sources of danger such as automobiles or matches.

Moreover, it is considerably more difficult to extinguish fears of evolutionarily primed stimuli such as snakes and spiders than conditioned fears to objects such as electrical outlets or guns.[48] The ancient origin of instinctual fears often leads to a tenuous connection between what sorts of objects and situations people fear at present and the corresponding senses of danger that they develop. People typically fear the "wrong things" in terms of the objective probabilities of suffering harm. Few individuals objectively calculate danger by formulas that involve the actual probability of experiencing some injury and the resulting severity of harm from it.[49]

Social Fears

Mismatched fears are not limited to particular objects or situations. Other people might be our greatest source of support and security, but they are also one of the most common causes of anxiety.[50] Humans are social animals who both depend upon and compete with others in their social group. Social relations are thus fraught with implications for the individual's reproductive success and, especially in earlier environments, survival. Consequently, many inherited dispositions to fear derive from the qualities of social relationships. It would seem that much current social anxiety is not a product of disordered psychological mechanisms but instead is due to mismatches between our natural social-anxiety mechanisms and an environment featuring far more interaction with and evaluation by strangers, weak social affiliations, competition for status and resources, and inequality than would have been the case in prehistory.

One especially powerful source of social anxiety involves entering settings where one is unknown to others and must interact with unfamiliar people. In the distant past, people lived in small bands of one or two hundred people, all of whom were well known to one another. Ancestral social structures were small, close-knit, egalitarian groups where intimates hunted, gathered, mated, and raised children. Group members shared ethnicity, lifestyles, and belief systems. Social success involved cooperating and reciprocating relationships with well-known others. Dangerous neighboring groups and predators surrounded the familiar world of intimates. Unfamiliar people often posed genuine threats to the sorts of small, tightly bound groups of intimates in which the human genome developed. Strangers were not encountered in daily activities; their appearance would typically have been the occasion of suspicion, flight, or violence.[51] Interactions with strangers would have been rare but, when they occurred, often entailed threats to well-being. In such circumstances, wariness of relationships with those outside of the group was a wise strategy. Fear of strangers would probably have been useful in such environments; thus, people who were afraid of unfamiliar people were more likely than the fearless to live and pass on their genes to descendants.

Social structures have radically changed and now involve numerous encounters with people one doesn't know. Fears of people who do not share one's own social traits are far less adaptive in situations that feature many fleeting relationships with unknown others from highly varying backgrounds. Consider that the most frequent current sorts of social fears involve speaking in front of groups to people one doesn't know, meeting new people, and talking with strangers.[52] Such inherited danger cues about meeting and interacting with strangers are no longer contextually appropriate; nonetheless, individuals are naturally prepared to be more anxious and inhibited with strangers than with intimates. A normal psychological mechanism is operating in an environment that is not the same as the environment for which it was designed.

The power of inherited fear of strangers is shown in the fact that infants universally develop fears of strangers when they are around 8 months old, an adaptation that makes evolutionary—if not current—sense.[53] Studies that show heightened amygdala activity among subjects exposed to flashes of pictures of people from other races that are too brief for conscious processing support this buried, innate basis of stranger fear.[54] Such fears appear to be inherited: even babies as young as 3 months old prefer faces of their own race compared to those of other races.[55] "The temptation," according to geographer Yi-Fu Tuan, "to see the other as hostile and subhuman is always present, though it may be deeply buried."[56] The fear of outsiders that typifies social groups thus seems biologically primed.

People also remain fearful of social evaluation. Isolation was a highly threatening experience during prehistory, and in a limited group the opinions of one held by even a very few individuals could matter to one's survival. A person who was not part of a collectivity would not have been able to survive if cut adrift from the group. Fears of ostracism were natural and adaptive when people depended on tightly connected and long-term ties and where their social status depended on their position in a group. People still fear peer evaluation even though they now have virtually endless choices regarding what individuals and groups they interact with. For example, many people become anxious about going unaccompanied to a social event despite the lack of any objective danger involved. One writer describes a typical experience: "I walked into the party alone. Surveying the group of unfamiliar faces, I felt nervous. I stood on the periphery with no one to talk to. It seemed as if everybody was looking at me and, at the same time, as if nobody was looking at me."[57]

Despite the decline of dependence on groups, people retain their concern for self-presentation and proneness to anxiety about social evaluation that make an individual feel unattractive within a group. The single most common current fear is public speaking, particularly in front of people who are not well known. This would not have surprised the ancient Roman philosopher Seneca, who noted, "the most eloquent orator's scalp tightens as he prepares to speak."[58] High levels of anxiety that arise when people must interact with strangers or enter new situations often indicate fear mechanisms triggered by contexts that were far more likely to be dangerous in the prehistoric world than they are at present.

In addition to fear of strangers and novel situations, social fears often stem from positions of dominance and subordination that entail differences in power, status, and wealth. The most primitive source of social comparison lies in assessing one's own strength relative to that of others. The ability to compare relative strength and rank must be part of the survival skills of any animal that needs to avoid dangerous conflicts. The nature of dominance hierarchies generally makes subordinates more nervous than dominants.[59]

Fears would have been adaptive among weaker parties thanks to inhibiting aggression toward a dominant who might respond with attacks that could lead to death or serious injury. Primatologist Jane Goodall characterizes the approaches of subordinate chimpanzees toward dominants as involving slouched postures, readiness to flee, and eye gaze avoidance.[60] They do not relax until the dominant offers them reassurance. Such avoidant behaviors not only ensure that the submitter will not confront the dominant but also are conducive to restraining attacks from more powerful others. The high mortality rates of less dominant primates who are poor submitters to more powerful ones testify to the adaptive nature of submission among the weak.[61]

Humans inherited from more ancient primates a biologically prepared tendency to develop appeasement strategies that helped deflect aggression from potential enemies regardless of whether they still retain their useful capacities.[62] Yet the strategies we inherited—such as gaze aversion—to indicate lack of threat and to deflect aggression are considered signs of social anxiety disorder today. Social anxiety involves behavioral inhibition, desires to escape from interactions, and cues such as eye gaze avoidance and blushing that typify the responses of threatened subordinates.[63] It also involves constant alertness to the status threats involved in social situations combined with readiness to withdraw from them quickly. Social anxiety often arises among individuals who see themselves as low in a relevant status hierarchy or who feel at risk for losing status through being viewed as undesirable.[64] Talking to people in authority remains one of the most common sorts of social fears.[65] The social discrepancies between females and males in most cultures also are consistent with the much higher levels of social anxiety among women, who in most cultures hold lower status than men. Adolescent girls, for example, report more concern than boys over negative social evaluations as well as greater desire for social approval.[66] Intense fears of social evaluation in particular contexts, especially when the subjects of scrutiny are of lower status than the evaluators, are evolutionarily normal.

* * *

Social scientists often decry the fact that people currently worry about things that are not, in fact, likely to harm them. For example, three-quarters of American parents express fears that a stranger might kidnap their children, despite the fact that non-family members kidnap only about 200 to 300 children a year in a country of over 300,000,000 people.[67] Most missing children are runaways from abusive or rejecting parents or are abducted by their own estranged parents. Likewise, modern Americans are far more afraid of flying in an airplane than of driving in a car, although air travel is many times safer (not a single death occurred in U.S. airspace in 2007 or 2008, while automobile accidents accounted for over 40,000 fatalities in each of those years).[68] Similarly, fears of being raped or murdered are astronomically higher than are warranted by actual rates of rape or murder.[69] Moreover, the kinds of people, such as the elderly, who are especially afraid of these two dangers have the least likelihood of experiencing them.

Humans bring emotional systems that were developed in the Stone Age to social structures involving intense amounts of interaction with strangers, novelty, and hierarchy. Our emotional mechanisms are not dysfunctional *per se*, but they are in certain respects poorly structured to face the social organization of the modern world. The over-responsiveness of naturally selected fear mechanisms is the price modern humans pay for maintaining brains developed in circumstances that required many immediate responses to physical threats and to the social exigencies of managing life in small groups of closely connected intimates who rarely interacted with strangers. High levels of anxiety are the unavoidable result, even now. The resultant natural anxieties are problematic in another sense—they can deflect our attention from, or at least fail to alert us to, far more dangerous objects and situations that do exist in our current environment.

Are Mismatches between Biologically Designed Anxieties and Current Environments Disorders?

This section addresses a basic challenge to the evolutionary approach to normality and disorder. The evolutionary view emphasizes how the foundation for distinguishing normality and abnormality lies in how and why we are biologically designed to be the way we are. By its nature, this understanding refers to the history of our species and how it was shaped by natural selection, as expressed in the harmful dysfunction (HD) analysis of disorder in which a dysfunction is a harmful failure of an evolved function. While some anxiety seems an obviously normal response to an understandable threat whereas some seems inexplicable and evidence of a disorder, many other instances of anxiety seem to entail mismatches between the way we are biologically designed and our current environment due to how that environment has changed since we were evolutionarily shaped. The harmful dysfunction analysis implies that such mismatches are disorders only when they are failures of biological design; the fact that undesirable, impairing, and harmful mental conditions are maladaptive in our current environment does not make them mental disorders, as long as they are part of human biological design and thus part of our species-typical nature.

An often-suggested and obviously appealing alternative to the harmful dysfunction approach is to judge what is natural, and hence what is disordered, by whether a condition is good for us in the current environment that we actually confront. This view—which we called the "impairment view"—deems a mental condition that is maladaptive in the current environment to be a mental disorder.[70]

We have observed that many common fears are unreasonable in the sense that they do not represent real dangers in our modern environment, even though they were naturally selected due to real dangers that our ancestors faced. These fears represent mismatches between human nature as shaped in early environments and the demands of modern reshaped social environments. Such "mismatched" fears are neither wholly inexplicable like many disorders nor wholly understandable in terms of immediate danger, leading to a question about how we should label them. Should such mismatches be considered disorders?

For example, if fear of speaking to a large group of strangers was a naturally selected fear, the HD analysis would imply that it is not a disorder when we have such a fear despite being a problem for some due to the modern necessity (for some) of speaking before groups of strangers. In contrast, the impairment criterion would imply that this fear, which is highly inconvenient in our culture and can interfere with job performance, is maladaptive in our current environment and thus a disorder.

Such mismatches represent such a common and widespread set of fears—often identified as "disorders"—that it is worth questioning the rationale for accepting these conditions as part of human nature and not pathologizing them. This issue is especially pressing as the pace of social and technological change becomes ever more rapid. As human beings reshape their own environments (and perhaps will face radically altered environments in the future due to factors ranging from computerized interaction and climate change to human migration into space), mismatches between what we are and what it would be beneficial for us to be will become more frequent. Indeed, science fiction has long portrayed the possibility that we may need to alter our biological natures through genetic manipulation to survive in harsh future environments, such as in outer space, the ocean depths, or a future ultra-polluted Earth. More subtly and immediately, social and technological changes constantly make new demands on us and favor certain human features over others. So, the question arises: When changing environmental circumstances make parts of human nature maladaptive, why not call that a disorder?

The impairment criterion has a powerful appeal. At the very least, maladaptive traits seem like a category between health and disorder. Moreover, such conditions might warrant treatment to reduce the mismatch for the convenience of individuals and society. Indeed, one might argue that it is a matter of social justice to provide such treatment to normal individuals whose traits disadvantage them within the value system of our society. So, why restrict disorder to those conditions that have sources outside the range of biologically selected trait levels? Who cares about what features were biologically selected thousands or even millions of years ago? What harm results from assimilating such impairing, enduringly maladaptive mismatches to our concept of medical disorder, especially because we might want to treat such problems?

There are three powerful arguments against pathologizing mismatches and classifying them as mental disorders. The first reason is a practical one. Many concepts exist in order to define the general nature of a problem, locate its cause, and direct further action. "Disorder" is such a concept. Labeling a condition as a disorder suggests that the problem originates in something going wrong inside the person relative to biological design. Obviously, many things can go wrong inside the person that are not failures of biological design and thus are not disorders, such as ignorance, lack of skill, or lack of talent. These suggest a different approach to solving the problem, such as standard educational techniques. Therefore, mismatches should be distinguished from disorders because the type of causation is broadly different and suggests a different approach to finding useful interventions.

Think back to the example of an individual placed in an alien environment such as under water or in outer space without a breathing apparatus. Why is labeling such a problem as a breathing disorder so absurd? The answer is that the nature of the causal process leading to the problem does not fit the concept of disorder. In general, the way we classify such problems tends to correspond with the way we think the problem is to be explained—the concepts themselves include broad causal hypotheses. Disorders are problems that need to be explained by some way in which naturally designed functioning has gone wrong, so the first priority would be to look to the inner workings of the individual's mental processes to identify what has gone wrong.

But when individuals suffer a mismatch between their biologically designed nature and their environment, the immediate causation of the problem lies not within them but in the mismatch itself. When the causation of the problem lies in an unexpected environment that makes our biologically designed natures no longer beneficial, that is a challenging problem, but not a problem of the kind posed by standard disorders. Moreover, researchers who strive to uncover the causes of such states in disturbances of brain circuitry or information processing within the individual will be misled: perfectly normal brains produce evolutionarily natural anxiety that results from mismatches with current conditions.

The second reason for separating impairing mismatches from disorders builds on the causation issue but links it to deeper strands within the history and nature of psychiatry. The problem is that the impairment criterion potentially transforms psychiatry into social control. The criticism of psychiatry as a medicalized form of social control, as well as the issue of distinguishing the truly medical nature of psychiatry from social control, was at the heart of the dispute between psychiatry and the "anti-psychiatry movement" in the 1960s and 1970s.[71] A relevant analysis of the concept of mental disorder must address the question of what distinguishes psychiatric diagnoses from the control of socially undesirable conditions.

To answer this question, the concept of mental disorder (and medical disorder more generally) must contain some component that provides a non-arbitrary baseline independent of social values. Otherwise, health may be just another socially manipulable value category, leaving the anti-psychiatrists' challenges unanswered. The impairment criterion for disorder runs afoul of these requirements for an adequate analysis, since the impairment view implies that one can create mass disorder simply by changing the social environment. Under the impairment approach, whenever human beings fail to satisfy social demands, they can be classified as disordered. This potentially leads to the justification of abuses such as the Soviet pathologization of political dissidents. The impairment criterion does not provide the needed baseline because social values are a large part of the cultural environment that the individual's features must "match" in order for the individual to be healthy.

Consider the following thought experiment: There is a character in a Woody Allen movie who was simply incapable of figuring out how to get the clock to work on his VCR. Many of us can empathize with that character. Now, imagine that technological advances proceed at such a pace during your lifetime that only young people growing up with a new technology can function effectively in society. But, just like a generalized version of the Woody Allen character, your capabilities fall below a new threshold needed to make standard technologies work. Does that mean that you and masses of other people now have developed a disorder as social demands change? If so, then more people can be given the disorder at will simply by raising the demands of society's technology or otherwise changing social values in ways that some people cannot satisfy.

The impairment principle also is inconsistent with the recognized distinction between cosmetic and medically necessary surgery. The fact that one's nose or weight does not fit the values and aesthetic of one's society is a problem and perhaps a very distressing one, but it represents a mismatch that is not a medical disorder. For example, Carrie Prejean, a winner of the Miss California USA contest, was thought to have insufficiently well-endowed breasts to fulfill current American preferences. Six weeks before competing for the Miss USA title, the pageant paid for, and she accepted, breast implant surgery.[72] This points to a further problem with the impairment criterion: the "mismatch" can be judged relative to the demands of a certain type of success, and thus the match that is demanded can be to an ideal prototype that requires extensive "treatment" even for those who might be thought exceptional to begin with.

If social demands become determinative of disorder, psychiatry becomes about social control and we cannot answer the crucial questions about disorder that motivated the analysis of the concept of disorder in the first place. The Soviet dissidents were, after all, mismatched in their longing for freedom with their current political environment. In contrast, the biological design approach to disorder offers some conceptual way to keep track of when individuals are disordered versus when social values are changing and making new and challenging demands upon humans. These distinctions should not be lost because they have potential implications for acceptance of variation, pluralism, and human freedom.

Finally, common intuitions about mental disorder are inconsistent with the impairment criterion but correspond to the harmful dysfunction analysis. People generally do not think that mismatches are mental or physical disorders. Consider the following:

- Taste preference for fat and sugar was helpful when calories were scarce but often leads to problems in our generally food-rich current environment, yet such taste preferences are not disorders.
- The fight-or-flight reaction to threat with rapid arousal was helpful when the occasional suddenly looming threat could be fatal, but can damage our bodies and minds in highly stressful environments; in itself, however, it is not a disorder.
- Sexual desire for individuals other than one's spouse or pair-bonded partner appears to have been adaptive in terms of reproductive potential in earlier times but is problematic in our monogamous and reproductively controlled social environment. However, it is not considered a disorder—even when such desires are experienced by moral leaders such as former President Jimmy Carter, who admitted "lusting in his heart" for other women.
- Men have higher levels of aggression than women, and this appears to have been adaptive in environments in which male aggressiveness may have been

crucial for hunting, defense of territory, protection from predators, and other aspects of survival. High levels of male aggressiveness have become maladaptive in today's controlled world yet are not considered to be disorders; the notion that men suffer *en masse* from a disorder of "testosterone poisoning" is taken to be a joke, not a serious proposal, because male testosterone levels are biologically shaped.

- There are subtle features of our mental faculties, such as biases in cognitive processing that lead us to focus on immediate threats and to have more trouble attending to gradual and less visible dangers such as climate change. These biases were advantageous at a time when direct threats were the main ones and we could do little about the larger but less visible dangers. In today's world these biases threaten our ability to act against a new range of dangers, but they are not disorders.

These are just a few of many examples of traits that are considered inconvenient or even harmful but are not disorders because they are part of how we are biologically designed. Of course, any of these features might become disordered when the feature itself goes beyond the range that is thought to be biologically selected, as in compulsive sexuality or uncontrollable aggression. But the basic mismatch exists across a wide range of conditions that are not considered disordered—our concept of disorder just does not work according to the impairment principle.

Mismatches between biologically designed traits and social demands may warrant intervention as a preventive measure or as the cultivation of life skills to minimize stress and optimize fairness. However, they are not best classified as mental disorders. Mental disorders as the concept is currently understood—and should continue to be understood, for the reasons above—involve the failure of evolutionarily designed functions, not just the failure to perform in a desirable way in current social circumstances.

Dickinson and Madden Again

With the above discussion in mind, we return to the examples we presented in the first chapter of John Madden's fear of flying—which we portrayed as a mismatch and thus, by our present argument, not a disorder—and Emily Dickinson's fear of seeing even old friends, which we judged a disorder. We address the puzzle of why one is a disorder and the other is not.

We suggested that Dickinson's anxiety about socializing appeared to be inexplicable in terms of our understanding of biological design, thus possibly best understood as a disorder, whereas Madden's fear of flying was understandable in terms of biological design, therefore not a disorder. But a closer look might lead one to wonder if this distinction can be maintained under the weight of similarities between the two examples. Social anxieties are just as widespread and seemingly normal as fears of heights and closed spaces, and just as anachronistic as flying fears in our society, where disapproval by one's group is not likely to get one killed or ejected into the wild. Both Dickinson's and Madden's fears lead them to limit their actions in ways that impair them. Both individuals, despite the manifest irrationality of their fears, are incapable of relying on their reasoning or other inhibitory power to suppress their emotional expression or to summon up the courage to overcome or ignore their fear. Nor have their fears weakened (or "extinguished") over time with maturation or experience, as typically happens to children's stranger anxiety and fear of the dark.

Despite all these similarities, there is a basic reason why Dickinson's anxiety is more plausibly a disorder than is Madden's. This has to do with the nature of the environmental context to which they respond with anxiety. Natural social anxiety is primarily experienced when one faces strangers or authority figures, presumably because the danger of a negative evaluation and its harmful consequences existed in such a situation—that is, social anxiety is a form of performance anxiety. However, such anxiety makes no sense as a protective feature with family or friends. They are unlikely to give you a negative evaluation of this sort or, even if they do, to act on it in a way that harms you. People who are incapable of giving a public speech or a dramatic performance without using medication typically feel no significant anxiety when talking to family or close friends.

Emily Dickinson's condition seems inexplicable not simply because she is on the intense end of social anxiety, but because this fear has become so overly generalized and misdirected that it impairs even more basic social functioning with her intimates. It is not just the intensity but the specific object of her fear that reveals a likely breakdown in biologically designed functioning and leads to the judgment that something has gone wrong. Human beings have always had alliances with sympathetic others within a group; friendship is so much an integral part of our lives that Aristotle suggested that no one would want to live life without friends.[73] Thus, the desirability of being able to function with one's friends without undue interference from anxiety is just as much a part of the forces that shaped us as the need to protect ourselves from strangers. One might expect that human beings, being social animals, would be biologically designed so that anxiety is suppressed in close relationships, and this is what we generally see. Emily Dickinson's anxiety seems to have gone awry and become misdirected in a way that undermines such essential functioning.

In this respect, Madden's fear is quite different. Although intense, it is aimed at an artificially created trigger—flying in an airplane—that did not exist during our shaping as a species and that biological design could surely not have foreseen as a useful environment in which to be comfortable. Unlike the need for closeness to acquaintances, there is nothing like the need for air travel in our biological past. Of greater importance, flying combines several features that we are biologically designed to shun, such as being trapped in a small space where escape is impossible, being crowded together with others, lacking control over our movement, and being taken to an altitude impossible for hominids before our era, each of which by themselves produce fear in large numbers of people. It makes sense that this unprecedented artificial environment would trigger fear, and it does so in large proportions of the population. Some, like Madden, decide on balance and in light of their other traits that they will not engage in this anxiety-provoking activity.

True, other people either feel this biologically based fear less intensely, or they manage to control or inhibit it despite its intensity so as to allow them—albeit with considerable discomfort—to travel by air. There are three keys here to understanding the non-disordered status of Madden's fear. The first is the remarkable degree of normal variation in intensity that exists in the population even when it comes to biologically shaped fears, just as there is great normal variation in features such as IQ, height, and personality traits such as shyness. The second is the need to consider the effects of normal variation in more than one feature, in this case, both the additive intensities of the several fears that flying commonly triggers and Madden's limited capacities for inhibition of those fears. Finally, Madden may be more subject to the psychological and physical aversive aspects of anxiety or pain in general and thus have more motivation to avoid it. The aversion to flying is an aversion to something we were not biologically designed to do and that contains many features we were biologically designed to avoid. Unlike Dickinson, Madden has natural fears that are not adaptive in current circumstances. While Madden is not in this respect disordered, one would perhaps want to add that in this matter, for whatever reasons, he lacks the virtue of courage.

CONCLUSION

Natural anxiety is ubiquitous. It results from the many threats that humans experience on a daily, or even hourly, basis as well as from structural and historical threats that affect entire populations. Moreover, many natural fears are not grounded in responses to any *current* environmental danger but are manifestations of ancestral fear mechanisms. What are commonly viewed as irrational, unconscious anxieties or as individual responses to idiosyncratic conditioning stimuli during childhood are often universally shared fears that have been programmed into the human genome. These include, for example, novel situations (especially when individuals are alone), separation from loved ones, meeting strangers, darkness, heights, enclosed spaces, and the sorts of animals that were dangerous in ancient environments. It is thus unsurprising that so many people fear spiders and snakes, although these fears cannot be seen as reasonable in current environments. Fears that are unreasonable under current circumstances can nevertheless be firmly grounded in our genetic heritage.[74] Moreover, evolution designed humans to have low thresholds of anxiety in reaction to these cues, so people naturally have high levels of anxiety. Because anxiety is so widespread, an enormous potential exists to pathologize natural as well as disordered anxiety conditions.

Yet, from the point of view of the requirement that a disorder must involve a dysfunction—a failure of a mechanism to perform as evolution designed it to perform—there are few dysfunctions of anxiety mechanisms. By far the majority of conditions that meet current psychiatric criteria for diagnosing anxiety disorders are conditions that were adaptive in ancestral circumstances, such as fears of crawling insects, meeting strangers, or public speaking, and that now emerge in an environment where they are no longer useful. In the modern world, such formerly adaptive fears can create much impairment, as when an individual cannot perform well in his occupation because of fear of public speaking or flying. Others arise from personally meaningful experiences in earlier life that are no longer adaptive but are difficult to extinguish because evolution designed the amygdala to maintain memories of early encounters of fear. Neither sort of case indicates a dysfunction of internal fear response mechanisms.

Conversely, a huge amount of anxiety arises when normally functioning fear mechanisms encounter environments for which they were not designed. Because the past rather than the present sets the criteria for designed functioning, terms involving qualifiers such as "groundless," "excessive," "irrational," or "unreasonable" are often applicable to anxiety reactions, even when they are perfectly normal parts of our biologically designed nature.

Distinguishing high normal anxiety from anxiety disorders is often extremely difficult if not impossible given our current limited knowledge of anxiety mechanisms and their evolution and the complex considerations of cultural and individual variation, yielding a substantial degree of fuzziness to the concept of anxiety disorder. The large degree of indeterminacy in whether anxiety states are natural fears or anxiety disorders means that no intrinsically sharp boundary lines demarcate normal from pathological fears. This fuzziness allows a variety of social, cultural, professional, and economic interests and values to influence where dividing lines are set between normal and pathological displays of anxiousness. These borders have changed substantially over the course of history.

CHAPTER 4

A Short History of Anxiety and Its Disorders

From the classic Greek invention of medical practice through the recent history of Western medicine, theory and diagnosis have always recognized both normal and pathological forms of anxiety. Physicians realized that many diverse types of disorders are frightening or threatening to one's well-being and thus are naturally associated with degrees of anxiety. They therefore often listed anxiety among the symptoms of a variety of disorders. Nevertheless, classical psychiatric thought did not recognize a distinct category of anxiety disorders—that is, conditions in which the primary problem is that anxiety processes themselves have failed to function properly in one way or another. Instead, anxiety became a pivotal independent category of psychiatric diagnosis only at the end of the nineteenth century, when Sigmund Freud began to focus on this condition.

This chapter traces how disordered forms of anxiety started as symptoms or epiphenomena of other disorders, entered the spotlight of diagnostic categories with the advent of Freud, and became an elaborated set of categories in the *DSM-III* that are now considered to be the most prevalent type of mental disorder in the modern world.

ANCIENT CONCEPTIONS

Throughout history, commentators have tried to separate natural fears from anxiety disorders while at the same time recognizing the elusive boundaries between these states. A long tradition stemming from the ancient Greek and Roman philosophers lists fear as one of a small number of basic natural passions or emotions, along with love, joy, desire, hatred, and sorrow.[1] For example, Socrates defined fear generally as "the expectation of evil."[2] The Roman philosopher Epictetus noted two major social situations in which performance fears are natural. The first occurs in front of groups of people, especially strangers: "A musician, for instance, feels no anxiety while he is singing by himself; but when he appears upon the stage he does, even if his voice be ever so good, or he plays ever so well."[3] The second arises when people wish to please their social superiors or authority figures: "Zeno, when he was to meet Antigonus, felt no anxiety. For over that which he prized, Antigonus had no power . . . But Antigonus felt anxiety when he was to meet Zeno, and with reason, for he was desirous to please him."[4] Fears that developed in the contexts of addressing large groups or being evaluated by more powerful people were not considered to be disordered because people naturally tend to fear humiliation, or worse, when under scrutiny.

In addition to describing fearful emotional reactions to specific situations, ancient commentators also recognized personality dispositions that were anxious but natural. The Roman writer Cicero, for example, distinguished an abiding proneness to anxiety from transitory states of anxiousness. "An anxious temper," wrote Cicero, "is different from feeling anxiety."[5] Just as some people were more vulnerable to sickness than others, people with anxious temperaments were more likely to have numerous sorts of fears—but these enduring personality states and the anxiety states they tended toward were not themselves viewed as sicknesses or disorders, although they might make people more vulnerable to developing melancholic disorders (among others).

Initial medical writings distinguished such normal fears and normal-range anxious personality dispositions from anxiety conditions that were medical disorders. Hippocrates occasionally presented melancholic cases that featured irrational fears as the dominant characteristics:

> Anxiousness—a difficult disease. The patient thinks he has something like a thorn, something pricking him in his viscera, and anxiety (perhaps loathing or nausea) tortures him. He flees from light and from people, loves the dark, and is attacked by fear. His diaphragm swells, and he feels pain at the touch. He worries and sees frightening visions, fearful dream images, and occasionally dead people.[6]

A second case resembled what would now be considered a social anxiety disorder:

> Another through bashfulness, suspicion, and timorousness, will not be seen abroad; loves darkness as life, and cannot endure the light, or to sit in lightsome places; his hat

still in his eyes, he will neither see, nor be seen by his good will. He dare not come in company, for fear he should be misused, disgraced, overshoot himself in gesture of speeches, or be sick; he thinks every man observes him.[7]

Hippocrates's descriptions indicated that, unlike fears that were related to threatening or potentially humiliating situations, anxiety disorders were unmoored from any realistic or naturally expectable context that could explain the extreme intensity of the anxiety. Later, in the middle of the third century BCE, Andreas of Charystos provided a more formal term—"pantophobia"—for patients who suffered from unmotivated fears of everything, thereby offering the first diagnostic category aimed specifically at an anxiety disorder.[8]

Nevertheless, while it is possible to identify scattered cases that are similar to those of modern anxiety disorders, early medical writings did not generally conceive of anxiety as a distinct condition. Instead, they viewed anxiety as one component of the broader condition of melancholia (i.e., depression). Hippocrates's initial definition of melancholia emphasized the joining of fear and sadness: "When fear and sadness last a long time, this is a melancholic condition."[9] He noted how "meditations and worries exaggerated in fancy" nearly always accompanied or caused sadness.[10] In the Hippocratic corpus, melancholia referred to a mix of anxious concerns, nameless fears, blackness of mood, suicidal impulses, and sullen suspiciousness.

Indeed, physicians did not clearly distinguish anxiety conditions as discreet disorders, in contrast to conditions such as melancholia, mania, or schizophrenia, until the latter part of the nineteenth century. Instead, anxiety was either subsumed as an amorphous type of melancholic disorder that was associated with psychic agitation, or it was seen as interchangeable with deep feelings of sorrow. "In the clinical descriptions of melancholia over the centuries," notes historian Stanley Jackson, "fear and sadness were usually central features."[11]

WRITINGS FROM THE SIXTEENTH THROUGH THE NINETEENTH CENTURIES

Hippocratic assumptions that fear and sadness tended to occur together in melancholic disorder served as the basis for Western psychiatric thought for many centuries. For example, in his classic work *Anatomy of Melancholy*, British vicar Robert Burton (1577–1640) defined melancholy as "a kind of dotage without a fever, having for his ordinary companions fear and sadness, without any apparent occasion."[12] Burton emphasized how "fear and sadness" are inseparable characteristics of melancholy, how they distinguished melancholy from insanity, and how their occurrence "without any apparent occasion" served to separate disordered from ordinary emotions of fear and sadness. Only groundless fears that were not related to an external threat were disordered. Burton also noted the presence of anxious personality dispositions, which might be susceptible to a variety of melancholic conditions in "such bodies especially as are ill disposed."[13]

Burton mentioned many sources of normal fear, including the possibility of death, losing intimates, and public humiliations. Love was an especially common natural source of concern: "Every poet is full of such catalogues of love-symptoms; but fear and sorrow may justly challenge the chief place."[14] Love affairs naturally produce joy and elation. Uncertain, unrequited, or deceptive love relationships, in contrast, are parts "of a lover's life . . . full of agony, anxiety, fear, and grief."[15] The negative as well as the positive aspects of love stem from its contexts: "Now if this passion of love can produce such effects if it be pleasantly intended, what bitter torments shall it breed when it is with fear and continual sorrow, suspicion, care, agony, as commonly it is, still accompanied! What an intolerable pain must it be!"[16]

Anticipating Darwin, Burton noted several characteristics that lead to normal somatic signs of anxiety:

Bashfulness and blushing is a passion proper to men alone, and is not only caused for some shame and ignominy, or that they are guilty unto themselves of some foul fact committed but . . . from fear, and a conceit of our defects; the face labours and is troubled at his presence that sees our defects, and nature, willing to help, sends thither heat, heat draws the subtilest blood, and so we blush.[17]

Burton went on to note that blushing is especially likely to occur in situations when people were among their "betters or in company that we like not."[18] Social anxiety was a widespread, normal fear: "It amazeth many men that are to speak or show themselves in public assemblies, or before some great personages; as Tully confessed of himself, that he trembled still at the beginning of his speech; and Demosthenes, that great orator of Greece, before Philippus."[19] In addition, Burton related the tendency to blushing to normal personality dispositions, noting, "They that are bold, arrogant, and careless, seldom or never blush, but such as are fearful."[20]

Burton indicated that some forms of anxiety are natural and not disorders, connecting them to threatening situations or to anxious temperaments. He distinguished such normal fears from morbid disorders, which are "immoderate" and "consume the spirits" and thus could become causes of melancholy.[21] He contrasted Tully's natural fear of public speaking with Augustus Caesar's fear of the dark, which was a morbid fear that was unrelated to its context or to the adult developmental stage when it afflicted Augustus. He also described a form of generalized anxiety disorder: "they cannot be quiet an hour, a minute of time, but even against their wills they are intent, and still thinking of (some terrible object), they cannot forget it, it grinds their souls day and night, they are perpetually tormented. . . ."[22] Several forms of anxiety disorders were based on paranoid delusions about some unreal threat, while others—analogous to today's post-traumatic stress disorder—came from experiencing some especially terrible events or objects, "which often drive men out of their wits, bereave them of sense, understanding, and all, some for a time, some for their whole lives, they never recover it."[23] Such descriptions emphasized how some disordered conditions feature anxiety that has become unhinged from particular situations and circumstances.

Commentators who followed Burton also emphasized the differences between natural fears and mental disorders. Welsh physician Nicholas Robinson (1697– 1775) described a particular kind of melancholy that involved "impertinent and groundless Fears, that render Life not only uneasy to themselves, but greatly perplexing to all their Friends about them."[24] Robinson's description not only made clear that disorders involve "groundless" fears but also indicated that sufferers as well as those around them recognized the "perplexing" nature of these fears. Such anxiety was usually linked to recognized types of melancholy that were distinct from deranged or psychotic forms of madness. For example, Dutch physician Herman Boerhaave (1668–1738) and Scottish physician George Cheyne (1671– 1743) each described a form of melancholic dejection that included anxiety and a number of associated physical symptoms, without any signs of madness (i.e., psychotic ideation).[25] Thus, anxiety disorders were in effect recognized as a type of mental disorder that did not contain the traditional features of psychosis.

Nevertheless, before the nineteenth century, medical writers rarely singled out pathological forms of anxiety in and of themselves as distinct medical conditions. Rather, they integrated such anxieties into the descriptions of those states of melancholia or hypochondria that involved an unusual degree of worry, preoccupation, and complaint about bodily illnesses that had no known organic basis. The emphasis on melancholia was largely grounded in the continuing importance of humoral theory, dating back to the ancients, which attributed depression to an excess of black bile. The major focus of melancholic conditions was on mood states of sadness and not on the fear or anxiety symptoms or on bodily pains, fatigue, insomnia, or other non-mood elements of the disease that might characterize anxiety. Sadness over actual or prospective loss, and anxiety about potential threat, were seen as naturally linked within the same overall condition. Thus, discrete conditions of anxiety got relatively short shrift.[26]

At the end of the eighteenth century, however, an emphasis on understanding the central nervous system replaced notions of humoralism as the major source of theories of mental disturbances.[27] The term "nervous disorder" became a residual medical category encompassing both psychological conditions, such as anxiety and depression, and physical symptoms, including fatigue and digestive problems. According to Scottish physician Robert Whytt (1714–1766), such disorders referred to "all those disorders whose nature and causes they were ignorant of," but "that it would be extremely hard, either rightly to describe, or fully to enumerate them," including patients' complaints of pathological anxieties.[28] Physicians considered the varying mixes of symptoms falling under nervous disorders to stem from pathological activity of the nervous system, so that they tended to enter the domain of general medical practice rather than psychiatry or religion. "Nervous disorders," notes historian Edward Shorter, "did not belong to psychiatry."[29] Instead, general physicians, neurologists, or spa doctors treated such conditions. Indeed, the term was attractive in part precisely because a "nervous" condition meant that the source of suffering was viewed as an organic illness over which the mind had no control. Especially as it became clear that nerves worked by conduction of electrical impulses, the conception of nervous disorders allowed for the eventual separation of the conceptualizations of melancholic slowing and anxious activation into conditions of, respectively, decreased versus increased activity of the nervous system.

THE EMERGENCE OF NEURASTHENIA

By the middle of the nineteenth century, people who experienced depression, anxiety, or compulsive behavior were seen as having some sort of nervous condition. Psychosomatic complaints among women would often be called "hysteria"; those among men were labeled "hypochondria."[30] At this time, a climate of medical and lay uncertainty developed about which conditions were really organic and which were psychological. Anxiety symptoms were not generally accompanied by the derangement associated with diagnoses of mental disorder, yet were unquestionably connected with considerable suffering. The climate was ripe for some organically anchored disease term that would explain psychiatric-looking symptoms that were not severe enough to be considered as signs of madness. Such a condition could serve as a bridge between psychological disorders that did not involve extreme mental debility and those that were not due to identifiable organic causes but that seemed to entail some malfunction of the nervous system.[31]

In 1869, the American neurologist George M. Beard (1839–1883) coined the term "neurasthenia" to describe a general exhaustion of the nervous system mixed with somatic anxiety-like symptoms, taking medicine a step closer to the diagnosis of anxiety disorders. This condition was not found among hospitalized patients but was extremely common in physicians' offices and society at large. According to Beard, an enormous range of presenting complaints could indicate neurasthenia:

> If a patient complains of general malaise, debility of all the functions, poor appetite, abiding weakness in the back and spine, fugitive neuralgic pains, hysteria, insomnia, hypochondriases, disinclination for consecutive mental labor, severe and weakening attacks of sick headache, and other analogous symptoms, and at the same time gives *no evidence of anaemia or of any organic disease*, we have reason to suspect that the central nervous system is mainly at fault, and that we are dealing with a typical case of neurasthenia.[32]

Neurasthenics complained about headaches, insomnia, diffuse physical pains, and general lethargy, which are often symptoms of anxiety. This extraordinarily broad condition was flexible enough to encompass among its many manifestations the various phobic, obsessive-compulsive, mild depressive, and generalized anxiety states that would later become the psychoneuroses. The major value of neurasthenic labels for patients lay in the fact that they allowed their ailments to be dissociated from psychiatric conditions, linked with nervous conditions, and treated by nerve doctors and in spas. A diagnosis typically led to recommendations of bed rest for women and vigorous exercise in natural settings for men.[33]

Beard believed that the frantic lifestyle of the upper social classes in industrial society, which induced general emotional arousal and intellectual effort, precipitated neurasthenia, although the disorder itself was rooted in the nervous system and resulted from an inheritable constitutional vulnerability interacting with modern social demands. Because neurasthenia explained subjective bodily and psychological symptoms in terms of an objective physical disease that had no relationship to madness, it became an influential prototype of functional nervous disease during the late nineteenth century. "There was," according to Edward Shorter, "probably no similar instance of a single label having such an impact in the history of medicine."[34]

Although neurasthenia was initially considered a highly variable condition that could refer to general nervousness, hypochondria, depression, or chronic fatigue,[35] by the end of the nineteenth century the label was primarily associated with fatigue-like conditions. The primary sufferers of this condition also changed from the well-to-do to less educated groups that resisted accepting the newly emergent psychogenic paradigm and that preferred a physical explanation of their problems.[36] The rise of more precise psychiatric diagnoses that separated anxiety symptoms from melancholic and fatigue conditions, as well as the embrace of Freud's psychogenic theory, partially removed the physiological rationale for anxiety symptoms and separated the causes of anxiety from exhaustion, signaling the death knell for neurasthenic diagnoses in Western countries. Beard's broad diagnosis descended into obscurity in American and European medicine, although it remains widely popular in other parts of the world to this day.[37]

THE GROWTH OF ATTENTION TO PATHOLOGICAL ANXIETY

Physicians from Hippocrates to those of the latter half of the nineteenth century had occasionally described types of anxiety conditions that were more specific than neurasthenia, such as phobic and obsessive-compulsive problems. Yet, from the emergence of mental asylums in the eighteenth century until the latter decades of the nineteenth century, psychiatric classifications typically stemmed from the problems of inpatients who suffered from psychotic conditions such as schizophrenia, mania, or severe melancholia. The need for more precise classifications of mental disorders arose only when the insane were hospitalized in centralized facilities where it became apparent that they all didn't suffer from the same condition. Anxiety disorders were not important aspects of early taxonomies of mental disorders because they were not connected with insanity and were rarely severe enough to warrant hospitalization. Such conditions seldom created danger to others, as schizophrenia or manic depression might, or danger to self or severe withdrawal from social roles, as melancholia often did.

Physicians, however, often noted the presence of anxious conditions. For example, in 1798 Benjamin Rush (frequently called the "father of American psychiatry") described a large number of distinct types of phobias. Rush distinguished phobias from normal fears: "I shall define phobia to be a fear of an imaginary evil, or an undue fear of a real one."[38] Later, in 1872 the German psychiatrist Carl Westphal delineated the syndrome of agoraphobia—the "impossibility of walking through certain streets or squares, or possibility of so doing only with resultant dread of anxiety."[39] By 1903, Pierre Janet had described a variety of anxiety conditions; for example, Janet coined the term "social phobia" (*phobie des situations sociales*) to refer to patients who were afraid of being observed while speaking, playing the piano, or writing.[40]

Despite these developments in the descriptive psychiatry of anxiety conditions, most psychiatrists still considered anxiety as relatively peripheral to psychiatric nosology, subsuming anxiety disorders under the general category of depressive conditions. For example, the most distinguished diagnostician of the era, German psychiatrist Emil Kraepelin (1856–1926), devoted considerable attention to *Angst* a general state of fear, dread, terror, and apprehension. He also described a condition of *Schreckneurose* (fright neuroses) that could "be observed after serious accidents and injuries, particularly fires, railway derailments or collisions, etc."[41] These conditions, however, were composed of a variety of phobic, obsessional, anxious, depressive, and somatic symptoms. As in the 2500 years of medical tradition before him, Kraepelin generally considered anxious symptoms as aspects of many types of psychiatric disturbances rather than as indicators of any specific disorder.

Moreover, in stark contrast to Freud's radical new theory, the psychoneuroses in general were at the bottom of Kraepelin's diagnostic hierarchy, which ranged from organic disorders at the top, to schizophrenia, manic-depressive illness, and then neurotic illnesses.[42] Similarly, although British psychiatrist Henry Maudsley (1835–1918) concurred with Westphal that agoraphobia was a separate syndrome, his influential text *Pathology of Mind* (1879) still classified phobias as a subtype of melancholic disorders.[43] In France, despite his delineation of anxiety conditions, Pierre Janet advocated for a unified family of disorders that encompassed a variety of anxious, depressive, and psychosomatic conditions.[44] Indeed, the eminent English psychiatrist Aubrey Lewis noted that in Great Britain and the United States, "The word anxiety was hardly used in standard medical and psychiatrical textbooks until the late 1930s."[45]

When psychiatrists established community practices independent of inpatient mental hospitals at the end of the nineteenth century, they began to attract non-psychotic clients who suffered from a diffuse collection of psychosomatic, bodily, and nervous complaints variously labeled as "neurasthenia," "hysteria," or "hypochondriasis." Prior to this period, severely anxious persons would have consulted practitioners who avoided psychiatric labels and treated anxiety as an amorphous type of medical state rather than as an independent psychiatric condition.[46] Many sufferers also related their anxiety to spiritual problems and consulted clergy for solace. Until the turn of that century, anxious conditions were rarely considered to be discrete, lacked sharp boundaries, and were generally linked to other somatic and mental disturbances. The ascendance of Sigmund Freud's writings and theories dramatically changed the status of anxiety.

FREUD AND ANXIETY

Mainstream psychiatry in the early twenty-first century is more likely to ridicule than to revere Sigmund Freud, who attempted to place meaning rather than physiology at the heart of the understanding of psychopathology. Many psychiatrists in our brain-physiology-oriented era mock his theories, dismiss his therapy, and view the period when psychoanalysis dominated the profession as an unfortunate hiatus in the progress of psychiatric thought.[47]

Whatever justification might exist for the scorn some heap on Freud's broader views is certainly not warranted for his contributions to the study of anxiety.

Although psychodynamic theory and therapy in general have little current influence in psychiatry, Freud's work on anxiety remains seminal.[48] Indeed, he made anxiety the central phenomenon in the field of psychiatry, explicated the differences between normal fears and anxiety disorders, developed a model of anxiety with elements anticipating both biologically oriented and cognitive-distortion theories, realized the lasting impacts of early fearful experiences, and outlined the major types of anxiety disorders that remain the basis for current diagnosis and classification.

Targeting Beard's overly bloated, vague, and inclusive conception of neurasthenia, in 1894 Freud coined the term "anxiety neurosis" for generalized, free-floating anxiety symptoms. On the basis of his clinical experience and evolving theorizing, he suggested that this condition should be separated from the more general state of neurasthenia.[49] Freud divided the "psychoneuroses," including anxiety and conversion hysterias, phobias, and obsessive-compulsive disorders—which stemmed from psychic causes where meaning played a role—from the "actual neuroses," including anxiety neurosis and neurasthenia that he associated with direct somatic (specifically sexual) causes. He initially posited that many of these anxiety conditions resulted from repressed sexual energy or from chronic sexual frustration, which often resulted from the withdrawal method of birth control widely practiced at the time.

Freud's thinking about anxiety subsequently changed, however, and he came to believe that anxiety did not arise directly from inhibited or frustrated sexual desire but instead was primarily a signal of perceived danger that, when too terrifying, became a fundamental cause of repression to avoid the overwhelmingly painful idea: "It was anxiety which produced repression and not, as I formerly believed, repression which produced anxiety."[50] Thus, phobias, free-floating anxiety, and other anxiety states consisted of anxiety that was displaced from an original terrifying, but repressed, idea to a substitute idea.

Anxiety, Freud explained, refers to the unpleasant emotional and physiological sensations that emerge when people are in dangerous situations or when they expect such situations will occur. It consists of psychic components of threat, irritability, and inability to concentrate, and somatic components of heart palpitations, breathing problems, tremors, sweating, and gastrointestinal disturbances.[51] These symptoms contrasted with the psychic pain and mourning that characterized depression.[52] In addition, anxiety was a future-oriented emotion where the concern is about some anticipated possible dangerous situation, while depression usually involved loss and was thus oriented in the past. Nevertheless, the situations giving rise to anxiety and depression were related. "Pain," Freud noted, "is thus the actual reaction to loss of object, while anxiety is the reaction to the danger which that loss entails and, by a further displacement, a reaction to the danger of the loss of object itself."[53]

Freud distinguished several major types of psychoneurotic anxiety disorders, in the first instance on the basis of their different kinds of symptoms. One type was a "freely floating," general apprehensiveness that was not tied to any particular situation and so was not grounded in appropriate external fearful circumstance.[54] This is now recognized as "generalized anxiety disorder." Freud observed that such undirected anxiety often transformed itself into directed worries and phobias. A second type, phobic anxiety, consisted of anxiety attached to a distinct object that people viewed as an external danger and experienced identically with realistic anxiety. However, because of unconscious internal conflicts the fear was exaggerated out of proportion to the actual danger that this object posed.[55] Phobias "have the character of a projection in that they replace an internal, instinctual danger by an external, perceptual one."[56] Agoraphobia—fear of leaving home or of public spaces—was a particular style of phobic defense marked by attempts to prevent or avoid situations that can lead to extreme anxiety and panic attacks, similar to current diagnostic descriptions.[57] Finally, obsessional and compulsive neuroses, which Freud construed as anxiety disorders in which the pathological behaviors and thoughts are attempts to reduce anxiety, emerged as efforts to ensure that the unexpected will never happen, the unknown will never be encountered, and thus that anxiety will never arise,[58] a description that also anticipated later characterizations of obsessive-compulsive disorders.

Freud aspired to explain each type of anxiety syndrome by a distinct etiology and so sometimes used diverse causes or strategies of coping with anxiety to distinguish them. More commonly, though, he did not view these various conditions as independent, and he emphasized how they often occurred in combination with each other and with other forms of disorder. In either case, he conceptualized neurotic symptoms as the result of an attempt to escape intolerable anxiety caused by conflict that the individual could not resolve. Intense anxiety that lacked grounding in appropriate external contexts characterized all these disorders. Moreover, all were subject to similar treatments that were based on the working through of underlying emotional conflicts.

Freud's influence was substantial enough that during the period between roughly 1920 and 1970, psychoanalysts tended to interpret all neurotic symptoms as either manifestations or derivatives of anxiety. Freud and his followers not only put anxiety at the heart of their theories, they also reversed the previous hierarchy of psychiatric classification, relegating depression to a secondary status. Anxiety, in their view, lay behind most forms of neurotic behavior, including not only direct expressions in phobias, obsessions, panic, and generalized anxiety but also hysteria, sexual dysfunctions, and psychosomatic problems, among others. "Anxiety," Freud wrote in *Civilization and Its Discontents*, "is always present somewhere or other behind every symptom."[59] In Freud's work, the understanding of anxiety was the key that could unlock the mysteries behind all the psychoneurotic disorders.

The distinction between normal fears and anxiety disorders was at the heart of Freud's conception of anxiety. Most commentators maintain that Freud had a continuous theory of anxiety running from normal fears on the one end to anxiety disorders on the other.[60] It is true that analysts who followed Freud often viewed anxiety as continuous in this manner. In fact, however, Freud himself saw a clear theoretical distinction between realistic fears and neurotic anxiety, however difficult it might be to make this separation in practice. The key difference lay in whether a realistic, external threat was present or not. Fears of extreme severity could be normal when they were contextually appropriate responses to traumatic external threats. Conversely, mild symptoms could be neurotic when they were not related to realistic contexts. Both normal fears and anxiety disorders had gradients of severity, but they did not fall on different ends of the same continuum.

Freud held that fear is grounded in actual, external situations of danger and that the capacity to develop fear is innate and rooted in evolutionary predispositions. Some fears, he asserted, "might perhaps be accounted for as vestigial traces of the congenital preparedness to meet real dangers which is so strongly developed in other animals."[61] This sort of anxiousness seemed to be a remnant of a condition that had been biologically adaptive during human prehistory. The capacity for anxiety is a shared, natural trait common to all people, which serves to mobilize energy and overcome obstacles in the face of threatening situations. This inherited emotion signals the presence of some threatening situation and allows people to take defensive action. Fear has an "indispensable biological function to fulfill as a reaction to a state of danger."[62]

Freud emphasized two kinds of realistic fears (which he called "realistic anxiety") that are normal, biologically programmed responses to external or internal dangers: primary anxiety occurs when some actual situation overwhelms an individual; signal anxiety emerges when people expect impending danger. Signal anxiety allows the person to take defensive action before the situation actually happens.

Freud's unique idea was that—in contrast to realistic fears that were products of external situations—anxiety neuroses stemmed from some inner threat, such as feeling overwhelmed by some instinctual drive that one had to suppress. In neurotic disorders, fear mechanisms that were constructed to alert people to the presence of actual dangerous situations were activated in the face of unconscious dangers from internal sources.[63] Individuals then mistakenly treated unconscious mental threats as coming from some outside stimulus and therefore reacted as if non-threatening situations or objects were potentially dangerous. Thus, the dangers seemed as absurd and irrational to the person experiencing them as they did to others.[64]

Unconscious fantasies that arose during childhood often explained the emergence of such neurotic dangers.[65]

Freud's distinction between natural and neurotic anxiety did not lie in the nature of the anxiety itself, because normal and pathological anxiety share common manifestations. Nor did it lie in how much distress or social impairment the condition caused, because responses to external threats could be just as distressing and impairing as internal ones. Instead, the central difference was that, unlike fear that arises in response to realistic dangers, neurotic anxiety is a contextually inappropriate response to the degree of danger in the actual circumstances and so seems enigmatic and pointless.[66]

For example, Freud noted that while early pre-Oedipal childhood phobias were "very puzzling" (because there was not time for the child to develop the Oedipal conflicts that Freud theorized were behind virtually all neurotic anxieties), other fears, such as "the fear of being alone and the fear of strangers, can be explained with certainty" and were realistic.[67] Even extreme fears were normal when they arose and persisted in contextually appropriate situations. "A person suffering from anxiety," Freud emphasized, "is not for that reason necessarily suffering from anxiety neurosis."[68] Fear involved a proportionate response to an external stimulus; morbid anxiety represented a disproportionate internal response.

The difference between "realistic" fears and "unrealistic" anxiety disorders was often difficult to make and was always relative to particular stages of the life cycle in which different prototypical fears tend to predominate. According to Freud:

> The danger of psychical helplessness fits the stage of the ego's early immaturity; the danger of loss of an object (or loss of love) fits the lack of self-sufficiency in the first years of childhood; the danger of being castrated fits the phallic phase; and finally fear of the super-ego, which assumes a special position, fits the period of latency.[69]

The fear of castration loomed especially large as a source of normal fear for boys during the Oedipal period. Freud anticipated the objection that castration fear was not a real danger: "what is decisive is that the danger is one that threatens from outside and that the child believes in it."[70] The realistic nature of castration fears pointed to a central aspect of Freud's thinking about anxiety: what is realistic at any point of time is intrinsically tied to the stage of life development and the individual's meaning system. Many such fears were evolutionarily grounded: "available anxiety is here used simply to exaggerate the aversions which are implanted instinctively in everyone."[71]

Fears that were present during suitable life stages were not neurotic but natural; for example, "when a child is alone, or in the dark, or when it finds itself with an unknown person instead of one to whom it is used."[72] Fears of castration, darkness, or strangers that were normal when experienced during the appropriate periods in childhood became neurotic when they persisted and became unconscious sources of anxiety symptoms later in life. Neurotics "remain infantile in their attitude to danger and have not surmounted obsolete determinants of anxiety."[73] They reverted to states of anxious helplessness even though the sources of danger no longer existed. Most people, however, naturally aged out of their fears—although exactly why evolved fears would subside on their own with age remains a topic of controversy.[74]

The appropriateness of the object of anxiety in combination with the stage of the life cycle when a fear arises indicated whether fears were normal or abnormal. Freud used the now-famous case of Little Hans to illustrate in a nuanced way the distinction between neurotic versus realistic anxiety. On the surface, it might seem that a boy's anxiety that his father would castrate him would be classifiable as a neurotic anxiety. However, Freud believed that all 5-year-old boys normally love and want to possess their mothers and, as a result, fear their fathers' jealousy and retribution, and interpret this as a threat of castration. "If 'Little Hans,'" Freud wrote, "being in love with his mother, had shown fear of his father, we should have no right to say that he had a neurosis or a phobia. His emotional reaction would have been entirely comprehensible. What made it a neurosis was one thing alone: the replacement of his father by a horse."[75] Normal Oedipal fears became neurotic only when they were displaced from the real fear of castration and "directed to a different object and expressed in a distorted form, so that the patient is afraid, not of being castrated by his father, but of being bitten by a horse or devoured by a wolf."[76] The unconscious displacement of the original offensive idea allowed the boy, who simultaneously hated and loved his father, to recognize only his loving feelings while he displaced his hatred of the father onto the bad horse. Fathers were natural sources of fears of castration; horses were not, and horses could be more easily avoided than one's father—although such avoidance came at considerable cost to freedom of movement in Vienna in 1909.

Freud's conception of anxiety and his classification of the anxiety disorders, including his focus on the importance of this class of disorders as independent syndromes, strongly influenced subsequent thinking. His symptomatic depictions are entirely contemporary; for example, Freud's description of anxiety attacks contained ten of the twelve symptoms listed in the *DSM-III* diagnostic criteria for panic disorders.[77] Although his etiological speculations have generally been abandoned, many strands of his thinking, such as the importance of early development and trauma, still resonate with current research findings. The anxiety conditions he delineated—very much in syndromal *DSM* style—continue to lie at the heart of the set of anxiety disorders in current diagnostic manuals. In addition, his notion that the unreasonable quality of disorders separates them from normal anxiety is still central in present criteria. Although largely unacknowledged, Freud's thinking about anxiety remains seminal.

The study of specific psychoneurotic disorders typically had a low priority during the era when psychodynamic theory and practice dominated the psychiatric profession. Few researchers and clinicians in the period between about 1920 and 1970 were concerned with classifying the various forms of anxiety.[78] Psycho-analytically oriented clinicians, although possessing diagnostic categories passed down from Freud, pursued similar explorations of unconscious meanings with all neurotic patients and placed little weight on particular diagnoses. The classifica-tions that were used in this era strongly reflected Freud's views that emphasized the grounding of symptoms of anxiety of all kinds in unconscious, internal sources. Specific diagnoses rarely influenced treatment because analytic therapies were comparable across different conditions. In addition, clients generally paid directly for their treatment; therefore, third parties did not require a diagnosis for clinicians to receive payment. Analysts had little motivation to be concerned about diagnostic distinctions or to create sharp boundaries among various types of disorders.

Because public mental hospitals were required to account for the diagnoses of their patients, initial psychiatric classificatory manuals emphasized the kinds of conditions that patients in these institutions displayed. The first such manual in the United States, the *Statistical Manual for the Use of Hospitals for Mental Disorders*, was issued in 1918 by the American Medico-Psychological Association (which became the American Psychiatric Association in 1921) and went through ten editions before being superseded by the first *DSM* in 1952.[79] Among its twenty-two princi-pal groups, just one dealt with all of the psychoneuroses, including anxiety, the rest being reserved for the more severe conditions typically seen among institutional-ized patients. Descriptions of the various anxiety disorders in this manual were short and cursory and indicated uncertainty over diagnostic descriptions.

The *DSM-I*, which replaced the *Statistical Manual* in 1952, reflected the move-ment of psychiatric practice from state mental hospitals to outpatient treatment and thus paid more attention to the psychoneuroses. It also responded to the find-ings of military psychiatrists that almost all of the stress-related conditions they handled during World War II were incommensurate with the psychiatric nomencla-ture of the time.[80] The *DSM-I* split diagnoses that were not the result of organic impairments between psychotic disorders that "exhibit gross distortion or falsifica-tion of external reality" and psychoneurotic disorders that included a variety of diagnoses including anxiety, phobia, and obsessive-compulsive, depressive, disso-ciative, and conversion conditions.[81] However, like earlier manuals, it provided only perfunctory definitions of each disorder.

Inspired by psychoanalytic theory, the *DSM-I* used anxiety as the central conceptual principle behind all the psychoneurotic disorders. The first sentences of the summary description for the overall Psychoneurotic Disorders category stated,

> The chief characteristic of these disorders is 'anxiety' which may be directly felt and expressed or which may be unconsciously and automatically controlled by the utilization of various psychological defense mechanisms (depression, conversion, displacement, etc.). . . . "Anxiety" in psychoneurotic disorders is a danger signal felt and perceived by the conscious portion of the personality. It is produced by a threat from within the personality (e.g., by supercharged repressed emotions, including such aggressive impulses as hostility and resentment), with or without stimulation from such external situations as loss of love, loss of prestige, or threat of injury. The various ways in which the patient attempts to handle this anxiety results [sic] in the various types of reactions listed below.[82]

The manual's conceptions of the psychoneuroses strongly reflected not only Freud's theories about anxiety—as in the mention above of anxiety as a "danger signal"—but also his account of their etiology via defense mechanisms of anxiety. For example, the *DSM-I* says of phobic reactions, "The anxiety of these patients becomes detached from a specific idea, object, or situation in the daily life and is displaced to some symbolic idea or situation in the form of a specific neurotic fear."[83] Regarding "obsessive-compulsive reaction," the manual states, "In this reaction the anxiety is associated with the persistence of unwanted ideas and of repetitive impulses to perform acts which may be considered morbid by the patient. The patient himself may regard his ideas and behavior as unreasonable, but nevertheless is compelled to carry out his rituals."[84] In addition, the *DSM-I* formulated depression as a reaction to anxiety, stating, "The anxiety in this reaction is allayed, and hence partially relieved, by depression and self-depreciation. The reaction is precipitated by a current situation, frequently by some loss sustained by the patient, and is often associated with a feeling of guilt for past failures or deeds."[85] It also characterized dissociative and conversion reactions as results of defensive reactions to desires that were repressed because of the anxiety they created.

In the psychoneurotic category of "anxiety reaction," the *DSM-I* recognized the objectless, free-floating anxiety that had been pivotal to Freud's theorizing about the results of repression and the causes of neuroses: "In this kind of reaction the anxiety is diffuse and not restricted to definite situations or objects, as in the case of phobic reactions. . . . This reaction is characterized by anxious expectation and frequently associated with somatic symptomatology."[86] But the manual also recognized that the clinician must discriminate diffuse anxieties due to internal conflicts from normal reactions to threats and to stressful modern lifestyles: "The condition is to be differentiated from normal apprehensiveness or fear."[87] However, no guidance is provided as to how clinicians should make this distinction.

The *DSM-II*, published in 1968, did not make any major changes in the account of the anxiety disorders or in the pivotal role of anxiety in psychopathology. It maintained anxiety as the key aspect of the psychoneuroses, emphasizing that "[a]nxiety is the chief characteristic of the neuroses."[88]

ORIGINS OF THE *DSM-III* DIAGNOSTIC REVOLUTION

A variety of influences led to a dramatic reformulation of the anxiety disorders in the third edition of the *DSM*. By the 1970s, research-oriented psychiatrists using biological perspectives were challenging etiologically based categories that were grounded in unconscious psychogenic processes. It had also become clear that psychoanalysis had failed to progress as a science and could not be the basis for a research-based psychiatric profession. Many studies had shown that psychiatric diagnoses, which were based on the vague *DSM-II* criteria, were unreliable, with different psychiatrists arriving at different diagnoses based on the same evidence.[89] In addition, the deinstitutionalization of mental hospital patients and the rise of community treatments required psychiatry to place more attention on persons with psychotic forms of disorder, which were rarely amenable to analytic methods of explanation or treatment and seemed to demand biological accounts of etiology. Moreover, the National Institute of Mental Health faced intense political pressures to constrict its focus and fund projects that dealt with narrowly defined types of mental illnesses rather than with general human misery.[90]

The success of some psychotropic medications suggested that biological accounts were a promising avenue to explore in developing therapeutic advances. Furthermore, during the 1960s the Food and Drug Administration began to require evidence that medications not only relieved suffering but also were effective treatments for well-recognized categories of disorder.[91] These internal and external pressures propelled the psychiatric profession to develop a classification system with sharply defined categories that made clear distinctions among various types of mental disorders.

An even more basic challenge was how to formulate the diagnostic categories that these various pressures demanded. Since the late nineteenth century, general medicine had come to rely on well-defined, specific disease entities, so issues of professional legitimacy dictated that psychiatry also adopt a discrete, categorical system.[92] The problem it faced, however, was that little theoretical and empirical knowledge existed about how such a system should be constructed. It had long been known that, while etiology was the ideal way to classify disorders, in reality the causes of mental illnesses were unknown. As far back as 1782, British psychiatrist Thomas Arnold noted, "When the science of causes shall be complete we may then make them the basis of our classification, but till then we ought to content ourselves with an arrangement according to symptoms."[93] In the absence of causal knowledge, manifest symptoms would have to serve as the basis of a disease-based classification system. The amorphousness and non-specificity of anxiety conditions presented a particular challenge to diagnosticians.

The publication of the *DSM-III* in 1980, under the overall direction of Robert Spitzer, revolutionized psychiatric classification by presenting a symptom-based diagnostic system with necessary and sufficient criteria for the diagnosis of each disorder.[94] Spitzer insisted that diagnoses must be based on the presence of manifest symptoms without regard to etiology. One effect of this approach was that Spitzer's various task forces addressing particular categories of disorders eliminated the unproven psychoanalytic inferences that underlay the previous *DSM* classifications. Because they would be grounded in observable symptoms, the new diagnoses would enhance reliability and be more suitable for cumulative research across theoretical paradigms. Because it did not favor any particular clinical orientation, this diagnostic system was also politically valuable in securing the acceptance of the new manual by psychiatrists and other mental health professionals aligned with a variety of theoretical persuasions.

A major obstacle to the realization of a symptom-based classification system was the generalized concept of "psychoneurosis" that underlay and unified the non-psychotic classifications in the *DSM-I* and *DSM-II*.[95] This concept was unacceptable to research-oriented psychiatrists because it pointed to a specific etiology based in unconscious processes and led to categories that were vague and difficult to measure and thus prevented the development of a discipline grounded in the scientific method. The bitterest struggles in the establishment of the *DSM-III* involved the ultimately successful efforts of Spitzer and his associates to abolish the concept of the neuroses as an overarching category in psychiatric classification and to replace it with discrete diagnostic categories anchored in symptomatology without any presumption of the existence of an underlying theoretical unity. Because anxiety had been the central organizing principle of the neuroses, the defeat of the psychoanalytic approach inevitably led to a fundamental reformulation of the nature of the anxiety disorders and to a fresh neutrality about what had formerly been accepted beliefs regarding the role of anxiety in the etiology of psychopathology.

Establishing symptom-based diagnostic categories was a particular challenge when dealing with the anxiety disorders, since placement of boundaries between normal worries/fears and anxiety disorders was so difficult. The distinction between natural and abnormal forms of anxiety was firmly entrenched in psychiatric and psychoanalytic thought, as indicated in the *DSM-I*'s mention of the need to discriminate anxiety neurosis from normal fear and apprehension. Indeed, this distinction was virtually taken for granted at the time. For example, one of the most common psychiatric interviews during the 1970s, the Present State Examination, advised interviewers: "Do not, of course, include anxiety appropriate to the situation, e.g. going into battle, narrowly avoiding a traffic accident, realistic fear of punishment, anxiety during an examination, etc."[96] "Of course" emphasized the commonsensical notion that situationally based anxiety was not a sign of mental disorder but a natural result of threatening contexts.

The members of the *DSM-III* work group responsible for formulating the new criteria for anxiety disorders faced a daunting challenge. It would be very difficult to construct purely symptom-based categories when so many anxiety conditions were clearly contextually grounded. In the absence of a reference to context, the ubiquity of symptoms of anxiety would lead to the massive pathologization of these conditions. Consequently, the work group attempted to formulate criteria that, although not requiring an assessment of context, did nonetheless manage to distinguish between realistic, external fears and anxiety disorders.

The primary model for the new categorical diagnoses in the *DSM-III* was what later became known as the Feighner criteria (after the name of the first author of the article in which they were first published), which stemmed from the work of a group of research psychiatrists at Washington University in St. Louis.[97] The goal of the Feighner criteria was to develop a reliable system of psychiatric diagnoses for research purposes based on a small number of symptom-based categories. Three of the fourteen Feighner categories—anxiety, obsessive-compulsive, and phobic neuroses—were traditionally considered anxiety disorders, and a fourth—hysteria— was considered a psychoneurotic condition due to defenses against anxiety.

The most crucial feature of the Feighner criteria, relative to the reigning *DSM-I* and *II* tradition, was that the Washington University group formulated its definitions entirely in terms of symptoms, with no mention of their causes. The criteria maintained complete neutrality with respect to the etiology of the disorder. Some of these disorders, such as anxiety neuroses and phobias, have anxiety as a feature of the definition because anxiety is inherent in the symptom picture that distinguishes the disorder. For example, the criteria define phobias as "persistent and recurring fears which the patient tries to resist or avoid and at the same time considers unreasonable."

However, other anxiety disorders such as obsessive-compulsive disorder (OCD)—traditionally viewed as a way of controlling anxiety—were defined in terms of their manifest symptoms alone, without reference to the theory that their causes resided in a response to anxiety. Thus, OCD was defined as "recurrent or persistent ideas, thoughts, images, feelings, impulses, or movements, which must be accompanied by a sense of subjective compulsion and a desire to resist the event, the event being recognized by the individual as foreign to his personality or nature, ie, 'ego-alien.'"[98] Such a definition leaves it an open question as to why the obsessive and/or compulsive symptoms exist.

The Feighner definitions dealt with the normal/disordered distinction by using the patient's own beliefs about the reasonableness of fear and did not require assessment of the actual context of the fear. Thus, they distinguished phobic neuroses from ordinary fears by whether patients themselves considered their symptoms to be unreasonable and tried to resist or avoid them. Similarly, the criteria distinguish obsessive-compulsive neuroses from normal obsessions by the requirement that individuals recognize that the compulsions are foreign to their nature and so try to resist them.

One critical aspect of the Feighner criteria was that they basically abolished the disorder category of generalized, or free-floating, anxiety that was at the heart of analytic conceptions of the condition but that was difficult to distinguish from normal worries. Rather than allowing diffuse anxiety over a prolonged period of time to define a disorder, the criteria distinguished anxiety neurosis from normal anxiety by the necessary presence of repeated anxiety attacks that did not occur in circumstances that might otherwise explain such episodes:

> Chronic nervousness with recurrent anxiety attacks manifested by apprehension, fearfulness, or sense of impending doom, with at least four of the following symptoms present during the majority of attacks: (a) dyspnea [shortness of breath], (b) palpitations, (c) chest pain or discomfort, (d) choking or smothering sensation, (e) dizziness and (f) paresthesias [numbing, or prickling of the skin]. Anxiety attacks are essential to the diagnosis and must occur at times other than marked physical exertion or life-threatening situations, and in the absence of medical illness that could account for symptoms of anxiety. There must have been at least six anxiety attacks, each separated by at least a week from the others.[98]

This conception of anxiety neurosis is much closer to what the *DSM* now considers to be the category of panic disorder than to generalized anxiety disorder as earlier conceived.

A second critical feature of the Feighner criteria was the presence of a diagnostic hierarchy that provided rules for what conditions would take precedence when patients presented more than one disorder. A lower-ranking disorder would not be diagnosed in the presence of a higher-ranking disorder. Following Kraepelin, the hierarchy placed organic conditions at the top, followed by schizophrenia, affective disorders, and then the anxiety disorders. Anxiety neuroses were diagnosed only if they preceded the onset of other types of disorders by at least two years, while obsessive-compulsive and phobic neuroses were never diagnosed in the presence of another psychiatric disorder.[99] The logic of this hierarchy was that various manifestations of anxiety were so common in severe mental disorders that clinicians should diagnose a separate anxiety disorder only when other disorders likely to contain anxiety as a symptom were not present.

In addition to the Feighner criteria, the work of psychiatrist Donald Klein, a colleague of Spitzer's at Columbia and an important member of the *DSM-III* Anxiety Disorders Task Force, provided another important conceptual stimulus for the *DSM-III*'s approach to anxiety. Klein's primary interest was in whether the newly emergent anti-anxiety and anti-depressant drugs worked for some specific types of mental disorders but not for others. A positive answer to this question would indicate that particular brain receptors were associated with singular disorders, which thus might provide pointers to the sort of specific underlying mechanisms and etiologies that psychiatry had sought for hundreds of years. His research indicated that the anti-depressant imipramine prevented the recurrence of panic attacks and agoraphobia but not chronic anxiety.[100] Klein used these findings to argue that panic and agoraphobia were not simply more intense forms of anxiety but instead discrete conditions that should be split apart from general anxiety conditions. For example, panic could involve a form of suffocation alarm that acts through a different mechanism than other forms of anxiety. Therefore, he emphasized the intimate relationship of panic attacks and agoraphobia and their distinctiveness from other anxiety states. His discontinuous model provided a conceptual basis for challenging the assumed centrality of anxiety across all of the psychoneuroses as well as for justifying the construction of distinct anxiety conditions in the *DSM-III*.[101]

THE TRANSFORMATION OF THE ANXIETY DISORDERS IN THE *DSM-III*

Using the Feighner criteria and Klein's view as conceptual models, the *DSM-III* thoroughly transformed the categorization of the anxiety disorders.[102] Its revolutionary nature, contrary to common conceptions, does not stem from its expansion of the amount and range of pathology that is subject to mental health treatment.[103] It is true that it contained far more discrete diagnostic entities than were present in earlier manuals. However, the new aspect of the *DSM-III* involved the way the manual recategorized as discrete diagnostic entities the same conditions that were previously seen as more amorphous and loosely bounded.[104] In addition, the manual was distinctly new in its rejection of any attempt to use unconscious processes as the basis for classification. Nevertheless, its diagnostic criteria remained grounded in self-reports of inner states rather than on physician observations or objective measures of any sort.

The *DSM-III* abandoned the etiological claim that had unified psychoneurotic conditions as defenses against underlying anxiety. Instead, it divided the psychoneuroses—according to their manifest characteristic symptoms—into separate anxiety, affective, dissociative, and somatoform categories. To address the problem of multiple diagnoses given the omnipresence of anxiety, the *DSM-III*, similar to the Feighner criteria, used a loose hierarchical system of classification that put anxiety on the lowest tier. An anxiety diagnosis was not made if the anxious symptoms resulted from depressive or schizophrenic conditions.

The manual divided the general category of anxiety disorders into phobias, anxiety states, and post-traumatic stress disorder (PTSD), each with subtypes. It divided phobic states into two types of agoraphobia (with and without panic), social phobia, and simple phobia. Anxiety states encompassed panic, generalized anxiety disorder, and obsessive-compulsive disorder. PTSD contained two subtypes of acute and chronic or delayed. Finally, the *DSM-III* provided a residual category of atypical anxiety for "when the individual appears to have an Anxiety Disorder that does not meet the criteria for any of the above specified conditions."[105] No single category of anxiety was preeminent, nor did any category encompass multiple forms of anxiety. The result, according to British psychiatrist Peter Tyrer, was the "wholesale slaughter of anxiety neurosis as a diagnostic entity."[106]

The construction of discrete categories of anxiety disorder was not new with the *DSM-III*. Freud, for example, had made careful distinctions among anxiety conditions based on their symptoms. The novel aspect of the *DSM-III* was that each category of anxiety represented basically different conditions with "pure" symptom profiles and potentially distinct etiologies. Although Freud initially postulated different etiological pathways to different symptomatic presentations of anxiety, he had located the common basis of all neuroses in defenses against anxieties generated by childhood conflicts over sexuality during the psychologically vulnerable Oedipal period of development. The ways that the individual defended against the anxiety, and the pathways by which the symptoms formed, could lead in a variety of unpredictable directions, so for Freud a mixing of symptoms was not unusual or an occasion for attributing two different disorders.

For example, in his early presentation of his Oedipal theory in the famous case history of Little Hans, Freud argued that Little Hans's anxiety was initially undirected and free-floating due to repression of Oedipal sexual desires, but that it later became attached to horses after Hans witnessed an accident involving a horse, so that the anxiety then took the form of a horse phobia. Freud considered these two syndromal presentations (free-floating and phobic) to be etiologically different stages of the same disorder, the sort of judgment that is difficult to express in contemporary symptom-based diagnostic systems. The characterization of anxiety disorders by the types and contents of anxiety symptoms led undirected, free-floating anxiety without any content to fall into a different category from phobic fear of a specific type of object. Thus, if Hans's free-floating anxiety had endured for long enough before transforming into a horse phobia, the manuals that followed the *DSM-III* (which abandoned the diagnostic hierarchies in the *DSM-III*—see below) would consider that Hans suffered from two different anxiety disorders in sequence, with one a risk factor for developing the other. In this way, an extraordinary degree of diagnostic comorbidity, the presence of more than one distinct disorder, was born. In fact, the *DSM-IV Casebook* uses the Little Hans case to argue that Hans suffered from two anxiety disorders, phobia and separation anxiety—yet Freud sensibly saw that the horse phobia that kept Hans at home with his mother was part and parcel of the broader anxiety about separation from his mother.[107]

The same problem of excessive comorbidity occurred in separating depressive from anxiety disorders. While pure depressive disorders without anxiety symptoms—as well as pure anxiety disorders without depressive symptoms—can of course exist, it is also true that for 2500 years medical thought considered anxiety to be one possible symptom of depression, both in normal and disordered conditions. Freud explained the reason well, stating that depressive emotional pain is the reaction to the loss of an object, "while anxiety is the reaction to the danger which that loss entails and, by a further displacement, a reaction to the danger of the loss of object itself."[108] That is, loss causes depression, but an integral part of the emotional reaction to loss is fear of what the loss means for the future, as well as a more basic fear of being alone and losing attachment figures. Anxiety, therefore, is often part of the depressive response. Yet, the *DSM-III* diagnostic system separated anxiety symptoms and depressive symptoms into two separate domains, so that an individual mourning a loss with a mix of sadness and anxiety about the future would have two distinct conditions. In eschewing etiology even in this minimal sense, the *DSM* surrendered the sense of the history and meaning of symptoms that within the psychoanalytic approach served to explain the coherence of different kinds of symptoms within one overall disorder.

A critical decision for the *DSM-III* was how to deal with generalized anxiety disorder (GAD), which was the paradigmatic form of psychoneurosis under the dynamically oriented system, but which the Feighner criteria had redefined as panic disorder. Freud, for example, viewed the nervousness, apprehension, and free-floating anxiety characteristic of GAD as the nucleus of the anxiety disorders.[109] He did not explicitly formulate a category of panic disorder; he no doubt would have seen such a distinction as superfluous, because generalized and more punctuated undirected anxiety would typically be common manifestations of the same sorts of etiological processes. However, unlike the research-oriented

Feighner criteria, where the generalized category simply disappeared, the *DSM-III* had to make room for such a central clinical condition.

GAD posed a serious problem for the diagnosticians. It was extremely likely to co-occur in the presence of other anxiety states: almost everyone with a GAD diagnosis could also receive an additional anxiety diagnosis. Patients with GAD were especially common in general medical practice but were not frequently found in specialty psychiatry unless their condition was accompanied by more specific conditions such as phobias, OCD, or panic. Generalized anxiety also commonly accompanied many other psychiatric conditions including depression, schizophrenia, manic depression, substance abuse, and somatization, so that it often seemed to be more a secondary outcome of, or an accompaniment to, a different disorder than an independent condition. Moreover, GAD could be a product of a worrying personality disposition rather than a separate disorder.[110]

The *DSM-III* resolved the GAD problem by making it a residual category. It diagnosed GAD only when symptoms of phobic, panic, or obsessive-compulsive disorders were not present, leaving GAD's generalized anxiety as the only prominent anxiety feature:

> The essential feature is generalized, persistent anxiety of at least one month's duration without the specific symptoms that characterize Phobic Disorders, Panic Disorder, or Obsessive-Compulsive Disorder . . . The diagnosis is not made if the disturbance is due to another physical or mental disorder.[111]

Subsequent research in the period immediately after the publication of *DSM-III* came to focus on the other specific anxiety categories, leaving GAD as the unwanted stepchild of the anxiety disorders.[112] GAD, which on its face might be viewed as the core anxiety condition, became "an atavistic ghost of its predecessor that can hardly stand alone as a diagnostic entity."[113] The neglect was so thoroughgoing that the major study launched to measure the prevalence of the central diagnostic categories of the *DSM-III* in the community didn't even report rates of GAD in its initial publications.[114] A renewed research interest in GAD would await a reformulation of its diagnostic criteria in a later edition of the *DSM*, discussed below.

HOW THE *DSM-III* ATTEMPTED TO DISTINGUISH DISORDERED FROM NORMAL ANXIETY

This section reviews—without formulating any substantial critique—how the *DSM-III* attempted to address the issue of distinguishing normal from disordered fear and anxiety. The next chapter more critically examines the adequacy of the current criteria in distinguishing natural fears from disordered anxiety.

The *DSM-III* faced a central problem in how to deal with the essential difference between realistic, external fears and anxiety disorders. Making decisions about which conditions of anxiety were contextually grounded and which were disordered often required nuanced clinical judgments that threatened the reliability of diagnoses and, thus, the major principle of the manual. Yet, ignoring such a crucial distinction would threaten the legitimacy of the profession's diagnoses of disorders as true medical conditions rather than as mislabeled natural fears.

The *DSM-III* used a variety of techniques in its attempts to separate disordered from natural worries and fears for most of the anxiety disorders. To some degree, it built upon the Feighner criteria's notions that such features as the individual's desire to resist the fear, and recognition that the fear is unreasonable, distinguish pathological from normal anxieties. However, it also went beyond the Feighner criteria to require that the fear is in fact irrational, implicitly requiring a judgment about the fear's relationship to the contextual situation. The introduction to the section on phobic disorders (agoraphobia, social phobia, simple phobia) indicated:

> The essential feature is persistent and irrational fear of a specific object, activity, or situation that results in a compelling desire to avoid the dreaded object, activity, or situation (the phobic stimulus). The fear is recognized by the individual as excessive or unreasonable in proportion to the actual dangerousness of the object, activity, or situation.[115]

Recognizing that many irrational fears can be trivial, the criteria also required that the fear entail significant distress. The manual noted that impairment is often minimal because people can often easily avoid many phobic objects, providing the example of city dwellers who fear snakes but are unlikely to ever encounter them. A phobic diagnosis, therefore, did not require impairment but just the presence of irrational and compelling fears that created significant distress.

The *DSM-III* diagnostic criteria for social phobia incorporated these ideas for separating natural fears from anxiety disorder, as follows:

A. A persistent, irrational fear of, and compelling desire to avoid, a situation in which the individual is exposed to possible scrutiny by others and fear that he or she may act in a way that will be humiliating or embarrassing.

B. Significant distress because of the disturbance and recognition by the individual that his or her fear is excessive or unreasonable.

C. Not due to another mental disorder, such as Major Depression or Avoidant Personality Disorder.[116]

These criteria attempted to avoid any implication that ordinary shyness and avoidance of social occasions that might be uncomfortable, humiliating, or embarrassing were mental disorders. Moreover, social phobic disorders did not consist simply of persistent, irrational, and compelling desires to avoid these situations. In addition, they required both significant distress and the self-recognition of excessive or unreasonable fears.

The manual also recognized that panic attacks can sometimes be normal and adaptive responses to life-threatening situations, so that diagnostic criteria must therefore separate realistic from pathological attacks. The criteria for panic disorder required "[at] least three panic attacks within a three-week period in circumstances other than during marked physical exertion or in a life-threatening situation. The attacks are not precipitated only by exposure to a circumscribed phobic stimulus."[117] Thus, any panic attack that resulted from a life-threatening situation—like Kendler's dangling from a cliff, described in Chapter 1—did not indicate a disordered response.

Likewise, the category of obsessive-compulsive disorder distinguished disorders that feature involuntary, senseless, and recurrent obsessions and compulsions from fears that had rational grounding in social contexts, indicating "the activity is not connected in a realistic way with what it is designed to produce or prevent, or may be clearly excessive."[118] In this vein, the criteria also required, as a way of distinguishing disordered conditions from normal-range idiosyncrasies, that a compulsion include the individual's "sense of subjective compulsion coupled with a desire to resist the compulsion (at least initially). The individual generally recognizes the senselessness of the behavior (this may not be true for young children) and does not derive pleasure from carrying out the activity, although it provides a release of tension."[119] OCD remained the one anxiety disorder for which the symptoms themselves did not inherently include anxiety (other than anxiety about the condition as one possible "clinical significance" indicator that it was a disorder). Thus, there remained an implicit etiological theory behind the placement of OCD within the anxiety disorders—namely, that the control of anxiety-motivated symptoms tangentially slipped into the criteria by the observation that failure to perform the compulsive actions led to "tension." The issue of whether OCD really belongs in the anxiety disorders section of the *DSM* remains a topic of active controversy among those with different etiological beliefs.[120]

Post-traumatic stress disorder (PTSD) represented a special case, which we discuss in a later chapter. PTSD, by definition, could arise only in traumatic contexts "that would evoke significant symptoms of distress in almost everyone," so contextual qualifiers for the diagnosis would be redundant since the criteria already required the presence of extremely stressful circumstances.[121]

In contrast to the other anxiety disorders, the *DSM-III* did not make any serious attempt to distinguish generalized anxiety disorder from intense normal worries and anxieties. Criteria for GAD were purely symptomatic and did not require intensity disproportionate to the context in which they arose. Thus, anyone suffering anxiety for a given period of time might be diagnosed with a disorder. This was a critical conceptual failing that later editions corrected.[122] Arguably, however, given the context of GAD in the *DSM-III*, this gross flaw in the criteria had less of an impact than it otherwise might have had on diagnoses of the disorder. As noted, GAD was placed at the bottom rung of the diagnostic hierarchy and was not diagnosed when a different anxiety disorder or another type of mental disorder was present. Thus, most potential GAD cases would have received some other diagnosis.

The manuals that followed the *DSM-III*—the *DSM-III-R* (1986), *DSM-IV* (1994), and *DSM-IV-TR* (2000)—changed the specific criteria of many of the anxiety categories, usually in minor ways.[123] They also relaxed many of the diagnostic hierarchies that had minimized diagnostic redundancy; as a result, many of the anxiety disorders could also be diagnosed even when other anxiety and mood disorders were present. Although the basic categorical principles of the diagnostic system have remained unaltered since 1980, subsequent revisions of the manual did make several significant changes aimed at strengthening or otherwise influencing the distinction between normal worries and fears and anxiety disorders. We briefly review some of the most important changes here. The next chapter more carefully assesses the current criteria that have emerged from these revisions.

GAD underwent major transformations in the manuals that followed the *DSM-III*. The *DSM-III-R* abandoned the hierarchical rule that disallowed GAD diagnoses in the presence of other disorders. This could have led to a vast increase in GAD diagnoses, since the *DSM-III* criteria for this disorder were entirely symptom based with no contextual restraints, but the *DSM-III-R* placed strict contextual requirements on the GAD diagnosis:

> Unrealistic or excessive anxiety and worry (apprehensive expectation) about two or more life circumstances, e.g. worry about possible misfortune to one's child (who is in no danger) and worry about finances (for no good reason), for a period of six months or longer, during which the person has been bothered more days than not by these concerns.[124]

The qualifier "two or more life circumstances" ensured that anxiety grounded in a single context would not qualify for the disorder. Its intent seemed clearly directed at limiting diagnoses to only conditions that are not contextually grounded. In any case, the examples of limiting diagnoses to anxiety about children who are "in no danger" or about finances "for no good reason" distinguished realistic worries from anxiety disorders. Worries about physically ill children or burdensome debts unmistakably did not qualify one for a GAD diagnosis. The *DSM-III-R* also required that symptoms must endure for six months, instead of the *DSM-III's* one-month requirement. These features moderated the possibility that purely situational anxiety would be misdiagnosed as GAD. Although the *DSM-IV* required only "excessive" (but not unrealistic) anxiety, the associated text made it obvious that only disproportionate worry was disordered: "The intensity, duration, or frequency of the anxiety and worry is far out of proportion to the actual likelihood or impact of the feared event."[125] Likewise, the *DSM-IV* criteria strengthened the link of obsessions and compulsions with true disorders by requiring that they "are not simply excessive worries about real-life problems."[126]

The criteria for social phobia were an exception to the clearer distinctions between normal fears and anxiety disorders in the manuals that followed the *DSM-III*. The *DSM-III* had required "persistent, irrational fear of, and compelling desire to avoid, a situation in which the individual is exposed to possible scrutiny by others and fears that he or she may act in a way that is humiliating or embarrass-ing."[127] The *DSM-III-R* weakened the contextual constraints over social phobia, requiring only "persistent fear of one or more situations . . . in which the person is exposed to possible scrutiny by others and fears that he or she may do something or act in a way that will be humiliating or embarrassing."[128] These criteria no longer require that the fear must be irrational, although it is still required that the individual believes the fear is unreasonable. Moreover, some of the examples the definition provided of situations indicating social phobia were common *natural* fears, such as "saying foolish things or not being able to answer questions in social situations" or "being unable to continue talking while speaking in public."[129] These changes made the boundaries between natural shyness and social phobias far more amorphous than they had been in the *DSM-III*. As Chapter 6 will show, these changes led to an enormous rise in alleged rates of social phobias in the population.[130]

CONCLUSION

A major task of psychiatric diagnosis is to distinguish mental disorders from normal, unpleasant emotions. The diagnostic criteria for some major *DSM* diagnostic categories, in particular Major Depressive Disorder and some of the childhood disorders, suffer from blatant invalidity because they do not seriously attempt to separate ordinary emotions from mental disorders.[131] This is not as flagrantly the case for the anxiety disorder diagnostic criteria, which at least attempt to distinguish normal from disordered fear and anxiety. Nonetheless, many questions remain about the adequacy of the criteria in drawing this fundamental distinction. We now turn to a more focused assessment of the adequacy of the current diagnostic criteria for the anxiety disorders and how they might be improved.

CHAPTER 5

The Validity of the *DSM* Diagnostic Criteria for Anxiety Disorders

The previous chapter examined the development of the *DSM* diagnostic criteria for anxiety disorders in the watershed third edition and placed these criteria in the historical context of thinking about anxiety and its disorders. It detailed the challenges the developers of the *DSM* faced in distinguishing normal from disordered anxiety, given that human beings are shaped to feel intense anxiety in response to some environmental circumstances, and described the ways they tried to deal with these challenges. Given the virtually universal use of the *DSM* criteria in determining what is and is not a mental disorder in a variety of contexts— whether clinical treatment, counting of cases in the community, financing health care, training mental health professionals, or maintaining records—the validity of these criteria is essential for the accurate diagnoses of anxiety disorders. This chapter addresses how successfully the current *DSM* manual (the fourth text-revised edition, *DSM-IV-TR* [2000]) distinguishes normal versus disordered anxiety and considers some of the changes in these diagnostic criteria proposed for *DSM-5*.

The *DSM-III* and subsequent diagnostic manuals have many advantages over their predecessors in the way they conceptualize anxiety. Their symptom-based diagnostic criteria are far more explicit and precise than the amorphous definitions found in earlier manuals, so clinicians and researchers find them far easier to use. They provide a common language for effective communication about specific conditions. They enhance the reliability of diagnoses because symptom-based indicators are easier to measure. Unlike the initial *DSM-I* and *DSM-II* manuals, they do not prejudge the causes of anxiety disorders. Moreover, their reliance on theory-neutral definitions means that clinicians and researchers from all theoretical persuasions can find them useful.

Despite its strengths and the fact that the *DSM* has such authority that it is known as the "bible of psychiatry," the work groups that formulate the diagnostic criteria are in fact quite fallible. There is ample precedent that the *DSM*'s diagnostic criteria can be invalid, even in fairly obvious ways. The *DSM* has been revised several times, and those who reformulated the *DSM*'s diagnostic criteria in each succeeding edition have corrected many flaws in previous editions' criteria, often based on face validity and conceptual plausibility rather than on research findings. One of the main reasons for such corrections has been errors in making the distinction between disorder and non-disorder, which resulted in the inadvertent misclassification of some normal conditions as disorders. Despite such periodic corrections, the reported prevalence of certain anxiety disorders has increased dramatically without any persuasive basis except changing diagnostic criteria, suggesting that problems of false positives (i.e., misdiagnoses of normal conditions as disorders) remain. We hope that a critical examination of the *DSM*'s diagnostic criteria sets can contribute to efforts to improve the validity of the anxiety disorder criteria.

As we write, the *DSM* is undergoing a revision that is expected to yield a fifth edition—*DSM-5*—to be published in 2013. Thus, the criteria we consider here may in some cases soon be changed. Although the initial suggestions for revision of the anxiety disorders are not very substantial and mostly do not impinge on what we have to say about current criteria, they do in some instances address issues relevant to our discussion of the boundaries between disorders and natural anxiety. We thus consider in this chapter not only the current criteria but also those changes proposed for *DSM-5* (as of this writing) that might influence strategies for preventing false positives.

We consider three issues regarding the diagnostic criteria: First, we identify the general strategies the *DSM* uses to distinguish disordered from intense but normal anxiety. Second, we explore the extent to which, given these strategies, the *DSM* criteria validly distinguish or fail to distinguish disordered from non-disordered anxiety. Finally, we ask whether the strategies that the *DSM* employs to separate disorder from non-disorder are congruent with an evolutionary perspective on human nature and are sensitive to biologically designed anxiety functioning or, if not, whether they provide a cogent alternative to that view. After initially considering general issues that cut across diagnostic categories, we focus in more detail on three of the highest-prevalence disorders—specific phobia, social phobia, and generalized anxiety disorder—that between them account for much of the enormous reported prevalence of anxiety disorders in the community. We examine both their current criteria and some selected proposals for changes in *DSM-5*. Our overall goals are to assess the validity of the criteria in distinguishing normal anxiety from disordered anxiety and, where appropriate, to suggest ways that the diagnostic criteria can be made more valid than the current and proposed criteria and thus more useful for enhancing knowledge about the causes, prognoses, and treatments of anxiety disorders.

One caveat is that we do not fully reproduce or examine every feature of the *DSM* criteria; we consider only elements relevant to our focus on whether the criteria validly identify disorders. Thus, we ignore categories of anxiety disorders due to a general medical condition or substance use, which are clearly abnormal conditions. We also ignore the "anxiety disorder not otherwise specified" (NOS) category because it has no specific criteria. We also limit ourselves to adult disorders, ignoring many criteria provided specifically for children. Because we are interested exclusively in the boundary between disorder and normality ("conceptual validity"), we generally ignore questions of how best to divide disordered conditions into separate disorders and how to distinguish one disorder from another ("differential validity"). Finally, because the relevant work groups have not yet finalized criteria for *DSM-5*, we focus on their proposals presented in published literature reviews, which may represent only an approximation of the final changes. These reviews in any event represent the most recent and sophisticated public reconsideration of the criteria by those involved in the *DSM* process.

DSM STRATEGIES FOR DISTINGUISHING NORMAL FROM PATHOLOGICAL ANXIETY

Anxiety presents a serious challenge to the approach to diagnosis that underlies the *DSM* because it is apparent that even intense anxious symptoms often are normal responses to threatening situations and not signs of disorder. Consequently, purely descriptive, symptom-based criteria have limited utility when it comes to defining anxiety disorders. Emotions of fear, worry, or dread of various objects or social situations as well as accompanying physical symptoms such as restlessness, sleep disturbance, or elevated heart rate are often natural reactions to perceived and actual dangers. Consequently, in assessing intense anxiety, there are frequently two competing hypotheses: individuals may be experiencing normal anxiety in response to circumstances, or they may have a disorder that is generating pathological levels of anxiety. It is true that anxiety disorders will generally (but not always—see Chapter 3) include intense anxiety, but it is not true that intense anxiety generally implies an anxiety disorder, even though in a clinical context it is easy to mistakenly think it does.

The *DSM* employs a set of characteristic strategies to accomplish its goal of distinguishing truly pathological anxiety from normal intense anxiety. These strategies include requiring the presence of a sufficient number of symptoms from a defined group; mandating that the anxiety is "marked" and thus possesses a sufficient degree of severity or intensity; and indicating either thresholds for the persistent duration of the anxiety or that the anxiety is recurrent. Beyond these standard elements of number, severity, and duration of symptoms, the *DSM* correctly assumes that only symptoms that have distressing or impairing consequences are disorders, thus eliminating trivial, transient, and innocuous anxiety states from disorder status (this is known as the "clinical significance criterion"). Finally, to zero in on the pathological nature of the anxiety, the criteria commonly contain qualifiers such as "excessive," "unreasonable," "inappropriate," or "unexpected" that attempt to differentiate disordered symptoms from natural fears and worries. These terms indicate recognition that symptoms alone cannot separate anxiety disorders from natural concerns but must be evaluated in relation to the context in which they appear.

Despite the *DSM*'s useful multiple strategies for attaining validity, the criteria for anxiety disorders have a number of flaws and limitations that lead to a confusion between disorder and normal distress. These problems stem from the failure of the criteria to ground definitions in an evolutionarily informed conception of fear-generating mechanisms and the ways in which these mechanisms normally work and can break down.

INTENSITY, NUMBER OF SYMPTOMS, AND DURATION

One way that *DSM* diagnostic criteria sets attempt to distinguish disordered from non-disordered anxiety is to set thresholds for the intensity, number of symptoms, and duration required for diagnosis of a disorder. Some of the criteria sets characterize anxiety and other symptoms in a way that requires a high degree of intensity, usually by specifying a "marked" degree of anxiety. For example, in obsessive-compulsive disorder, the recurrent thoughts or actions need to cause "marked anxiety or distress." Panic attacks require "a discrete period of intense fear or discomfort." In agoraphobia, the feared situations "are avoided (e.g., travel is restricted) or else are endured with marked distress." Similarly, one of the acute stress disorder symptoms requires "[m]arked symptoms of anxiety or increased arousal."

In an additional attempt to confirm that there is high intensity of anxiety, diagnoses generally require severity in the form of multiple symptoms. For example, the criteria for generalized anxiety disorder require three or more out of six possible symptoms, panic attacks require four or more out of ten symptoms, and acute stress disorder entails five symptoms distributed over dissociative, re-experience, avoidance, and increased arousal categories.

The criteria also assign varying required minimal durations to some of the anxiety disorders. Acute stress disorder must last a minimum of two days. Panic requires "recurrent" attacks and at least one month of concern following some of the attacks, although there is no duration requirement for the attacks themselves. Similarly, obsessive-compulsive disorder requires "recurrent and persistent" thoughts or actions. The *DSM-IV* contains no specific duration requirement for specific and social phobias for adults, specifying only that the fear must be "persistent." However, there is a six-month minimum duration for children, due to how common transient intense fears are in children. It has been argued that "it is unclear . . . whether duration should differ for individuals under 18 or over 18," and it appears that the *DSM-5* might require six-month duration for all specific and social phobias.[1]

There is a basic problem with all three of these strategies for defining anxiety disorders: *normal* anxiety responses can feature intensity, multiplicity of symptoms, and extended duration. Consequently, these strategies do not suffice to identify pathology.

Regarding intensity, as we have seen, many normal fear reactions involve "marked" or "intense" anxiety, especially when the circumstances are extraordinarily threatening. Furthermore, while the presence of intense anxiety might seem to be a useful necessary—although not sufficient—condition for disorder, there are also mild and moderate disorders in psychiatry, just as there are in physical medicine. Extraordinarily intense anxiety can be a sign of disorder in some instances, and on average disorders are certainly more likely than normal responses to be highly intense within a given context. However, intensity and disordered status are ultimately two different dimensions. Normal responses can be moderate or intense, and disordered conditions can also be moderate or intense. Indeed, chronic moderate anxiety for no reason can be a serious disorder (imagine, for example, experiencing chronic moderate social anxiety even when sitting quietly with one's children or unobserved in the back of a lecture hall).

Requiring a multiplicity of symptoms is also a fallible indicator of disorder because intense anxiety, whether normal or disordered, can have many different symptomatic manifestations. Indeed, normal responses can have many symptoms, and disorders can sometimes have few. For example, panic disorder requires four or more symptoms of accelerated heart rate, sweating, trembling, shortness of breath, feeling of choking, chest discomfort, abdominal distress, lightheadedness, feelings of unreality, and fear of losing control.[2] This multiplicity requirement at best serves to ensure that the individual is experiencing a substantial anxiety response; it implies nothing about whether these experiences are normal or disordered because multiple somatic symptoms such as accelerated heart rate, sweating, trembling, and feeling dizzy also typify normal episodes of extreme fear or terror. What makes panic into a disorder is that the intense anxiety is unexpected and unrelated to any contextual threat, not the number of symptoms the intense anxiety contains.

As for duration, some time frames that the *DSM* specifies are short enough to be compatible with normal responses and are not distinctive of disorders, such as the two days required for an acute stress response. It is difficult to imagine why symptoms for acute stress disorder—including dissociative symptoms (e.g., numbing, sense of unreality), re-experiencing symptoms (e.g., via dreams or flashbacks), and avoidance symptoms (e.g., of situations that remind one of the traumatic event)—are assumed to imply a disorder after a period as short as two days immediately after a traumatic experience of threat or horror. Such responses are well within the range of normal responses to intense threats and seem potentially adaptive in allowing the individual to gradually process the event while maintaining vigilance for further danger and altering emotional memory to influence future behavior to avoid similar situations.

A further problem is that enduring threats can create chronic but quite normal anxiety. Contrary to the idea of context-free duration thresholds, chronic symptoms may be normal responses to chronic stressors.[3] Even for the most demanding *DSM* duration requirement of six months for GAD (which the *DSM-5* proposes to change to only three months), normal worries can last over long periods of time if they are responses to persistent marital, financial, or medical problems. Extended duration, as well as marked responses with multiple symptoms, can be compatible with normal anxiety responses. The pathological nature of anxiety must be shown in some other way.

CLINICAL SIGNIFICANCE

In addition to the general features of intensity, duration, and multiplicity of symptoms, the *DSM* attempts to discriminate disorder from non-disorder by adding a "clinical significance criterion" to the symptom sets. Each anxiety disorder diagnosis requires that the symptoms have some negative effect on the individual, such as impairment in social or occupational functioning or distress. The only exception is agoraphobia, in which the restriction on movement seems so likely to interfere with role functioning that an additional impairment criterion perhaps seems unnecessary.

DSM clinical significance criteria typically require significant distress or role impairment. However, these criteria vary slightly from disorder to disorder in ways adjusted to that disorder's peculiarities. For example, specific phobia criteria require that the fear "interferes significantly with the person's normal routine, occupational (or academic) functioning, or social activities or relationships, or there is marked distress about having the phobia," whereas acute stress disorder criteria mandate that "the disturbance causes clinically significant distress or impairment in social, occupational, or other important areas of functioning or impairs the individual's ability to pursue some necessary task, such as obtaining necessary assistance or mobilizing personal resources by telling family members about the traumatic experience."[4] In addition to "distress" and "impairment" criteria, panic disorder allows a month or more of concern about a repeat attack as one proof of clinical significance,[5] whereas OCD criteria allow as proof of clinical significance that the obsessions or compulsions are time-consuming (take more than one hour per day).[6]

One problem is that the "distress" component of clinical significance is close to tautological because anxiety in and of itself—whether normal or disordered—is inherently distressing. Thus, the requirement that there be "clinically significant distress" is largely redundant in the PTSD, acute stress disorder, and GAD categories (as well as some other categories) because satisfying the symptom criteria for those disorders almost inevitably involves distress. This flaw undermines the usefulness of the clinical significance criterion in these disorders because it is a disjunctive criterion ("either distress or impairment") and consequently is as weak as its weakest disjunct. If almost everyone with the symptoms satisfies one of the disjuncts for spurious reasons, then almost everyone will also spuriously satisfy the entire requirement, rendering the criterion useless. As now formulated, the clinical significance criterion basically provides a "free pass" to classify as pathological many intense anxiety conditions that may be normal.

Even aside from the fact that the tautological "distress" clause renders the impairment clause superfluous, the role interference clause does not help matters much because intense normal anxiety also can impair social or occupational functioning. Another troubling aspect of role impairment being used to indicate clinical significance is that this resonates with the classic anti-psychiatric concern that—under the guise of making medical judgments—psychiatry is actually intervening to ensure that people meet their social role obligations. There is, however, an important potential role for a restricted version of the impairment component of the clinical significance criterion that we consider later.

Can the clinical significance criterion be eliminated altogether from diagnostic criteria for anxiety disorders without decreasing validity, as is being considered for *DSM-5*? It might seem so, since other criteria generally require that a condition must involve "marked" fear or anxiety to be considered an anxiety disorder. Thus, virtually by definition—without the clinical significance criterion—a condition must involve harm in the form of distress to warrant diagnosis. Such distress by itself would be sufficient to warrant disorder attribution *if the distress is a symptom of a dysfunction.* The clinical significance criterion in its usual form is thus superfluous as a harm specifier due to the inherent suffering involved in anxiety and fear.

"UNREASONABLE" AND/OR "EXCESSIVE" CRITERIA

If basic features of the anxiety disorder diagnostic criteria sets such as intensity, duration, and multiplicity of anxiety symptoms do not ensure disorder because they can also be features of normal anxiety responses, and if the clinical significance criterion that was designed to eliminate false positives fails to validly discriminate disordered from non-disordered conditions because it is redundant with the symptom criteria and normally anxious people are distressed and sometimes role-impaired, then what strategies remain within the *DSM*'s approach to anxiety disorders that might provide the needed distinction? The *DSM*'s answer is to require the anxiety to be unreasonable, excessive, or inappropriate, and also, in some of the disorders, that the individual recognizes it as such. This is an important attempt to contextually evaluate the level of the anxiety in relation to the reality of the danger and thus to infer whether the symptoms represent a normal-range response to a threatening situation or result from a dysfunction.

A number of the criteria sets use terms such as "excessive" and "unreasonable" to characterize disordered conditions.[7] For example, obsessive-compulsive disorder requires that "[a]t some point during the course of the disorder, the person has recognized that the obsessions or compulsions are excessive or unreasonable"; that obsessive thoughts, impulses, or images at some point are experienced as "inappropriate"; that compulsive "behaviors or mental acts either are not connected in a realistic [i.e., reasonable] way with what they are designed to neutralize or prevent or are clearly excessive"; and that obsessions are "thoughts, impulses, or images (that) are not simply excessive worries about real-life problems."[8] GAD requires "excessive anxiety and worry (apprehensive expectation), occurring more days than not for at least 6 months, about a number of events or activities (such as work or school performance)."

Why the "excessive or unreasonable" criterion is needed is obvious from the great range of normal fears of truly dangerous objects and situations. The necessity for this criterion is also clear if one examines the anxiety disorder criteria sets in which this requirement does not appear. For example, the criteria for agoraphobia read in part as follows: "Anxiety about being in places or situations from which escape might be difficult (or embarrassing) or in which help may not be available in the event of having an unexpected or situationally predisposed Panic Attack or panic-like symptoms. Agoraphobic fears typically involve characteristic clusters of situations that include being outside the home alone; being in a crowd or standing in a line; being on a bridge; and traveling in a bus, train, or automobile . . ."[9] However, anxiety in situations in which escape is difficult or help is unavailable is perfectly normal if one has reason to expect that escape may be necessary or help may be needed. For example, people with various medical conditions routinely limit their activities and their travel on this basis, judging that it is better to be safe than sorry. These criteria don't have the logical heft to distinguish such disorders from normal-range anxiety. The question "what is necessarily disordered about that?" goes unanswered. This is why the *DSM* adds "unreasonable" and "excessive" to many criteria sets in the quest for diagnostic validity.

Some criteria sets also require that individuals themselves recognize that symptoms are unreasonable or excessive. This is questionable as a valid criterion for disorder due to the great influence of social pressures and personal desires on people's judgments, and, as we shall see, the *DSM-5* might eliminate such requirements.

The use of such qualifiers as "excessive" and "unreasonable" is a move in the right direction of incorporating context into the evaluation of whether anxiety is normal or disordered. Nonetheless, these criteria raise some fundamental issues about the normal/disordered distinction and create some false-positive problems of their own.

EXCESSIVENESS

Excessiveness and unreasonableness are closely related ideas. However, because they differ in nuance and have tended to be the focus of discussion in different disciplines—excessiveness within psychiatry, and irrationality and reason within the philosophy of psychiatry—we consider them separately. The central question is whether either of these qualifiers offers a cogent elaboration of, or alternative to, the evolutionary view of the distinction between pathological and non-pathological human distress. Excessiveness obviously suggests a mismatch of some kind between the level of the fear and the nature of the threat or danger in the current environment. But one must ask, "excessive relative to what?"

"Excessive" is highly ambiguous in meaning, depending on the kind of norm relative to which the excess is judged. It can refer, first, to statistically intense responses that are in the upper end of the intensity distribution, thus meaning "excessive relative to what most people feel under the same circumstances." There are two major problems with the "excessiveness" criterion when understood as referring to statistically higher-than-typical anxiety. First, people normally vary in the intensity of their emotional reactions, and this criterion would pathologize the upper end of the normal continuum of the personality trait of emotional intensity.

Second, the excessiveness could be a reaction to special circumstances that explain the greater intensity of response, but the criteria make no reference to context. For example, if there have been several snake attacks in one's area in recent weeks, one may feel "excessive" fear of snakes relative to the general level of fear.

Second, "excessive" is often used as a label for responses or feelings that are considered socially undesirable, so the term means "excessive relative to social norms." Such social judgments clearly should not determine what is and is not a psychiatric disorder. Indeed, one of the primary goals in defining psychopathology is to distinguish it from social desirability. A related possibility is that "excessive" means something like "harmful to the individual," in the sense that it causes some considerable degree of distress or distraction from usual roles or activities. In this case, "excessive" is an indicator not so much of disorder (in which an internal dysfunction causes symptoms) as of clinical significance due to harm to the individual.

Anxiety that is statistically intense, outside social norms, or harmful can still be non-disordered anxiety. There is, however, one way that the "excessiveness" criterion can validly indicate disorder. The criterion is valid if it means "excessive relative to the range of biologically designed responses within the existing context." That is, excessiveness could be judged by evolutionary criteria that take into account not only the immediate context and the individual's temperament but also the levels of anxiety that people naturally feel in response to evolutionarily shaped fears of snakes, spiders, and so on. Given this approach, "excessive anxiety" is a good way to characterize likely disordered anxiety.

One way the *DSM* expresses the notion of excessiveness is its occasional requirement that symptoms be seriously "out of proportion" to environmental stressors. (This is an approach, we shall see, that is proposed for *DSM-5*.) For example, the criteria for intermittent explosive disorder require that the "degree of aggressiveness expressed during the episodes is grossly out of proportion to any precipitating psychosocial stressors."[10] There is a 2500-year tradition of using disproportionality of a response to denote that the response is outside a normal-range response, given that many mental mechanisms are designed to generate responses that are in some broad sense calibrated to be proportionally related to the nature of the circumstances, as in sadness after varying degrees of loss or fear in situations of varying degrees of danger.

Interpreted as disproportionality, and depending on how "disproportionality" is defined, "excessive" is clearly a contextual criterion that would go a considerable way toward suggesting dysfunction if it refers to anxieties that are not within some biologically designed range of response that varies with actual danger and must be adjusted for species-typical fear as well as for local cultural shaping and individual normal-range personality variations. However, as we shall see, the proposals for *DSM-5* clarify that "proportional" is to be understood in narrower terms, as referring to proportionality not in light of overall biological design but rather to the actual danger in the perceived threat. Consequently, the status of the "disproportionality" interpretation of "excessive" will require further consideration below.

UNREASONABLENESS

What of the other central *DSM* characterization of disordered anxiety as "unreasonable"? In relying on fears being unreasonable as a way to identify pathology, the *DSM* embraces what is historically the primary alternative to our evolutionary view for judging normal versus disordered anxiety. From Aristotle onward, reason has traditionally been seen as the distinctive and highest human capacity.[11] Consequently, what is irrational or unreasonable has often been taken to be a criterion for mental disorder, and many commentators use the actual degree of danger the feared object poses to distinguish anxiety disorders from normal anxiety. For example, the prominent British psychiatrist Aubrey Lewis defined anxiety disorders as follows: "There is either no recognizable threat, or the threat is, by reasonable standards, quite out of proportion to the emotion it seemingly evokes."[12] This "reasonableness" conception of normal anxiety and proportionality plays a prominent role in current *DSM* diagnostic criteria.

However, this is a flawed tradition when applied to anxiety disorders; mental normality and reasonableness do not always coincide. True, reasonableness can to some extent be used to appropriately evaluate fears when those fears are primarily based on cognitive evidence of current threat, which is one common route to fear. For example, if one is intensely preoccupied with the possibility of a stock market crash during a period of prosperity when there is no current evidence for such a potential catastrophe, then the unreasonableness of the belief may indeed arouse some concern that a disorder exists (although one must be careful in such judgments, because people who seem unreasonable may be following divergent strands of evidence that others ignore or downplay—and they not infrequently turn out to be right!). But many fears are not so simply cognitively grounded and are not formed through weighing evidence that can then be judged as reasonable or unreasonable. Instead, they have more to do with how our species was shaped to experience fear.

Consequently, not all irrational or unreasonable anxiety is pathological. Natural selection did not sculpt human nature according to reasonableness in our current environment but, rather, according to what promoted reproductive fitness in the environment in which natural selection took place. The resulting biologically designed fears are part of human nature, but if the environment has changed, they do not always correspond to what is reasonable now. Nor are our emotions generally shaped to conform to reason. For example, it is unreasonable for people to think quite as highly of their own children as they do, to admire their lovers as much as they do, to be as suspiciously jealous as they are apt to be at times, or to be quite as optimistic about life as they are. These unreasonable distortions of attitude from the strictly rational assessment of the facts, however, are consistent with how biology shaped people to be, so such cognitive distortions are not disorders—indeed, people who lack these emotional tendencies and are too rational might be the ones responding in atypical ways.

Aside from the fact that some of our fears stem from our ancestral past but are mismatched to the realities of our present environment, there is another way that fear (as well as other emotions) can be irrational without being disordered. This consists of what traditionally has been considered a "disconnect" between emotion and reason—the idea that emotion and reason are opposed and that a degree of unreasonableness is built into experiences such as intense anxiety. The function of anxious feelings is to focus attention on some aspects of the facts and not others in order to facilitate action. When we experience intense emotions such as fear or anxiety or anger or jealousy—or joy or love or triumph—our thought processes become focused on certain aspects of reality to the exclusion of other aspects. Thus, when one feels intensely anxious, it is hard to think about anything but those concerns that arouse your discomfort. So, part of the anxiety of people waiting for their talk or performance to begin lies in thinking only about the prospects for disaster, the ways that things might go wrong. That is, emotion distorts thinking in terms of accurate appraisal of reality (or it at least changes our usual appraisal of reality; there is some evidence that depressed people in some respects make more accurate judgments because depression reduces the natural human bias toward optimism).[13]

Yet, this cognitive transformation is not pathological. It is not abnormal to feel inflated admiration for one's lover or child, or to feel an inflated sense of optimism and power after a hard-won achievement. Indeed, it is likely part of the function of emotion to focus on certain immediately salient issues and thus distort rational thinking, because under some circumstances it is disadvantageous to take all relevant considerations into account in a balanced way. Emotions limit information processing to certain adaptively crucial issues and set aside the broader picture. Such natural human tendencies should not be mistaken for psychiatric disorders.

We have considered how anxiety is at times naturally irrational or unreasonable when it stems from our evolutionary heritage in a way that was reasonable in the distant past but is mismatched with current reality. We have also considered how anxiety transforms our thinking to lead us to focus on just certain potentially threatening aspects of the situation and to reduce our ability to rationally assess all facets of the situation, yielding a natural and adaptive form of irrationality. With these forms of normal irrationality in mind, we now turn to an in-depth exploration of the

DSM-IV criteria for three common anxiety disorders, and some changes proposed for those categories in *DSM-5.*

SPECIFIC PHOBIA

Specific phobia refers to disordered fears directed at particular types of objects or situations. We have seen how attempts to distinguish normal fears from disordered fears on the basis of the reasonableness of the fear in light of the actual danger from the feared object or situation, as in the *DSM-IV's* criteria, flounder on the problem of how to deal with evolutionarily shaped fears that are currently unreasonable. For example, the early American physician Benjamin Rush distinguished "reasonable" objects of fear such as death from "unreasonable" objects such as "thunder, darkness, ghosts, speaking in public, sailing, riding, certain animals, particularly cats, rats, insects, and the like."[14] Yet all of Rush's examples—with the exceptions of cats and ghosts, which are examples of fears based on cognitive theories about the world that give rise to superstitions—are closely related to natural sources of danger or their equivalents that confronted our distant ancestors and shaped our natural dispositions to experience fear. They can thus arise today from normal as opposed to pathological functioning of fear response mechanisms, even though such fears are not usually proportionate responses to current external, realistic threats.

Such inherited concerns that are part of our nature but that are not necessarily realistic in our current environment challenge the common notion that "unrealistic" fears and anxieties are disorders. Taking such a challenge seriously is important for two reasons, besides the obvious one that clinicians have a professional responsibility to correctly label people as disordered versus normal as accurately as possible. One reason is that research that attempts to identify what is distinctive about anxiety disorders cannot proceed validly if it conflates groups having normal fears due to biologically designed functioning with those having disordered fears due to something going wrong with such functioning. The ultimate goal of understanding the etiologies of anxiety disorders cannot be achieved if we cannot distinguish such disorders from normal, non-disordered fears. Overly inclusive categories combining normal and disordered cases make it impossible for research or treatment studies to identify etiologies or treatments specific to disorder.

The second reason is that treatment decisions may partly depend on whether the anxiety is understood as an intense example of a normal fear or as a failure of anxiety mechanisms. For example, many medications for anxiety disorders target anxiety generally, whether normal or disordered, not just a specific fear. If the problematic fear is normal, one might be inclined to set a higher threshold for tinkering with overall normal anxiety functioning and enduring the side effects of a medication than if one believes that something has gone wrong with the functioning of anxiety processes that the medication might bring closer to normal.

We acquire intense fears in a variety of ways. One way is through reasoning and information that leads us to rationally conclude that there is a threat. Such evidence-based fears can disappear in a moment if our beliefs about the evidence change. Similarly, some intense fears, though perhaps not rational, seem to be based on processes of the kind behaviorists describe as "conditioning," wherein one becomes inclined to feel afraid of the circumstances in which one previously experienced fear or pain—such as developing a fear of the dentist after having bad experiences during dental treatment.

However, many other fears have an evolutionary basis and may be innate or easily triggered by minimal experiences. Such fears are to one degree or another "noncognitive," that is, irrational in the sense of not having their source in, or being easily subject to change by, reasoning about the actual danger—as well as sometimes not being easily changeable (or "extinguished," as behaviorists call it) by new experiences. For example, intense fears of snakes are usually not justified in modern environments unless one lives in an area populated with poisonous snakes. Considerable evidence, however, indicates that many people inherit or are predisposed to easily learn snake fears, which were adaptive during the period when the human genome was being formed.[15] And even if one is cognitively aware of the unlikelihood of a snake being poisonous, seeing a snake slithering in the grass nearby can cause an automatic anxiety reaction. Fears that are excessive and unreasonable at present might be aspects of inherited fear mechanisms that are operating as evolution has designed them to act. Such fears are normal even though irrational in many contexts (i.e., in response to snakes that are known to be nonpoisonous). Similarly, fear of exposed heights, of open spaces, of closed spaces, and of deep water appear to be based partly in biological adaptations rather than reasoning about danger or accrued negative experiences.

Psychologist Martin Seligman offers a vivid illustration of the point that humans are biologically shaped to have fears and aversions that may not be rational or easily swayed by experience. Building on the discovery that animals are biologically prepared to develop aversions to specific food tastes if the taste has been associated with becoming ill, Seligman offers an example from his own life of how such links may be strong even if they are not rationally defensible.[16] He tells the story of how, after he got sick following his eating a steak béarnaise dinner on an evening out with his wife and colleagues, he developed an intense aversion to béarnaise sauce, even though it was one of his favorite foods. He asked, "What is it about phobias that makes them . . . irrational?" His answer is that "[p]hobias are highly prepared to be learned by humans, and . . . probably are noncognitive."[17]

Seligman emphasizes that rational considerations do not easily penetrate the taste-aversion system. He knew that there was a wave of stomach flu going through his office among people who had not been at the dinner, and he knew that companions who had been with him at dinner and had also eaten the steak béarnaise had not gotten sick. Seligman himself had gone with his wife to an opera after dinner, so there was a considerable delay between eating the steak and the onset of illness. Despite all these factors weighing against the illness arising from the béarnaise sauce, and despite Seligman's reasoned opinion that it could not have been the sauce that caused his illness, he developed such a strong aversion to this sauce that he did not touch it again for over a decade. His conscious, rational theory of causation had little impact on the development or amelioration of his aversion. Rationality does not necessarily characterize or influence the development of normal biologically shaped fears and aversions. As Seligman puts it, "The noncognitive nature of prepared associations is illustrated by at least one observation: Knowing that the stomach flu and not the sauce Bearnaise caused the vomiting does not inhibit the aversion to the sauce. In addition, there are several experiments which suggest that, unlike unprepared conditioning, prepared conditioning is not readily modified by information."[18]

Presumably Seligman's béarnaise aversion, which endured for a decade and thus was certainly "persistent," could be diagnosed as a specific phobia if it caused him to be so distressed that he could not eat what was formerly his favorite dish. He certainly recognized that the aversion was unreasonable. Yet it would seem that this reaction reflects the operation of a normal human defense mechanism, which was evolutionarily adaptive, even if it occasionally impairs the pursuit of one's usual culinary pleasures. Presumably this is an adaptation to prevent the organism from ingesting toxic material a second time. To treat this aversion as a "disorder" would be to intervene in a perfectly normal and potentially adaptive set of brain mechanisms biologically designed to monitor blood for toxins and create aversion when there is a chance an earlier tasted food contained an illness-causing pathogen. To do research to identify the "etiology" or "pathogenesis" of such an aversion would be to seek to identify a perfectly normal set of brain mechanisms.

There is another way that our natural fears can be unreasonable. The particular object of a specific instance of the fear, whether now or in the past, may not be threatening at all. Instead, the fear may be directed at an overall class of objects of which there are occasional dangerous instances. The fear, however, naturally arises because taking the time to figure out whether a particular instance is dangerous before feeling fear could be fatal.

For example, it is of course unreasonable to be afraid of a snake that you know to be nonpoisonous (or an exposed height that is in fact safe, etc.). Yet people often experience anxiety at the sight of even a garter snake, despite knowing that such snakes are harmless (one of us can attest to this, having found himself swimming in a pool with a snake he believed to be a garter snake—yet feeling extreme anxiety and exiting the pool in record time). To the extent that there is any uncertainty about the snake's identity and whether it is poisonous—and there frequently may be such uncertainty—this is an understandable matter of "run away now, ask questions later." Analogously, many experts on mushrooms refrain from eating wild mushrooms because of the chance of a misidentification, despite their considerable expertise. But fear of snakes, to the degree that it is a biologically prepared sensitivity transcending reason and a quickly triggering fear based on naturally selected mechanisms, seems to have no built-in distinction between poisonous snakes that are reasonable to fear and nonpoisonous snakes that are not. The prepared fear seems biologically designed to be of snakes, period—biological design appears in this case to have erred on the side of caution, in accordance with the "smoke detector principle"—so such fears are not inherently abnormal despite their frequent unreasonableness in light of the actual nature of the feared snake. Presumably, when preparedness for snake fear was being naturally selected, delaying one's fear response while one drew a distinction between poisonous and nonpoisonous snakes was not the most adaptive way to respond to the situation of suddenly coming across a snake. This is not to say that there cannot be snake phobias that are true disorders; even a naturally unreasonable fear can inflate into a disabling fear that, for example, keeps one from moving about even in snake-free environments. But the unreasonableness is not evidence of a failure of biologically designed functioning, thus is not sufficient for disorder.

These elemental prepared fears are not easily overcome by reason, although they can shift with effort and experience. This points to a further reason why reasonableness and fear diverge: fear is often most useful when it is irrationally intense and its triggering threshold is irrationally low. In effect, the best way to design an organism to escape serious threats and live to reproduce is to make some of its normal, biologically designed fears unreasonably intense in terms of the actual likelihood of threat in any one instance, because there will be no further instances if the organism gets it wrong just once. Thus, the *DSM*'s "unreasonable" criterion for phobic disorders does not get at the appropriate difference between normal and disordered anxiety.

We now turn to the question of how adequately the current *DSM-IV* and proposed *DSM-5* diagnostic criteria for specific phobias deal with these issues.

The current *DSM-IV* core criteria for specific phobia are:[19]

A. Marked and persistent fear that is excessive or unreasonable, cued by the presence or anticipation of a specific object or situation (e.g., flying, heights, animals, receiving an injection, seeing blood).

B. Exposure to the phobic stimulus almost invariably provokes an immediate anxiety response, which may take the form of a situationally bound or situationally predisposed Panic Attack.

C. The person recognizes that the fear is excessive or unreasonable.

D. The phobic situation(s) is avoided or else is endured with intense anxiety or distress.

E. The avoidance, anxious anticipation, or distress in the feared situation(s) interferes significantly with the person's normal routine, occupational (or academic) functioning, or social activities or relationships, or there is marked distress about having the phobia.

We have already addressed the main features of the *DSM-IV*'s criteria and seen how its emphasis on excessiveness and unreasonableness of fear as indicators of disorder cannot adequately separate natural from disordered fears. We therefore turn directly to the proposed changes in the *DSM-5* criteria put forward in the work group's review paper, which provides the justification for their likely changes. After surveying some of the other issues addressed in the recommendations, we then consider whether the proposed changes help to overcome the ambiguities in the "excessiveness" criterion and the problem that the "unreasonableness" criterion often misclassifies natural, biologically shaped fears as phobic disorders.

Some of the proposed changes are not substantive but clarify, for example, that "marked" anxiety means "intense" anxiety. We have seen that the *DSM-5* work group also proposes that the vague "persistent" requirement be improved by applying to adult fears the same six-month duration requirement that is currently applied to children's fears before labeling them as phobias .[20] This change will help to guard against mislabeling as disorders various forms of transiently intense but normal fears in response to frightening events that then subside and perhaps extinguish on their own when the stimulating events end. It should reduce false-positive diagnoses of transient fearful reactions to events. However, the change does not address normally occurring chronic fears, a category that typically includes many evolutionarily shaped fears.

DSM-5 proposals for changing the clinical significance criterion for specific phobia. The *DSM-5* proposals also suggest revising the avoidance component of the specific phobia criteria. The *DSM-IV* criteria require that "[t]he phobic situation(s) is avoided or else is endured with intense anxiety or distress."[21] This leaves open the possibility that the feared object or situation is "avoided" simply because it is never present in the individual's environment. The proposed criteria alter the "avoidance" part of this criterion to require active avoidance on the part of the individual, thus implying at least some potential harm: "The phobic object or situation is actively avoided or endured with intense fear or anxiety."[22] The work group explains that "actively" is added to raise the diagnostic threshold. The change is best understood as reducing false-positive diagnoses by ensuring harm (even when the individual never confronts the feared object or situation) in the form of actively and negatively changing one's freedom of movement.

This is a useful albeit quite nuanced change. Often an individual has a fear in the abstract but is never confronted with the feared object or situation due to the individual's circumstances, thus never in fact experiencing any resulting anxiety. The individual need not take any special actions to avoid the feared situation (e.g., heights) or object (e.g., snakes) because such avoidance automatically results from the location or other circumstances. In such cases, it is difficult to see how the condition is harmful, and it makes sense to refrain from diagnosing a disorder unless the individual anticipates some future scenario in which the fear would be activated. Otherwise, there are all sorts of fearful situations one could conjure up that might trigger terror but that are never experienced (e.g., a primitive innate fear directed at a type of creature that no longer exists), and we would all have to be diagnosed with many phobias that have no bearing at all on our lives. Conversely, one cannot require actual confrontation with the feared situation or object because individuals may have substantially narrowed their desired range of activities in order to ensure that the feared situation or object is never confronted. Even if no further ongoing actions are necessary, such choices of environment could qualify as "active" avoidance.

The *DSM-5* proposals also consider the possibility of eliminating the current clinical significance criterion for specific phobias, or replacing it with the more standard clinical significance criterion requiring either distress or role impairment. We saw earlier that the standard *DSM-IV* clinical significance criterion has a fatal flaw when applied to anxiety conditions including intense anxiety: anxiety is inherently a form of distress, so of necessity any condition involving intense anxiety must involve great distress. The current *DSM-IV* clinical significance criterion for specific phobia is designed to avoid the tautological requirement that intense anxiety must involve distress, and also to avoid the problem that when the object of a fear is successfully avoided there may be no direct anxious distress. It attempts to evade these problems with a "distress" criterion that requires that the individual must be not merely distressed but distressed *about having the condition*. This is a clever strategy but unfortunately does not improve the situation. The problem with this current "distressed-about-the-condition" approach to clinical significance is that anyone seeking help is likely to be distressed about having the condition bringing them into treatment, and most people become distressed about painful or problematic conditions whether they are normal or disordered and whether or not they seek treatment. Requiring distress about having a condition does not set a meaningful threshold for distinguishing disorders from other problems in life. This flaw undermines the usefulness of the standard clinical significance criterion in these disorders because the criterion is disjunctive ("either distress or impairment"). If almost everyone with the symptoms satisfies one of the disjuncts—namely, distress about the condition—then almost everyone will also spuriously satisfy the entire requirement, rendering the criterion useless for distinguishing the normal from the disordered among those with the symptoms. Thus, both the standard clinical significance criterion and the current variant are not very useful in achieving their purpose of preventing false positive diagnoses due to their "distress" clauses.

So, if the "distress" criterion for an anxiety disorder offers no help in distinguishing normal from disordered anxiety, does the clinical significance criterion's impairment clause actually or potentially help identify disorders and increase the validity of diagnosis? The role-impairment component of the standard clinical significance criterion has the major flaw noted earlier: it does not distinguish role interference that suggests disorder from other types of interference. To suggest disorder on the basis of role impairment, the role performances that are being impaired must be part of what human beings are biologically designed to be able to do. Interferences in normally anxiety-provoking tasks do not suggest disorder. For example, some occupations depend on the individual's lack of claustrophobia (tunnel digger, chimney sweep), height fear (skyscraper construction worker, office-building window washer, mountain-climbing guide), or a combination of both (elevator operator, airplane pilot), even though it is normal to be "impaired" in pursuing such occupations due to common natural fears of these circumstances. Public-speaking or public-performance fears are entirely natural even if they can be impairing in some professions that require overcoming such fears.

In contrast, when a fear reaches such proportions that, even when there is no imminent threat, it interferes with other aspects of basic designed human functioning—as, for example, the inability to walk past even a leashed dog, the inability to climb to a moderately high secured perch due to fear of height, or the inability to comfortably speak to one's family—it is plausible that a non-selected range of impaired behavior has occurred and that a presumptive disorder exists. In other words, it is not interference with role functioning as demanded by our society *per se*, but the specific type of role and the type of fear that matter in deciding whether the impairment indicates disorder. If the fear is a natural one, and the impairment is in a role that challenges and requires the overriding of natural fears, there may be no disorder. However, if the impairment is in a role that is itself part of biologically designed functioning or its plausible extension within a given cultural setting, then a true dysfunction and disorder may be inferred. The role-impairment criterion, if rewritten to identify failures of basic functioning and separated from the distress criterion, could be of great help in distinguishing disorders from normal anxieties involved in many of our social roles.

The other alternative that the *DSM-5* work group explores is the elimination of the clinical significance criterion. LeBeau et al. argue that the other proposed changes in the diagnostic criteria would require that anxiety be intense, active, and durable in order to be diagnosed as a disorder, and this would be enough to protect against false positives without the clinical significance criterion. They note that the clinical significance criterion eliminates three types of fears. First, there are fears that might in theory be impairing but are so unimportant that they never arise for the individual. For example, someone would avoid air travel due to fear if the issue ever arose, but the need, preference, or opportunity for air travel never arises for that person. Second, there are objects or situations that arise so infrequently in the individual's environment that a fear has no impact on the individual's life, such as when a city dweller is afraid of snakes. Third, there are fears of circumscribed situations that the individual has found ways to avoid and accommodate so that they have negligible impact, as when an individual who is afraid of crossing bridges can find driving routes to all desired destinations without negotiating a bridge. LeBeau et al. claim that the proposed *DSM-5* requirements that fear be intense, active, and durable would eliminate such cases from diagnoses without the need for any clinical significance criterion.

The problem here is that LeBeau et al. fail to consider normal evolutionarily shaped fears that are intense, active, and durable, yet entirely normal. Fear of being in rough, deep water, fear of public speaking, fear of great heights that are relatively unprotected, fear of enclosed spaces, and many other fears that naturally emerge from our biologically shaped dispositions have all three of these properties. LeBeau et al.'s three example of false positives in which clinical significance is not really necessary all consist of fears of objects or situations that are basically unencountered, yet the real problem with the exploding prevalence estimates is the counting as disorders the real fears people naturally have and that they are forced to encounter and confront due to social and occupational demands. Among intense, active, durable fears, many are non-disorders, and thus far nothing in the *DSM-5* proposals even attempts to draw this basic distinction.

The DSM-5 proposal to replace "excessive or unreasonable" by "out of proportion to the actual danger." The single potentially most significant change in the *DSM-5* proposal from the perspective of eliminating false positives is the switch from the current characterization of phobic fear as "excessive or unreasonable" to a "proportionality" approach that requires that "[t]he fear is out of proportion with the actual danger posed by the specific object or situation."[23] The *DSM-5* working group explains, "The intent of this recommendation is to first operationalize what is meant by 'excessive or unreasonable,' as a fear that is out of proportion with the danger posed by the situation. In addition, it recommends that the designation of 'out of proportion' is a clinician-judgment rather than self-judgment."[24] The proposal thus eliminates the current requirement that "[t]he person recognizes that the fear is excessive or unreasonable." Instead, clinicians rather than patients should make such judgments, based in part on the fact that "[c]linical experience suggests that some individuals are judged by diagnosticians to exhibit excessive or unreasonable fears even though the individuals themselves would deny that that their fear is excessive or unreasonable."[25]

A "disproportionality" requirement, reflecting a classic approach to distinguishing disordered from normal emotions, has much to recommend it. Our previous book, *The Loss of Sadness*, argued that the central flaw of current criteria for depression is a lack of reference to context through just such a criterion that would specify that a disorder exists only if the feelings of sadness and associated symptoms are not better explained as a proportionate response to loss.[26] In some broad sense, the proportionality of a response to the nature of the circumstances must be part of what distinguishes disordered from normal reactions.

However, the effectiveness of the proportionality criterion in eliminating false positives depends entirely on how it is interpreted. One must ask: proportional to what? This is where the proposal goes astray, for "proportional" responses are defined as those that are "out of proportion to the actual danger posed by the specific object or situation."

This takes us straight back to all the problems we saw earlier with defining phobias as "unreasonable" or "irrational" fears. As we have seen, many fears are either innate or biologically prepared to be easily learned, and the health versus disorder status of these fears has little to do with their reasonableness or rationality. Fear of a snake or spider that is not poisonous may be irrational but not necessarily disordered. Judging disorder by whether the intensity of fear corresponds to the actual level of danger leads to an invalid approach in which many normal fears are mislabeled as pathology. One reason is that it is belief about danger (when not itself disordered, as in paranoid delusions), not objective danger, that determines when a fear is reasonable. For example, if, due to misleading information they have obtained, people believe that drinking soda invariably causes cancer, then their fear of these beverages may be disproportionate to the actual danger but nonetheless entirely normal.

The more subtle yet serious problem is that declaring fears that are disproportionate to actual danger to be disorders mistakenly pathologizes many evolutionarily shaped fears. Human beings are not biologically designed to have only fears that are proportional to actual—or even believed—danger, although cognitive assessment of danger is certainly one pathway to fear. Biologically designed and innately prepared fears are normal when functioning as designed, whether reasonable or not, as discussed in earlier chapters. Reasonableness may at times allow one to override innate fears (which may be considered a form of courage), but the fear itself is generated on other grounds entirely and may be experienced intensely despite its unreasonableness.

In addition, circumstances might have changed since the fear developed so that it is even more out of proportion. (To see such unreasonable fear in action, remember back to the first chapter where we described the reactions of people who go to the top of the Sears—now Willis—Tower in Chicago and confront the glass overhang, which allows them to stand over a sheer drop without any observable barrier except the clear glass floor on which one is standing.) Thus, the new criterion, while usefully building a proportionality criterion into the specific phobia criteria, fails to recognize that in many cases, disproportionality is not enough to indicate dysfunction. Considering intense fears that are disproportionate to actual danger as disorders pathologizes an enormous range of normal fear. Context and proportionality to actual danger do not suffice for an adequate psychiatric assessment of fear. The criteria must also consider the question of whether the fear is within the normal range of a biologically shaped feature of human beings.

The *DSM* could explicitly consider proportionality not only in relation to actual danger but also in relation to how human beings are designed to respond to the particular kind of object or situation. Without such a baseline to constrain diagnosis, an enormous potential to pathologize natural fears exists. It may well be unreasonable to be anxious about a spouse's affair (how actually dangerous is an affair? How dangerous even to lose one's spouse to another?), a snake in the wild (what percentage are actually poisonous?), or glass floors over abysses (virtually no danger at all). Yet such unreasonable responses are part of normal human nature.

Finally, we would note that phobias are one area where understanding is developed enough that the criteria might reflect etiological distinctions. The various etiologies of fear—e.g., rational judgment, conditioning, and innately programmed or easily triggered biologically prepared reactions—could require different criteria for recognizing when they go wrong. Perhaps this has not been recognized because of the current bias toward establishing physiologically describable etiologies: these psychologically distinct causes are not yet brain describable distinctions.

SOCIAL PHOBIA

Anxiety about being socially evaluated is perhaps the single most common and normal human anxiety. This is true even among many of those who have the greatest natural talent for, and success at, public performance and whom one might assume to be immune to such feelings. Consider, for example, the experience of Robin Meade, now a highly successful news anchor, who had just begun working as a weekend TV news anchor in Chicago when the following incident occurred:

> I looked down at the copy of the news story. My stomach clenched. My heart started palpitating. I think I held my breath without realizing it. The floor director gave me the cue, pointing at me as the camera came up on my face.
>
> I felt sweaty. Just as I opened my mouth to speak, the set seemed to fade into a gauzy haze. My breathing was jagged. The words came, but my voice was quivering so much it sounded like a kid singing into a big box fan on a humid summer day: "Bray-ay-ay-ay-king new-ew-ew-ews tonigh-igh-ight."
>
> My hands shook uncontrollably, and I was huffing and puffing as if I were running mile twenty five of the Chicago Marathon. These were not the controlled, measured tones of someone who had been doing this for a living for years. My heart pounded in my ears, and my face flushed. I was losing it, right there with who knows how many thousands of people watching.
>
> What the hell is happening? As I delivered the facts of the story, I didn't hear a thing that came out of my mouth. All I heard were my own thoughts. Oh, no, you're screwing up! Oh, no, your bosses are probably watching! You're going to get fired! How will you pay your mortgage? What will people think of you? And then, of course, Holy crapola, where is that sound bite? Can you see how the cause-and-effect relationship of my thoughts just engulfed me in doom and gloom? I couldn't keep my mind on the story. I totally slipped into imagining the future and the horrible repercussions of my screw-up.[27]

In fact, both intimates and professional associates did notice Meade's "screw-up," and it could easily have been disastrous for her career. Given the professional stakes, her fear was not entirely irrational, even if her anxiety about it did have the unfortunate consequence of helping to bring her close to the very outcome she feared—like athletes "choking in the clutch" and failing under pressure when the game does in fact depend on their performance. Yet there seems nothing disordered about such a reaction. For example, Meade was not anxious with her intimates after the show and was able to conquer her fears and go on to be a successful news anchor.

Like Meade, many people deeply and naturally fear public exposure to ridicule. Most would not be as capable of overcoming these natural fears or as ambitiously driven to do so as was Meade. Yet our society contains many occupations and settings that require individuals to risk humiliation in performing before or speaking to an audience of strangers. Consequently, fear of public speaking is one of the most prevalent fears in our society. However, the fact that fear of public speaking yields impaired occupational or academic functioning for many individuals due to the unique demand for such performances in our society does not by itself indicate that such fear of public speaking is a disorder. In contrast, when fear reaches such proportions that it interferes with basic designed human functioning, there is presumably a disorder—as, for example, when social anxiety does not allow someone to be comfortable with even his or her own family members, to speak in front of a group of friends, or to engage in social interactions where there is no significant chance of consequential evaluation or humiliation, such as sitting in a lecture hall watching someone else talk. Nor is interference with role functioning *per se* a sign of disorder; if the fear is a natural one, and the impairment is in a role that challenges and requires the overriding of that biologically designed fear, there may be no disorder. However, if the impairment is in a role that is itself part of biologically designed functioning or its plausible extension within a given cultural setting, then a true dysfunction and disorder may be occurring.

With these considerations in mind, we consider the core *DSM-IV* diagnostic criteria for social phobia (AKA social anxiety disorder) and the proposed changes in *DSM-5*. The criteria for specific phobia and social phobia overlap to some extent, and we do not repeat at length the arguments presented above for specific phobia when they apply equally to social phobia.

The core *DSM-IV* social phobia diagnostic criteria require:

A. A marked and persistent fear of one or more social or performance situations in which the person is exposed to unfamiliar people or to possible scrutiny by others. The individual fears that he or she will act in a way (or show anxiety symptoms) that will be humiliating or embarrassing.

B. Exposure to the feared social situation almost invariably provokes anxiety, which may take the form of a situationally bound or situationally predisposed Panic Attack.

C. The person recognizes that the fear is excessive or unreasonable.

D. The feared social or performance situations are avoided or else are endured with intense anxiety or distress.

E. The avoidance, anxious anticipation, or distress in the feared social or performance situation(s) interferes significantly with the person's normal routine, occupational (academic) functioning, or social activities or relationships, or there is marked distress about having the phobia.[28]

Perhaps the oddest thing about the *DSM-IV* definition of social phobia is that it classifies as disordered those people who are afraid in exactly those situations in which fear is most natural: "social or performance situations in which the person is exposed to unfamiliar people or to possible scrutiny by others." Consequently, the individual's fear "that he or she will act in a way (or show anxiety symptoms) that will be humiliating or embarrassing" is without any *prima facie* pathological content. Unfamiliar people are inherently more threatening than familiar ones, and humiliation is a potent threat to people when others—especially, say, their bosses or competitors—evaluate them.

As we discussed in Chapter 3, human beings likely evolved in conditions where they lived in small groups of familiars, and strangers could easily mean danger. Moreover, disapproval or rejection within such groups could be highly consequential for survival. In such small and highly interdependent groups, incurring the negative evaluations of others or confronting strangers carried real risks. Unsurprisingly, high anxiety about social evaluation and potential rejection, as well as about encountering new people, became a common part of our nature and remains so even though such anxiety is no longer as contextually suited to modern societies, where individuals often have many alternative social options if they are rejected or fail an evaluation. The *DSM*'s practice of diagnosing social phobias when people have marked and persistent fears when "exposed to unfamiliar people or to possible scrutiny by others" appears to label anxiety states as disorders that may not make sense in our current environment yet are biologically designed aspects of human nature.

The current clinical significance criterion for social phobia does little good in preventing the mislabeling of normal anxieties as disorders. This is because it is satisfied if the social anxiety "interferes significantly with the person's normal routine, occupational (academic) functioning, or social activities or relationships." Obviously, intense anxiety about some social situation that is either avoided or endured with intense distress virtually tautologically interferes with one's social functioning.

How much do the changes in the *DSM-5* criteria help remedy this basic problem? There is no proposal to change the basic mischaracterization as a disorder of fear of scrutiny by unfamiliar others in even one type of social performance situation that may lead to humiliation or embarrassment. These are situations in which people naturally are anxious. The *DSM-5* review does not question whether fear of just one kind of situation alone (e.g., initiating conversations with strangers, dating, speaking to authority figures) is sufficient for disorder; nor does it address the very broad sweep of the possible types of situations that can qualify a condition as a social phobia, including naturally anxiety-provoking situations such as performing in front of others, giving speeches, and interacting with strangers; and it fails to confront the central puzzle of what is disordered about experiencing anxiety in situations in which one might be negatively evaluated and humiliated. Like the specific phobia review, it thus largely ignores many of the most obvious false-positive challenges to the current *DSM* approach to social phobia.[29]

Some of the proposed changes are similar to those proposed for specific phobia and suffer from similar limitations. These include a proposal to add a six-month duration requirement due to recognition that transient periods of change of social context may naturally involve heightened social anxiety: "Severe social anxiety may occur temporarily in different stages of life in which new social roles are required (e.g., entering school, entering puberty, going to college, getting married, having children, getting divorced) and can be viewed as an adaptive response if it resolves within 6 months. Therefore, it is recommended that the duration criterion F of 6 months, which in DSM-IV applies only to persons under 18, be extended to all ages."[30] This does set a useful lower bound for duration before diagnosis. However, social fears that arise during role transitions in new social hierarchies are not the only kinds of normal social fears. Many natural social and performance fears can be long-term standing fears, which the change in the duration requirement does not address.

Again, as in the specific phobia proposals, the social anxiety work group recommends that the requirement that "[t]he person recognizes that the fear is excessive or unreasonable" be eliminated and replaced by clinician judgment to optimize validity: "Our clinical impression is that some adult SAD patients do not recognize the "irrationality" of their fears. . . . Our recommendation for DSM-V is that it is sufficient that the clinician recognizes the fear as exaggerated."[31] These modest improvements, however, are unlikely to correct the category's core false-positives problem.

As in the criteria for specific phobia, the major proposed change for preventing false positives is the recommendation that the "excessive or unreasonable" requirement be reworded to read, "The fear is out of proportion with the actual danger posed by the social situation."[32] This produces greater consistency across the criteria for specific and social phobias, but at the cost of introducing a bewildering element in assessing the proportionality of the anxiety to the actual danger: what exactly is the danger in the social situations about which people tend to become socially anxious?

The problems with the "proportionality" approach to social phobia warrant some elaboration. In early societies in which the human genome evolved, negative evaluations had real risks in situations in which one's very life depended on cooperation with a small group of individuals. Humans thus seem to have been shaped with a generally high though normally varying threshold for risking social humiliation. Modern societies, however, consist of many varied social circles. The actual danger from the social judgments of any particular individual is generally quite small. Thus, social anxiety often seems quite irrational in the current environment (even if it was rational at some point in the past) and in fact is likely highly out of proportion to the actual danger social scrutiny poses. In a sense, social anxiety is doubly disproportionate to real danger. First, it was likely originally overly intense to avoid deadly mistakes, in accordance with the "smoke detector principle"—this is a case in which, if you wait to accurately assess the danger, it is likely too late. Second, even the level of danger that did exist when social anxiety evolved has now largely disappeared; today, even strange humans are usually pretty safe. Social anxiety is thus one of those features of human nature that is biologically designed to be disproportionate and has become more so due to environmental change. Thus, social phobia is a category where the "proportionality" criterion is likely to yield enormous numbers of false positives due to normal variations in human nature being mislabeled as disorders because they are out of tune with social demands.

Actual danger is simply not the issue in social phobia. Indeed, danger is a slippery concept when dealing with the things that matter most to people, such as other peoples' opinions of them, or social humiliation with its vast potential effects on social resources and self-esteem. How would one evaluate the actual danger of having someone whom one admires come to think badly of you? In the case of social phobia, the proportionality criterion is useful only if relativized to biologically designed proportionality.

In sum, the proposed *DSM-5* criteria for social anxiety disorder—despite some helpful changes—don't fix what is essentially wrong with the current criteria. They allow the spurious pathologization of large swaths of normal-range social anxiety and will continue to yield unreasonably high prevalence estimates for this disorder.

GENERALIZED ANXIETY DISORDER

Freud's original idea when he developed the early precursor of today's generalized anxiety disorder (GAD) category was of a condition marked by chronic, intense, free-floating, and undirected anxiety.[33] This sort of state is pretty clearly a disorder in anxiety-generating processes. Remarkably, not only has the *DSM* abandoned this conception, but such a condition would not even fulfill its current GAD criteria. Indeed, there is no such disorder in the manual at this point. Instead, both the *DSM-IV* and proposed *DSM-5* approach exchanged a condition marked by intense, chronic, and free-floating anxiety for one defined by multiple worries about various concerns. This conception can potentially lead to massive false-positive diagnoses because, whereas the sort of undirected anxiety Freud described is *prima facie* a disorder, intense worries about specific areas of concern such as children, health, and finances are often not disordered, whether they are entirely realistic or somewhat overly vigilant and concerned.

The current core GAD criteria are as follows:

DSM-IV Generalized Anxiety Disorder Criteria[34]

A. Excessive anxiety and worry (apprehensive expectation), occurring more days than not for at least 6 months, about a number of events or activities (such as work or school performance).

B. The person finds it difficult to control the worry.
C. The anxiety and worry are associated with three (or more) of the following six symptoms (with at least some symptoms present for more days than not for the past 6 months). Note: Only one item is required in children.

   1. Restlessness or feeling keyed up or on edge
   2. Being easily fatigued
   3. Difficulty concentrating or mind going blank
   4. Irritability
   5. Muscle tension
   6. Sleep disturbance (difficulty falling or staying asleep, or restless unsatisfying sleep)

D. The anxiety, worry, or physical symptoms cause clinically significant distress or impairment in social, occupational, or other important areas of functioning.

Both the current GAD diagnostic criteria and the proposed *DSM-5* changes ignore the opportunity to address the fundamental anomaly in the evolution of a free-floating condition into one marked by worry about multiple problems: GAD is now a worry disorder, not an anxiety disorder. The *DSM-5* work group's review makes clear that they consider worry about various problems the core feature of GAD, which is reflected in their proposed name change for the category: "One option is for GAD to be re-labeled in DSM-V as generalized worry disorder. This would reflect its hallmark feature."[35] Indeed, the review starts with the definition not of anxiety but of worry ("Worry (n), a troubled state of mind arising from the frets and cares of life ...").[36]

The *DSM-5* work group treats its reconceptualization of GAD as if it is an empirical discovery rather than a definitional coup:

> It has been suggested that GAD could be considered the basic anxiety disorder because worry as its defining feature reflects a basic process of anxiety. At the same time, current theory and research suggest that GAD is distinguished by a specific component of anxiety—worry—that is generalized to a number of future events and activities, is excessive and is negatively enforced avoidant coping strategy that is associated with symptoms of feeling restlessness, feeling keyed up or on edge, and muscle tension, and with consequent behaviors (avoidance, procrastination, reassurance) that attempt to reduce worry and/or emotional/affective distress.[37]

In fact, worry is not a fundamental or necessary feature of anxiety. By "cognitivizing" GAD based on the notion that anxiety must be based on specific worries, the criteria build in an etiological theory that makes GAD much more like the rumination that forms part of depression. Consequently, factor analyses now tend to place GAD closer to depression than to other anxiety disorders, leading to proposals to classify GAD with the mood disorders.[38] GAD-type symptoms and depression do often occur comorbidly—indeed, since antiquity, anxiety was generally considered one symptom of depression until the *DSM-III* artificially separated depressive and anxiety symptoms. But GAD also was originally conceived as the prototypical (non-depressive) anxiety disorder. The clarity of the disorder's conceptualization suffers when GAD is redefined as "generalized worry disorder." In turning GAD into a multiple-worry disorder rather than a chronic free-floating anxiety disorder, a novel category with questionable validity as an anxiety disorder replaced a clear disorder of anxiety with high face validity.

Aside from perpetuating the problem of conceptualizing GAD as a worry disorder, the proposed *DSM-5* changes to specific *DSM-IV* criteria don't help resolve the problems with these criteria—and in several instances make matters worse. Criterion A specifies that the individual must be worried about more than one problem, a feature not proposed for change, but this is entirely compatible with normal worry. The work group proposes that the domains of worry that are listed as typical of this disorder, which are now limited to work and school performance, should be expanded to "family, health, finances, and school/work difficulties."[39] The problem is that, as the review makes clear, these tend to be the most common domains of worry not only for disordered individuals but for people in general. Multiple worries of such kinds are not in themselves pathological. This leaves the "excessiveness" requirement—discussed below—to do all the work of defining a valid disorder.

Andrews et al. propose eliminating the current GAD criterion that "The person finds it difficult to control the worry." This change likely does not impact validity much because anxiety, like other emotional states, is not biologically designed to be within voluntary control—although worry as a cognitive phenomenon may, more than most feelings, be subject to voluntary control through redirection of attention. When people say that their anxiety is "out of control," they likely mean that the anxiety is sufficiently intense that they cannot easily ignore it. Generally, given the unpleasantness of anxiety, anyone with intense anxiety, whether normal or disordered, will likely lack control over the anxiety to some degree. As the work group notes, research comparing GAD sufferers to others shows that "belief that worry is uncontrollable and dangerous was not unique to the GAD group."[40] Consequently, requiring that the individual finds it difficult to control the anxiety/worry is of questionable discriminative value because it is not at all clear that normal anxiety/worry is voluntary and under an individual's control to begin with (was Kendler able to control his anxiety when dangling from a cliff?). Inability to control worry does not necessarily signal that something has gone wrong. They also note that the degree to which GAD sufferers perceive their worry as out of control is likely closely related to the degree that they perceive it as "excessive." After all, if one is in control of an emotion, why would one voluntarily allow it to be excessive? Thus, whatever minimal work the "out of control" criterion does is largely accomplished by the "excessive" criterion.

The work group proposes to reduce the number of anxiety symptoms needed for GAD from the current three to one symptom (they suggest either "restlessness or feeling keyed up or on edge" or "muscle tension"[41]), but they are apparently considering a much broader set of options from the current list. The problem with this idea lies in the non-specificity of a single symptom in implying intense anxiety. Symptoms such as restlessness, feeling keyed up, muscle tension, fatigue, concentration difficulties, irritability, and sleep disturbance are general distress symptoms not distinct to disorder or to anxiety. A higher threshold is more diagnostically prudent.

The work group also recommends that the required duration of the anxiety symptoms should be reduced from six to three months in the *DSM-5*. This change could significantly decrease the validity of the criteria. Even the longer criterion is inadequate by itself to eliminate false positives, since normal worries can easily last for six months when the stressors that cause them last that long. This group acknowledges that changing required duration from six months to three months could be perceived as increasing false-positive problems: "Reducing the duration threshold to 3 months (or more) could increase the prevalence of GAD and attract similar criticisms to the DSM-III 1-month threshold."[42] However, rather than worrying about the false positives due to mistaking normal anxiety for disorder that this change might generate, the work group argues that the new emphasis on worry rather than free-floating anxiety gives GAD a core other than intense anxiety *per se* that makes up for the weakened duration requirement in ensuring validity: "A reduced duration threshold could also face similar criticisms as the 1-month DSM-III threshold, which reduced the discriminant validity of GAD relative to ordinary anxious reactions to life events and did not reflect the chronic course of GAD. However, these critiques of the lower threshold were made at a time when GAD lacked a defining feature. . . . Given that the GAD diagnosis now has worry as a defining feature and a lower duration threshold would largely recognize the same type of patient experiencing similar distress and impairment as those with DSM IV-defined GAD, it is recommended that the duration requirement of GAD in DSM-V be 3 months. . . . [T]his shorter duration requirement reflects some of the chronicity of the disorder while increasing the validity of the diagnosis by recapturing clinically significant cases"[43]

The claim that switching the core GAD feature to worry from undirected anxiety will control false positives is made without evidence that excessive worry is any less prone to false positives based on duration than is excessive anxiety. In fact, one would expect *more* false positives, not fewer, given that chronic undirected anxiety is clearly pathological whereas having multiple worries is commonly not pathological. Yes, the identified patients are "clinically significant" and they are similar in type to patients experiencing GAD in the sense that they have multiple worries over a period of time. But citing this as evidence of validity reveals a deep confusion about the nature of false-positive diagnoses of anxiety disorders. The essence of the problem of false positives is that intense anxiety is manifestly "clinically significant," and the challenge is to distinguish those "experiencing similar distress and impairment as those with DSM IV-defined GAD" who are not disordered from those who are. If these similarities did not exist between disordered and normal anxiety, there would be no false-positives problem undermining validity of diagnosis. In a category as potentially subject to false positives as the "worry" version of GAD, reducing the duration requirement from six months to three months can only make things worse.

What, then, of the pivotal requirement that the worry be "excessive," which the work group does not propose to alter? Virtually all of the changes discussed so far weaken the criteria and allow more cases to be diagnosed. The "excessive" requirement is the only bulwark against an increase of false positives due to such changes.

We saw earlier that "excessive anxiety" has the problem of heterogeneity of potential interpretations, including such highly invalid construals as statistically deviant or socially undesirable levels of anxiety—indeed, the work group itself notes, "Excessiveness is an ambiguous term."[44] However, it appears this group interpreted the concept as either extreme anxiety or anxiety that is disproportionate to the problems at which the worry is directed: "Anxiety and worry (apprehensive expectation) focused on multiple future activities or events that is extreme or disproportionate to those events is the defining feature of GAD and distinguishes GAD from normal worry and other anxiety and mood disorders."[45]

Extreme anxiety is of course compatible with normality—in fact, the central issue in defining GAD is how to distinguish normal intense anxiety from disordered intense anxiety. As to proportionality, we have argued that the interpretation of excessive anxiety as anxiety that is disproportionate to the actual danger posed by the problem is useful in eliminating certain kinds of false positives when the worry is based on rational assessment of threat. Proportionality, however, does not approach a valid criterion that takes into account the degree of irrational anxiety that we experience within the parameters of normal biological design. Human beings are not designed to respond proportionately to many kinds of danger, which may include, for example, problems with children, work, or health. Disproportionality of worry may or may not be a sign of disorder, depending on the nature of the worry as well as circumstances and individual temperament and history. With no constraints on "excessive," these criteria are subject to abuse as a social regulator of normal responses.

A final obstacle that impedes progress in achieving valid GAD criteria is the confused perception of clinical significance as a criterion for disordered responses that might be able to replace the dysfunction criterion. The idea is, first, that anyone experiencing significant distress and worry *prima facie* has a disorder: "The validity of the diagnosis has been questioned because some individuals experience GAD-like symptoms and significant distress, and appear to warrant a clinical diagnosis, but they do not meet the DSM-IV GAD criteria."[46] Second, the work group flirts with the notion that the clinical significance criterion might potentially trump the excessiveness criterion in identifying abnormality, and thus GAD might encompass all those with distressed worry: "If the excessiveness criterion were omitted from the GAD definition in DSM-V, the classification would continue to identify a group that experiences clinically significant distress or impairment as measured by endorsement of criterion E. However, the identified group would experience milder symptoms than if they were diagnosed by DSM-IV criteria. . . . This broader classification (i.e., including respondents who report either excessive or nonexcessive worry as having GAD) would also increase the number of children and adults with GAD by approximately 27 to 40%."[47]

In fact, as in the other categories examined above, the proposed distress-or-role-impairment clinical significance criterion is vacuous as an indicator of disorder. The fact that anxiety and worry involve distress and less effective role performance is not in itself evidence of disorder. Indeed, deleting the clinical significance criterion would likely have minimal impact on validity due to the criterion's extreme weakness. For better or worse, if psychiatry is to make progress by identifying valid etiological categories, there is no way around struggling with the "dysfunction" requirement for disorder.

HOW CAN THE CRITERIA BE IMPROVED?

The disordered quality of anxiety disorders—unlike, say, psychotic disturbances—is not necessarily apparent from symptoms alone. In the face of widespread anxiety in normal life, the challenge for the *DSM* with respect to anxiety disorders is to formulate diagnostic criteria that are broadly descriptive in nature (i.e., symptom-based and theory neutral) and that validly distinguish anxiety disorders—where something has gone wrong with a person's psychological functioning—from intense but normal anxiety responses. The *DSM* uses a variety of strategies to address the problem of validly distinguishing normal from disordered anxiety, and these techniques together go some way toward distinguishing disorder from non-disorder.

However, given how common normal anxiety is, even partially flawed criteria can yield large numbers of mistaken diagnoses. Perhaps the most fundamental challenge is that the criteria do not take into account what is evolutionarily normal human anxiety. The result is a hodgepodge of methods for trying to separate the normal from the disordered, each of which, or even all of which, may fail to be valid in a substantial number of instances. The evolutionary approach by no means resolves all ambiguities. Even with evolutionary grounding, there remains an enormous fuzzy area within which lines must be drawn based on a variety of pragmatic considerations. Nevertheless, to the degree that we can, it is essential to consider how we are likely biologically designed, for even our primitive understanding can have an immense impact on the conception of anxiety disorders. This is especially so in light of the limitations of the various methods the *DSM* uses to distinguish normal from disordered anxiety.

The requirement that anxiety be marked or intense is useful, but in the end intensity and disorder are two different dimensions, for there are intense normal reactions and moderate disordered ones. Duration and multiplicity of symptoms are similarly of limited validity, in the case of duration because chronic threats can cause chronic normal anxiety reactions, and in the case of multiple symptoms because the kinds of symptoms required in several categories are also the kinds of symptoms found in normal responses. Clinical significance requirements of distress or role impairment are also of limited validity because intense anxiety is by its nature distressing and impairing.

Finally, the "excessiveness" criterion is too vague and unclear to be of much help. It could be interpreted as a statistical or a social-norm criterion, which in either case would not validly indicate disorder, or as a redundant "intensity" criterion. It potentially gains effectiveness if interpreted as a veiled "disproportionality" criterion interpreted very broadly to mean "excessive relative to what is the biologically designed range of response to the given circumstances." The *DSM*'s requirement that disordered anxiety be "unreasonable" or "disproportional" in the sense that it is out of proportion to the actual danger may increase validity for some range of cases in which the etiology of fear is via cognitive processing, but it fails to reflect the reality that the nature of biological design is such that much normal anxiety often does not meet the reasonableness test and is not proportionate to actual danger.

DSM criteria such as "excessiveness" or "unreasonableness," whatever their flaws might be, helpfully indicate to clinicians that anxiety symptoms alone are not sufficient for diagnoses of anxiety disorders. The criteria, however, would be even more helpful if they would place symptoms in the context of life situations and treat only those that are disproportionate to these given contexts. For example, a popular psychiatric text, Donald Goodwin's and Samuel Guze's *Psychiatric Diagnosis*, cautions:

> Sometimes, however, patients do experience anxiety attacks in response to a fear-provoking situation such as facing an angry employer or giving a public speech. In these cases the clinician must decide whether the anxiety is grossly out of proportion to the fear-provoking stimulus, as well as make a diagnosis based on the over-all history.[48]

The *DSM* "proportionality" criterion reinforces the necessity of clinical judgment in distinguishing normal from disordered anxiety. However, in the case of anxiety disorders, the challenge goes beyond proportionality to danger to encompass judging proportionality in the context of biological design considerations.

What, then, are some strategies for improving the validity of the criteria?

- Review the symptom criteria to ensure that the intensities and specific types of required anxiety symptoms not only reflect intense anxiety—which is shared by normal and abnormal states—but also to the degree possible to specifically reflect disordered anxiety.
- Don't rely on what people think about their symptoms, which is an odd approach to validation that has no significant place in the rest of medicine because people's views of their anxieties are not really relevant to whether their anxieties are disorders. In this respect the proposed *DSM-5* criteria represent an improvement over current criteria.
- Eliminate distress as a clinical significance criterion because all intense anxiety, whether normal or disordered, is distressing.
- Reframe the "role impairment" component of clinical significance to ensure that the activity being impaired is one for which the capacity is biologically designed. For example, in social phobia, an anxious response that makes one unable to be with intimates without distress is more valid as a disorder indicator than anxious responses to socially sanctioned but humanly novel challenges that naturally evoke fear, such as public speaking, performing in front of groups of strangers, or situations when much depends on an evaluation of one's performance. Such a modified role-impairment feature of the clinical significance criterion has a crucial role to play, not so much in identifying harm but in inferring dysfunction in specific phobia diagnoses. Normal, biologically shaped fears can easily satisfy all the other specific-phobia criteria. Sometimes, the only way of differentiating a phobic disorder in which a naturally shaped fear has become so strong as to be best considered a disorder from an intense normal fear is by the impact of the fear on other aspects of normal functioning, based on the speculative assumption that such fears

that override other basic functions in a sustained way are outside of the evolutionarily selected range of fear. For example, if one cannot walk on high mountain ledges without intense fear that interferes with a desired family outing, that is likely non-disordered; one or more of such intense fears are likely part of almost everyone's "fear map" due to their distribution in the population. In contrast, inability to walk up a single flight of stairs due to height fears is plausibly over the threshold of impairment for disorder given our species' need to roam over varying terrain. If many fears labeled as specific phobias are in fact instances of biologically prepared, normally distributed fears, it may be that the best evidence that something has gone wrong is not the intensity of the fear itself but the fear's interference with other basic, biologically shaped functions, manifested in role impairment.

- Interpret "excessiveness" relative to the baseline of the range of biologically designed responses.
- Limit the use of the "unreasonable" requirement because many biologically designed fears are unreasonable in current environments. Especially with the phobias, it should be made clear that many normal fears are not rationally based. Unreasonableness should play a role only in evaluating fears that are based on information and reasoning, but it appears that few anxiety disorders are based on such etiological pathways independent of biological preparedness.
- Use "disproportion" in a way that indicates how humans are designed to respond to dangerous contexts, not to the actual amount of danger that inheres in some situation.
- Most radically of all, take into account the known etiologies of intense fear—including information, conditioning, preparedness for rapid learning from minimal cues, and innate programming. We know enough about the etiologies of fear that theory neutrality is no longer necessary or justifiable, for no one set of criteria can easily encompass the divergent approaches necessary to evaluate the disorder versus normal status of fear of different kinds.

CONCLUSION

The *DSM*'s good-faith efforts to separate anxiety disorders from normal fears are seriously flawed. In clinical practice, the resultant problem of conflating natural anxiousness with anxiety disorders is somewhat minimized because patients generally seek help only after judging that their conditions are not merely natural responses to threatening situations. Otherwise, they may choose to cope with the problem themselves or rely on informal social support. However, whether normal or disordered, individuals may well seek help when they are distressed, when social norms lead them to think that they should not be feeling what they are feeling or that it is embarrassing to feel it, or when their anxiety is an obstacle to some goal such as occupational advancement. Consequently, it remains a critical issue to get the normal/disordered distinction right.

The problem of invalid diagnostic criteria becomes much more serious when the *DSM*'s criteria are transferred to the study of fears and worries in the community. The flaws in the validity of the criteria for distinguishing normal anxiety from disordered anxiety mean that the potential exists to massively overestimate how many people have anxiety disorders. These flaws have come home to roost in epidemiological studies that claim that huge numbers of people suffer from anxiety disorders. Because epidemiological studies guide policy considerations, the problems the *DSM* anxiety disorder criteria have caused for the validity and interpretation of epidemiological surveys warrant careful examination, which we undertake in the next chapter.

CHAPTER 6
Fear and Anxiety in the Community

Many individuals who qualify for a diagnosis of an anxiety disorder never-theless do not seek professional treatment. Indeed, this is true of psychiatric disorders in general. Nor do the rates of treatment by professionals accurately reflect in any simple way the true prevalence rates of disorders in the community, because such rates depend heavily on the types of treatment services available in the community, the methods by which they are accessed and paid for, the attitudes of the individuals within the community toward psychiatric treatment, and many other factors. To find out the true prevalence rates of psychiatric disorders in the population in order to guide policy and estimate health-care needs, one must use epidemiologic studies that psychiatrically evaluate representative samples of community members.

Numerous studies have tried to present an accurate picture of the extent and distribution of psychiatric problems in the population at large.[1] The key problem for studies striving to measure mental pathology in the community is how to define the nature of a psychiatric case among people who have not defined themselves as mentally ill or who have not had a mental health professional make this judgment. This is particularly problematic when it comes to anxiety disorders. Psychiatrists since ancient times have realized that worry can be a realistic response to threat, an expression of a nervous personality disposition, an accompaniment to a variety of other psychiatric disorders, or a symptom of an anxiety disorder. As eminent psychiatrists John Wing, J. Cooper, and Norman Sartorius observe of a worried patient:

> In clinical terms, an individual may worry because he has something to worry about, because he is a worrier, because he has phobias, because he has depressive preoccupations, (or) because he has persecutory delusions . . .[2]

The distinction between realistic worries and anxiety disorders is often a difficult one to make, yet it is especially important when the object of study moves from treated patients to untreated people in the community. Most patients who have sought treatment have already judged that their responses are beyond the normal range, not merely proportionate responses to threatening contexts. In contrast, anxious people in the community have the full range of normal anxieties, but most have not sought psychiatric treatment because they relate their symptoms to worrisome situations or to their own nervous dispositions and so consider them normal rather than seeing them as disorders that warrant clinical attention.[3] Sorting out the disorders from the natural anxieties based on a questionnaire or short interview is not easy. Anxiety symptoms can have a variety of meanings, and diagnosticians traditionally thought that nuanced clinical assessments were necessary to accurately judge the meaning of a particular collection of symptoms and, especially, to judge whether the symptoms represent an anxiety disorder or a normal response to psychosocial stressors; thus, it was thought that psychiatrists would have to interview all the participants in an epidemiologic study to ensure its validity.

Since the advent of the *DSM*'s descriptive, symptom-based diagnostic criteria in the 1980s, psychiatric epidemiology has embraced the opportunity the *DSM* revolution presented to transfer symptom-based descriptions of each disorder from clinical treatment to community cases.[4] The translation of *DSM* criteria into diagnostic algorithms that computers can assess meant that massive epidemiologic studies could be carried out by lay interviewers who administered questionnaires that ascertained whether the respondent had experienced certain symptoms; no professional psychiatric judgment was needed, dramatically reducing the cost of such studies.

The application of the *DSM*'s criteria for anxiety disorders to the general population has produced startling results. Based on community studies that appeared before 1980, the *DSM-III* reported, "It has been estimated that from 2% to 4% of the general population has at some time had a disorder that this manual would classify as an Anxiety Disorder."[5] Recent studies, based on the *DSM-IV* criteria, indicate that nearly 30% of the population reports one of these disorders over their lifetime, roughly a tenfold increase.[6] Studies that use the best longitudinal methodology find even higher rates, reaching over 40% for just the age group from 18 to 32 years old.[7] European studies using similar criteria find comparable results.[8]

These figures have had major influences on policy discussions, mental health treatment programs, scientific studies, media stories, advocacy reports, the development of aggressive screening efforts, and the promotion of psychoactive drugs. Documents in each of these areas routinely cite the results of community studies to show that anxiety disorders are a public health problem of vast proportions, that few sufferers receive appropriate professional treatment, that untreated disorders incur huge economic costs, and that more people need to take medication or seek psychotherapy to overcome their suffering. Findings about the large numbers of untreated anxiety disorders have reshaped mental health policy, justifying efforts to address an unmet need for professional treatment through proactive screening efforts in primary medical care, schools, and workplaces that strive to identify the vast number of people with untreated anxiety disorders.[9] Because anxiety is so common and emerges so early in life, and has increasingly come to be characterized as a risk factor for suicide comparable to depression, it has become a linchpin of epidemiological efforts to aggressively search for and control negative emotions.

We observed in Chapter 5 that the *DSM* manuals since 1980 have attempted to formulate diagnostic criteria that separate anxiety disorders from realistic worries about life problems. The question thus arises: How is it possible that, despite such efforts, the translation of the *DSM* criteria to community populations has produced such enormous numbers of people with anxiety disorders? Do these prevalence estimates represent real disorder in the population? We believe instead that, in addition to flaws inherent in the *DSM* criteria themselves (which we considered in Chapter 5), the enormous prevalence rates result from faulty translations of the *DSM* criteria into criteria used in epidemiological studies. In this chapter, after some initial comments on the history of epidemiological studies of community mental disorder, we closely examine how community studies handle the *DSM* criteria for two of the most common anxiety conditions—generalized anxiety disorder (GAD) and social phobia.

HISTORY OF COMMUNITY STUDIES

Interest in the prevalence and distribution of mental illness has a long history in the United States.[10] Before the 1950s, however, studies of rates of mental illness usually focused on institutionalized populations, sometimes supplemented with surveys of general medical practitioners, clergymen, and other community leaders.[11] These studies rarely focused on anxiety, which was not a primary condition among hospitalized patients. Overall rates from epidemiological studies conducted before World War II indicated that about 3.6% of the population suffered from some kind of mental disorder, including anxiety disorders.[12]

Starting in the 1950s, inspired by the new insights into mental disorder achieved in the treatment of soldiers during World War II, epidemiologists undertook large studies of untreated community members. Because it was far cheaper, these studies used lay interviewers rather than mental health professionals to gather information from community respondents and relied on respondents' self-reported symptoms rather than open-ended clinical interviews. These studies also developed standardized scales of psychopathology that could be scored without the use of any clinical judgments.

The measures these studies used did not diagnose particular disorders, which were not of primary concern to psychiatrists at the time, but assessed the general level of psychiatric symptoms. In contrast to earlier community studies, most of these symptoms were related to anxiety. The most common scale of the era, the Langner scale developed for use in the Midtown Manhattan Study, illustrates the prominent role of anxiety symptoms at the time.[13] Among its twenty-two items, twelve involved symptoms of anxiety: restlessness, nervousness, worries getting you down, being the worrying type, feeling hot all over, heart beating hard, shortness of breath, fainting spells, acid stomach, cold sweats, fullness in the head, and trembling hands. Six others were more related to depression: couldn't get going, low spirits, feeling apart, nothing turns out, nothing seems worthwhile, and feeling weak. The remaining four—poor appetite, trouble sleeping, memory all right, and pains in the head—could fit either category. "The prominence of anxiety in psychoanalytic formulations of psychiatric disorders," notes epidemiologist Jane Murphy regarding the symptom scales of the 1950s and 1960s, "meant that depression, at least neurotic depression, was thought of as an epiphenomenon to anxiety."[14]

The *DSM-II* had explicitly emphasized that anxiety neurosis "must be distinguished from normal apprehension or fear, which occurs in realistically dangerous situations."[15] Nevertheless, none of the scales in wide use at the time tried to make contextual distinctions about whether symptoms were appropriate responses to given situations. Yet the symptoms they used were widespread and normal indicators of distress, not necessarily indicators of anxiety or other disorders. Researchers unjustifiably assumed that each symptom indicated some degree of psychiatric impairment. In light of their failure to consider the context in which symptoms developed, these studies unsurprisingly found extraordinarily high rates of what they considered to be mental disturbance. On one extreme, less than 20% of members of community populations were classified as "well" (they reported no symptoms).[16] On the other extreme, surveys found that a majority of respondents who had undergone stressful events such as natural disasters, marital separations, or job loss reported anxious symptoms.[17] The absence of context in the community studies that predated the *DSM-III* provided a template for studies that would use the new diagnostic criteria after 1980.

Although community studies during the 1950s and 1960s failed to separate natural from disordered anxiety conditions and so largely ignored the point that context might separate disorder from non-disorder, their dominant assumption was that external social conditions led to anxiety. They were especially likely to view anxiety as the outcome of poor socioeconomic conditions rather than as an individual pathology.

In general, it did not seem so important to distinguish contextually responsive anxiety from out-of-context anxiety at that time because, in the wake of the experiences during WWII with war neuroses, the dominant psychiatric ideology held that virtually all negative symptoms are brought about by environmental stressors of one kind or another. Therefore, while these studies greatly overstated the number of disordered conditions based on symptoms, they also focused on the social environment as the source of mental disorder and so did not pathologize individuals.

A small number of studies had tried to measure specific anxiety disorders, as opposed to generalized distress, in community populations before the 1980s. They found relatively low rates of these disorders at a particular point in time, ranging from less than 1% to 4.7% of the population.[18] One study conducted in the 1970s found point prevalence rates of 2.5% for generalized anxiety, 1.4% for phobic disorders, 0.4% for panic disorders, and no cases of obsessive-compulsive disorder in a sample of 500 persons.[19] Another found only a 0.6% rate of agoraphobia in the 1960s.[20] These figures led to the *DSM-III*'s estimate that about 2% to 4% of the general population suffered from an anxiety disorder.[21]

The symptom-based diagnoses of the *DSM-III* provided epidemiologists the tools—and the motivation, given the renewed emphasis on differential diagnosis—to specify and to measure distinct disorders in community populations. Epidemiologists simply translated the *DSM* criteria into closed-format questions about what symptoms respondents had experienced. This yielded a questionnaire that non-professionals could be trained to administer, allowing data to be collected from large numbers of people in a cost-effective manner. To obtain reliable prevalence estimates, different interviewers must ask questions in exactly the same way, because even minor variations in question wording, interviewer probes, or instructions can lead to different results. As one study notes, "The interviewer reads specific questions and follows positive responses with additional prescribed questions. Each step in the sequence of identifying a psychiatric symptom is fully specified and does not depend upon the judgment of the interviewers."[22] The resulting unvarying interview format excluded any discussion with the respondent about reported symptoms and their context. Computer programs using the *DSM* criteria then determined whether a disorder was present. The rigid equivalence of structured interviews improved the consistency of symptom assessment across interviewers and research sites and the consequent reliability of diagnostic decisions.

The initial epidemiological studies that used the *DSM-III* criteria did not find strikingly high rates of anxiety disorders. The first such study, the Epidemiologic Catchment Area Study (ECA) conducted in the early 1980s, presented the first nationwide estimates of anxiety disorders in samples generated from five U.S. cities (Baltimore, Durham, Los Angeles, New Haven, and St. Louis). Using six-month prevalence across three of these sites (New Haven, Baltimore, St. Louis), it found rates of 0.8% for panic, 3.8% for agoraphobia, and 1.7% for obsessive-compulsive disorder.[23] Rates of social phobia ranged from 1.8% to 3.8% across the four sites where it was assessed. The best estimates from all sources of data during the 1980s were that the annual prevalence of anxiety disorders ranged from about 4% to about 8%.[24] Another summary from the same period estimated a comparable range of 2.9% to 8.4%.[25] These estimates were higher than, although still in the range of, the *DSM-III* estimate of 2%–4%. Nevertheless, they were high enough to lead anxiety expert David Barlow to exclaim in 1988 that "These are startling figures."[26] These "startling" figures were soon to seem quite modest.

ANXIETY IN THE NATIONAL COMORBIDITY SURVEY

Since the early 1990s, the National Comorbidity Survey (NCS) has been by far the most preeminent epidemiological study of mental disorders. It is the only nationally representative study specifically of the general population's mental health, was brought up-to-date in a second replication study (NCS-R) during the early 2000s, and has become the model for similar studies in Europe and worldwide. Its methods of assessing psychiatric cases in community populations have become the standard in epidemiological studies.

There is general agreement among epidemiologists that the NCS's translation of the criteria of the *DSM* diagnostic categories for use in community populations has solved epidemiology's perennial problem of defining what a psychiatric case is.[27] In 1992, for example, prominent epidemiologist Lee Robins exulted that "the problems of measuring prevalence have been largely solved. Diagnostic interviews have been developed which are based on official diagnostic criteria and are so well-standardized that they can be administered very reliably by lay interviewers and scored by computer."[28] One of the major European collaborators with the NCS, psychologist Hans-Ulrich Wittchen, asserts, "The last two decades have witnessed an unprecedented progress for epidemiological research."[29] In contrast to earlier epidemiology, which was "plagued by . . . preoccupation with studying social class issues and psychosocial correlates," current epidemiology has made evident "that mental disorders are very frequent disorders of the brain, affecting almost every other person over his/her life course."[30] The NCS findings are cited in virtually every research article about anxiety (and other mental disorders). The principal investigator of the study, Ronald Kessler (a sociologist by training), is the world's most cited mental health researcher.[31] The NCS has had far more influence than any other psychiatric epidemiological study ever conducted. It is thus worth looking at its construction of the anxiety disorders in detail.

The NCS finds extraordinarily high rates of anxiety disorders. The rates of anxiety disorders reported in the initial NCS considerably exceeded those of all earlier studies that measured specific kinds of anxiety disorders. Although the NCS and the ECA were conducted only ten years apart, the prevalence of anxiety disorders in a one-year period rose from 9.9% in the ECA to 15.3% in the NCS; lifetime rates soared from 14.2% to 22.8%.[32] The NCS Replication study (NCS-R) indicated even higher rates of anxiety disorders: 18.1% of the population suffered some anxiety disorder over the past year, and 28.8% reported one of these disorders over their lifetime.[33] As noted, these results were between seven and fifteen times higher than those presented in the *DSM-III* in 1980.

These rates make anxiety disorders by far the most prevalent class of psychiatric disorders; aside from major depression, simple phobias (12.5%) and social phobias (12.1%) were the two most widespread particular disorders of any type.[34] These two types of phobic conditions along with GAD compose about two-thirds of all anxiety conditions. Moreover, rates of anxiety disorders in the United States far exceed those in the rest of the world. For example, a World Health Organization survey of mental disorders in fourteen countries showed that France, the second-highest country in terms of anxiety disorders, had a rate of only 12% compared to the 18.2% figure in the NCS.[35] The lowest level of anxiety disorder, found in China, was only 2.4%.

Kessler is not concerned about the very high amount of mental disorder the NCS supposedly uncovers. "Although the published reports of these high prevalence estimates were initially met with a good deal of skepticism," he notes, "subsequent clinical reappraisal studies showed that they are accurate."[36] Is Kessler's optimistic view that these rates provide superior estimates to the consistently far lower previous estimates warranted? No theory of these disorders—whether biological, psychological, or social—posits any factor that could possibly account for such huge leaps in prevalence in such a short period of time. What explains the extraordinary rise in the prevalence of distinct anxiety disorders from studies conducted during the 1960s, 1970s, and 1980s to those of the 1990s and 2000s?

We believe that the rise in prevalence rates primarily results from, first, seemingly small changes in the wording of questions and, second, how the boundaries between normal fears and anxiety disorders are set—often in ways that have no strong warrant. We use two anxiety conditions to illustrate the way the NCS constructs anxiety disorders. The first, generalized anxiety disorder (GAD), is potentially the most ubiquitous kind of anxious condition. Very high proportions of people who experience a seriously threatening life event could easily meet purely symptom-based criteria that lack the contextual and duration constraints of the *DSM*. The symptoms of the second condition, social anxiety disorder (SAD), can naturally emerge from entering potentially embarrassing social situations or situations where people fear evaluation, especially among those who have anxious, but not disordered, personalities. Community studies such as the NCS must take particular care to use criteria that separate anxious symptoms that reflect actual worries or anxious personality dispositions. Instead, we argue, the NCS uses criteria that turn the ambiguous borders between natural and disordered symptoms into categorical differences that expand the realm of pathology and shrink the domain of normality. In Chapter 5, we examined in detail the limitations of current and proposed *DSM* diagnostic criteria for these two disorders, and we now examine how these criteria were translated in the NCS and how they came to yield the extraordinarily high community prevalence rates that are now accepted as fact within the mental health professions. We then complete our examination of the construction of epidemiological prevalence estimates with an examination of recent estimates of the rates of mental disorders following major disasters.

GENERALIZED ANXIETY DISORDER

Generalized anxiety disorder (GAD), which involves diffuse chronic anxiety, is an especially problematic diagnostic entity. Originally defined as a separate disorder of "anxiety neurosis" by Freud, its symptoms are both the most likely of any anxiety condition to result from realistic concerns and the most likely to co-occur with other anxiety disorders. The *DSM-III* initially dealt with the latter problem by establishing decision rules that made GAD a residual entity that would not be diagnosed in the presence of other disorders. Because of its frequent comorbidity, this decision meant that GAD was a rare condition despite the very broad symptom criteria and lack of contextual anchoring. If GAD is assessed without the hierarchy rules, its prevalence leaps—for lifetime GAD, to about 8.5% of the population.[37]

The *DSM-III-R* and *DSM-IV* changed the hierarchical system so that GAD could be diagnosed concurrently with other disorders. This could have led to a substantial increase in prevalence. However, these manuals also increased, from one month to six months, the length of time that symptoms must endure before diagnosis is warranted. They also introduced a contextual criterion that made it clear that the symptoms must be out of proportion to the actual likelihood of the feared event.[38] These changes were designed to minimize the possibility of mistaking natural, contextually appropriate fears for anxiety disorders. However, when transported into community studies, the flaws in the contextual criteria fueled a substantial increase in reported GAD prevalence.

The NCS's translation of the *DSM-III-R* criteria uses a two-step method for constructing cases of anxiety (and all other) disorders. At the beginning of the interview, it asks a series of gate questions that serve as screens for future inquiries.

These questions try to assess the core features of each disorder.[39] Generalized anxiety disorder (GAD) is representative. Respondents who answer "yes" to any one of the following three questions would later be asked questions based on the detailed criteria for GAD: "Did you ever have a time in your life when you were a 'worrier'— that is, when you worried a lot more about things than other people with same problems as you?"; "Did you ever have a time in your life when you were much more nervous or anxious than most other people with the same problems as you?"; or "Did you ever have a time lasting one month or longer when you were anxious and worried most days?" Only persons who affirm that they have experienced the symptoms in any one of the gate question are asked detailed questions about particular disorders later in the interview.

The gate questions have the practical function of saving time, energy, and respondent goodwill. If all respondents were asked every question, interviews would go on for hours, leading people to simply answer "no" to questions in order to avoid being asked further questions. In addition, the gate questions for all disorders are grouped together at the beginning of the interview, so respondents have not yet become so exhausted or bored by the interview that they would be tempted to answer in the negative as a way to avoid further questioning. This structure maximizes efficiency because only respondents who answer the gate questions in the affirmative are asked detailed questions about particular disorders. But the NCS makes no corresponding effort during the early stem-question phase of the interview to screen out people who had experienced anxiety symptoms that were proportionate responses to actual life situations.

The gate questions should ensure that everyone who has experienced some anxiety disorder will also be asked the detailed questions at the second stage of the interview. Given the broad nature of the screening questions, very few people who have experienced an anxiety disorder are likely to answer "no" to all three. While the first two questions do ask if people worry more than others with the same problems, they neither ask about the context of worries, explore the nature of the reference group respondents use for their comparison, nor try to distinguish higher-than-average levels of anxiety from anxiety disorders.

In any case, the third question—"Did you ever have a time lasting one month or longer when you were anxious and worried most days?"—would override denials of excessive levels of anxiety compared to others. This question ensures that anyone who has been anxious for a month or more, regardless of whether such worries were excessive to a given context or to what respondents think others' levels of worries would be, would proceed to the second-stage questions. In effect, everyone who has been worried for a month at some point in their lives would become a candidate to receive a diagnosis of GAD. The failure of the gate questions to distinguish normal fear from anxiety disorders, however, is not necessarily a problem at this stage because diagnostic decisions about disorder are based only on later sections of the interview.

All respondents who affirm experiencing any gate question for a particular disorder are asked a long series of detailed questions about the symptoms of each disorder, its initial onset, and the amount of distress and impairment that it caused. GAD is again illustrative. The specific criteria for this disorder have changed considerably across the *DSM-III*, *DSM-III-R*, and *DSM-IV*. Nevertheless, its core aspect is persistent anxiety, nervousness, and worry that is accompanied by somatic symptoms of anxiety and is to some extent uncontrollable; that is, the person cannot stop worrying at will.[40] The questions about GAD ask about experiences of ten common anxiety symptoms during the respondent's worst period (e.g., heart pounding, sweating, trembling, difficulties in concentration and sleeping). Additional questions ask about how much emotional distress and interference with social roles the symptoms created. Respondents are also asked if they think their worries resulted from "physical causes such as physical illness or injury or the use of medication, drugs, or alcohol," but they are not asked if their worries arose within any other contexts. Finally, the interview asks about the causes of worries, but not to see if symptoms arose because of understandable reasons—rather, in order to ascertain the content of what people with GAD worry about.

The NCS asks if respondents have "ever" experienced symptoms of anxiety, so just one such episode qualifies for a lifetime diagnosis. The vast majority of people have experienced a traumatic event at some point in their lives that could expectably produce a large number of distressing anxiety symptoms.[41] (Examples such as health, financial, familial, social, or work-related anxieties are provided in Chapters 1–5.) Worries that arose from such situations would expectably be distressing, impairing, and uncontrollable, but if they are proportionate responses to threatening contexts, they would have dissipated once the threat passed. Psychiatry has always distinguished fears that are contextual and abate when the threatening situation is over from worries that are not context-bound. It is therefore problematic that the NCS makes no attempt to establish the context in which worries arise, endure, and disappear so as to separate contextually appropriate anxiety from disordered anxiety conditions.

The only NCS question that might establish a boundary between normal and disordered symptoms is the one that attempts to capture the *DSM*'s requirement that the individual's worry be excessive: "Do you think your (worry or anxiety/ nervousness or anxiety/anxiety or worry) was *ever* excessive or unreasonable or a lot stronger than it should have been?" This question makes respondents themselves the judge of whether their symptoms were "excessive" or "unreasonable" and thus whether they have made proportionate responses to some external threat or might have an anxiety disorder. The "excessiveness" or "unreasonableness" criterion in the

NCS is supposed to be parallel to the *DSM* criteria used in clinical practice described in Chapter 5. It presumably functions to distinguish people who respond to situational stressors with proportionate (not excessive or reasonable) responses from those whose responses are disproportionate to contexts (excessive or unreasonable).[42] But there are major differences between the *DSM* and the NCS criteria.

Whereas the *DSM-III* GAD criteria had simply required generalized, persistent anxiety symptoms for one month irrespective of the context, the *DSM-III-R* criteria introduced some major improvements by requiring that the clinician use judgments that a respondent's anxiety is unrealistic or excessive and is about "two or more life circumstances," with examples of worries about children *who are not in danger* or about finances *when there is no good reason to worry*.[43] In the NCS, however, although respondents are asked whether the worries they have experienced involved excessive or unreasonable anxiety, respondents themselves determine whether their worry is excessive or unreasonable; no clinical judgment provides a check on their answers. In addition, the interview does not provide any examples of "excessive" or "unreasonable" worry that would indicate what standard the person's symptoms must exceed. Respondents are required to judge their own excessiveness and unreasonableness but receive no guidelines for what these terms mean or what comparison group they should use for their answers.

"Excessive" thus could easily be interpreted to mean greater than what respondents consider to be socially appropriate or usual, or what they themselves think they ought to feel.[44] Likewise, "A lot stronger than it should have been?" is extremely vague and could refer to a respondent's own personality type or to cultural norms as well as to the life circumstances in which the anxious symptoms arose. The NCS makes no attempt to separate high-range but normal levels of anxiety from anxiety disorders, nor does it use any questions that are comparable to the *DSM* criteria that indicate that anxiety is disordered only in the absence of some realistic, external threat.

It is also noteworthy that the *DSM-III-R* implicitly requires that the anxiety comprising GAD must be unrealistic or excessive in a persistent way across worries, requiring "[u]nrealistic or excessive anxiety and worry (apprehensive expectation) about two or more life circumstances . . . for a period of six months or longer, during which the person has been bothered more days than not by these concerns."[45] In contrast, the NCS translation asks only whether the respondent's worries were "ever" excessive, etc., so that threshold is very low indeed—just one instance of one worry within the broader period of anxiety being considered excessive will satisfy the criterion. It is clear that even those without an anxiety disorder but undergoing chronic worrisome stress might consider that at least once they might have become overwrought to an excessive extent. This subtle change in the criteria could itself lead to a substantial inflation of estimated prevalence of disorder.

Consequently, despite the *DSM* effort to create valid diagnostic criteria and the NCS's inclusion of the *DSM* contextual and multiple-worry requirements within its translation of these criteria, the criteria remain seriously conceptually flawed and limited in their capacity to distinguish normal from disordered anxiety states. In principle, it should not be especially difficult to develop valid contextual criteria for GAD. Respondents could be asked whether their periods of anxiety corresponded to particularly worrisome situations, such as a child being seriously injured, a period of unemployment, or a spouse's affair, and whether the anxiety ended when the situation was over. GAD would be present when symptoms emerged or persisted in the absence of a threatening context or were excessive in relation to the situation in which they arose.[46] It is possible that such methods would lower reliability, but they should result in more valid indicators of cases of GAD.

The estimate of the lifetime prevalence of GAD, though very substantial at about 6% of the population,[47] is relatively modest by NCS standards when compared to the prevalence of other anxiety disorders. Recently, NCS researchers have published some papers that explore the implications of broadening the GAD criteria to include a wider range of anxiety conditions, thus increasing GAD prevalence. These papers offer supporting arguments and generally seem to express a position sympathetic to such changes, although they call for further study of the optimal cut point for GAD diagnosis. While it is uncertain whether these proposed changes will find their way into *DSM-5* and subsequent epidemiological surveys, we complete our discussion of GAD by reviewing the arguments these papers present. They are important because they offer an *in vivo* glimpse into how such proposals are argued and evaluated, why they are seen as desirable or appropriate, and the degree to which such proposals respect the need to distinguish disordered anxiety from normal anxiety.

The first target is the "excessiveness" criterion mentioned above. The NCS researchers suggest eliminating this question, which would abolish even the weak measures of context it provides, the argument being that the subjectivity and ambiguity of these criteria lower the reliability of diagnoses and unjustifiably decrease rates of GAD.[48] Instead of trying to develop alternative criteria that would more clearly separate anxiety stemming from external threats from disordered anxiety, the researchers would eliminate the excessiveness requirement completely so that all anxiety symptoms, regardless of whether they were more excessive than they should have been, would be considered to indicate disordered anxiety.

This position provides a vivid illustration of the primary flaw in the way symptom-based criteria have been pursued: the focus on reliability overrides considerations of validity and as a result undermines the entire purpose of the diagnostic system. Missed altogether is the fundamental point, expressed in the *DSM*'s definition of mental disorder, that a syndrome—even if distressing and impairing—is not a disorder unless it is caused by an internal dysfunction. Indeed, the researchers argue that contextual measures should be abolished because all symptoms that cause distress or impairment are clinically significant and therefore should be professionally treated regardless of how situationally grounded they might be.[49] Dropping the excessiveness requirement would increase GAD prevalence by about 40%.[50]

The NCS researchers do not note the implications of calling people "disordered" who specifically say that their worries were never more excessive or unreasonable than they should have been. To the extent possible—given the questions they are asked—such people are explicitly responding that their anxiousness was proportionate to the situation in which it arose. For the NCS investigators, however, all worries of a serious enough level, even if proportionate responses to real threats, should be considered disorders.

The NCS researchers also suggest a second change to the GAD criteria that would lower the duration requirement of symptoms from six months to one month.[51] According to Robert Spitzer and Janet Williams, the *DSM-III-R* had originally increased the required duration for GAD from one to six months because the one-month requirement in the *DSM-III* "makes it difficult to distinguish this category from relatively transient stress reactions."[52] When the NCS decreases the duration requirement in this way, GAD prevalence increases by 50%–60%. When researchers relax both the duration and the excessiveness requirements, lifetime and one-year rates of GAD more than double: from 5.6% and 3.0% to 12.8% and 6.2%, respectively.[53] Researchers using data from an earlier epidemiological study found that lifetime rates of GAD increased *fivefold*, from 9% to 45%, when they lowered the duration threshold from six months to one month.[54]

It is possible that some individuals with anxiety lasting less than six months might have an anxiety disorder. But if one contemplates lowering the duration threshold, thus making it harder to distinguish between disordered and normal anxiety, it would obviously be desirable to simultaneously increase the assessment of context so that one would have some alternative means to differentiate symptoms with different implications. Perversely, the NCS group instead suggests both decreasing the duration requirement and eliminating the excessiveness criterion, ignoring the problem of false positives. In considering such changes, the primary argument is that subthreshold GAD is similar in certain respects to current GAD in such factors as risk of a later disorder and role impairment when anxious. One would expect highly anxious individuals to share some such features, whether the anxiety is normal or disordered. But there is no attempt to distinguish risk of disorder from actually having a disorder, and there is no attempt to distinguish similarities that might be expected in both normal and disordered anxiety—for example, role impairment—from effects that might distinguish disorder from normality.

The NCS researchers argue that the *DSM* criteria for anxiety should be comparable to those for major depressive disorder (MDD). The *DSM* does not require MDD symptoms to be excessive, instead treating all symptoms that don't result from bereavement as indicators of disorder and requiring only a short duration of symptoms.[55] As with MDD, the NCS group asserts that criteria for anxiety should be based purely on distressing and impairing symptoms without regard for the objective life circumstances of the individual. They believe that these changes would increase not only reliability but also validity because nonexcessive cases and those of shorter duration display distress and impairment.[56] However, the criteria for MDD are themselves clearly invalid and an inappropriate model for other categories.[57] They imply that all sufficiently distressing negative emotions (aside from certain cases of bereavement) are pathological, regardless of their relationship to social contexts.[58] Even emotions that are proportionate to their contexts and are not long-lasting, as well as those that arise from chronically poor socioeconomic circumstances, would be diagnosed as mental disorders if the NCS investigators have their way.[59] Such a policy would reverse thousands of years of psychiatric history regarding anxiety, up to and including each edition of the *DSM*, without any adequate grounds for doing so.

Adopting the NCS suggestions to abolish the excessiveness requirement and lower the duration requirement for GAD would likely lead to a massive pathologization of normal worries and concerns. The findings from a study of mothers of children with chronic illnesses such as cystic fibrosis, cerebral palsy, and myelodysplasia are illustrative.[60] This study used a diagnostic instrument, the Diagnostic Interview Schedule, which was based on the purely symptom-based *DSM-III* criteria with no excessiveness criteria and a duration requirement that symptoms last a minimum of only one month. It found that a *majority* of these mothers— 56%—had a lifetime diagnosis of GAD. Even 45% of the control group of mothers with healthy children received GAD diagnoses under these criteria.

This study of mothers with chronically ill children shows how criteria that make no allowance for the context of anxiousness produce spectacularly high rates of supposed anxiety disorders when they are applied to groups that face clearly threatening situations. Purely symptom-based criteria would mistakenly label mothers who are naturally worried about the health and future of their disabled children as people who have an anxiety disorder. As we have seen, most people experience comparable situations at least once over their lifetimes. If the NCS suggestions are adopted and their proposed criteria accurately applied, it is possible that a majority of the population would have GAD at some point in their lives.

The NCS suggestions would also have potentially disastrous consequences for research about the causes of anxiety disorders. People with perfectly normal fear mechanisms would be lumped together with those who have anxiety disorders.

The resulting group of "disordered" individuals would encompass some individuals with anxiety disorders and others who have no disorder at all. Research striving to find common risk factors would founder on the tremendous heterogeneity of a group with GAD diagnoses, some of whom are responding naturally to realistic concerns while others are genuinely disordered. Such a step would greatly expand the amount of diagnosed pathology at the cost of accurate diagnoses, treatment, and understanding.

SOCIAL ANXIETY

Social anxiety provides another example of how the NCS attempts to separate realistic fears from anxiety disorders. This distinction is especially important because shyness is a ubiquitous condition: some 90% of Americans self-report that they sometimes feel shy.[61] Shyness is grounded in evolutionarily natural feelings of unease in the face of threats to reputation or social status.[62] As detailed in Chapter 4, since ancient times, commentators have recognized that anxiety about entering certain social situations was widespread. "Almost everyone," noted Charles Darwin, "is extremely nervous when first addressing a public assembly, and most men remain so throughout their lives."[63] In addition, as Cicero indicated, "An anxious temper is different than feeling anxiety."[64] Many non-disordered people have introverted temperaments. Social anxiety disorders, in contrast, either arise in inappropriate contexts or involve greatly disproportionate anxiety intensity relative to their triggering situations.[65] The difficult separation of natural shyness from anxiety disorders must involve situating the anxious feelings in the particular contexts in which they develop.

Social anxiety was not mentioned in the *DSM-I* or *DSM-II*. When it appeared for the first time, the *DSM-III* defined social phobia as a persistent and irrational fear that one would act in a humiliating or embarrassing way while under the scrutiny of others, accompanied by a compelling desire to avoid such situations.[66] This manual noted, "The disorder is apparently relatively rare."[67] The first study that measured the prevalence of the disorder in the early 1980s indicated a lifetime prevalence rate of 2.5%.[68] A standard text published in 1988 indicated, "Social phobia occurs in from approximately 1.2% to 2.2% of the population."[69] What, then, accounts for its huge rise since then to 13.3%, more than one out of every eight people?

The two NCS screening questions for social anxiety do not attempt to separate extremely common, but normal, fears from possible disorders: "Was there ever a time in your life when you felt very afraid or really shy with people, like meeting new people, going to parties, going on a date, or using a public bathroom?" and "Was there ever a time in your life when you felt very afraid or uncomfortable when you had to do something in front of a group of people, like giving a speech or speaking in class?" The content of these questions guarantees that people who become uncomfortable in just the sort of situations in which anxiety was designed to arise will be considered as potentially disordered.

The more detailed second-stage questions about social anxiety ask if respondents have ever experienced one of six fears: public speaking, talking in front of a small group, talking with people when you might have nothing to say or might sound foolish, using a toilet away from home, writing while someone watches, and eating or drinking in public. About 40% of people report at least one of these six fears.[70] The problem of defining what should be considered a case of social anxiety disorder is especially difficult given that nearly all of the situations in which people report feeling anxious are those where anxiety would be natural. Table 6.1 shows the most frequent social fears.[71] By far the most common fear is of public speaking.[72] "A substantial proportion of people with social phobia," write the NCS researchers, "meet the criteria exclusively because of speaking fear."[73] Talking in front of a small group of people and fearing sounding foolish while talking with people were the only other fears endorsed by a sizable proportion of respondents. In other words, most social anxieties occur in exactly the kinds of situations that invoke evolutionarily normal fears of risking social status.

As with GAD, the only attempt to separate normal social anxiety from an anxiety disorder comes later in the interview when respondents are asked, "Do you think the fear was ever excessive, or unreasonable, or much stronger than it should have been?" However, recognizing the fear as excessive or unreasonable can depend on personal or social values as well as on social desirability. "You could have a scar on your face that makes you extremely self-conscious," according to psychologist Jerome Kagan in reference to the NCS criteria, "or you could live in a place where you feel that you're less educated than everyone else around you."[74] What matters is

Table 6.1. LIFETIME PREVALENCE OF SOCIAL FEARS IN NCS

Public speaking	30.2%
Talking in front of small group	15.2%
Feeling foolish when talking	13.7%
Using a toilet away from home	6.6%
Writing while someone watches	6.4%
Eating or drinking in public	2.7%
Any	38.6%

Adapted from Kessler, Stein, & Berglund, 1998, p. 614

whether the fear is actually excessive or unreasonable in relationship to the context in which it emerges. In effect, the NCS does not make a serious attempt to separate natural fears of embarrassment or humiliation from disordered ones; it considers all high-end responses to be disordered. Likewise, people with naturally anxious temperaments but not disorders could make positive responses to these questions.

Among those respondents who report their social anxiety as excessive, the NCS uses the intensity of anxiety and the accompanying distress or interference in functioning to separate social anxiety disorders from normal shyness. It considers to be disorders all conditions that are highly distressing and that interfere with functioning. The problem is that even intense and impairing anxiety in situations that threaten social status and that are potentially embarrassing can arise from evolutionarily natural processes. This is especially true for people with high-range but normally anxious temperaments. Adequate epidemiological studies must separate pathological from species-natural social anxiety.

Subtle changes in the wording used to measure social phobias account for the apparent epidemic of this disorder that began in the early 1990s. The *DSM-III* criteria used in the earlier ECA community study during the early 1980s had required "[a] persistent, irrational fear of, and compelling desire to avoid, a situation in which the individual is exposed to possible scrutiny by others and fears that he or she may act in a way that will be humiliating or embarrassing."[75] The NCS, using the revised *DSM-III-R* criteria, stated that the person need have only an "unreasonably strong fear" of situations such as meeting new people, talking to people in authority, or speaking up in a meeting or class. These seemingly minor changes resulted in an increase of lifetime prevalence from 2.5% in the ECA to 13.3% in the NCS, a nearly sixfold increase in prevalence over the course of a decade.[76] Another example of how small changes in wording created very large changes in prevalence is that 6.5% of respondents answered in the affirmative to the ECA question about having extreme distress when "speaking in front of a group you know" versus a prevalence rate of 14.6% when using the NCS question regarding "speaking in front of a group."[77] As an evolutionary perspective would predict, people are much less likely to be anxious among intimates.[78] The result is that social anxiety has become the third most frequent "disorder" of any kind in the general population.

The high frequency of social anxiety in the community is not the only reason for its importance in the NCS. It is a particularly crucial condition because it has the earliest reported age of onset of any type of disorder. Over 80% of respondents with an anxiety disorder report that social anxiety was their first lifetime disorder.[79] Thus, it is the linchpin for the NCS efforts to prevent the emergence of mental disorders. "Early-onset social phobia," write Kessler and colleagues, "is a powerful predictor of the subsequent onset and course of a wide range of secondary mental and substance use disorders."[80] Their reasoning is that if an earlier age of onset of one disorder is a risk factor that predicts the onset of future disorders, then preventive efforts with the primary disorder can presumably also help in averting the secondary disorder. Therefore, if anxiety disorders can be prevented at an early age, subsequent depressive and substance abuse disorders can also be avoided.

The contextual nature of natural fears helps explain the finding that anxiety symptoms precede symptoms of other types of disorder. Psychologists and psychiatrists have long linked the emergence of normal fears to early stages of the life cycle. Consider Darwin's observation:

> May we not suspect that the vague but very real fears of children, which are quite independent of experience, are the inherited effects of real dangers and abject superstitions during ancient savage times? It is quite conformable with what we know of the transmission of formerly well-developed characters, that they should appear at an early period of life, and afterwards disappear.[81]

Recall as well that Freud emphasized how normal anxieties were grounded in childhood:

> The danger of psychical helplessness fits the stage of the ego's early immaturity; the danger of loss of an object (or loss of love) fits the lack of self-sufficiency in the first years of childhood; the danger of being castrated fits the phallic phase; and finally fear of the super-ego, which assumes a special position, fits the period of latency.[82]

Other psychiatrists, such as Isaac Marks, show how certain kinds of fears universally emerge among young children.[83] Fearful situations are especially prominent during childhood and adolescence. Threats to reputation or status that naturally give rise to social anxiety, for example, typically begin with the emergence of status hierarchies during the school years.

When asked about the first emergence of symptoms, respondents in community surveys might naturally recall fears and worries that arose at young ages. This finding does not necessarily indicate that anxiety *disorders* emerge at temporally earlier periods and then predict the emergence of other types of disorders. Normal fears are especially likely to emerge among young children and adolescents, so when respondents retrospectively ponder when their first distressing emotions occurred, they are likely to give primacy to symptoms of anxiety.[84] Threatening contexts that lead to normal fears emerge at the earliest ages, but their temporal primacy does not indicate causal primacy. Indeed, prospective research does not find that anxiety is temporally prior to depression.[85] One might even think that a child's sensitivity to threat might be an adaptive trait. The NCS researchers, nevertheless, use the early appearance of anxiety symptoms as grounds for assertive proactive efforts to uncover anxiety as the key to preventing the emergence of other disorders.

Where and how researchers draw the line between disordered and non-disordered conditions have enormous effects on prevalence rates. Clear cases of social anxiety disorder involve people with dysfunctional internal mechanisms that create such intense anxiety that they cannot interact with intimates or enter social situations that are not likely to be embarrassing or threatening to social status, such as purchasing goods in a small shop or sitting in an anonymous lecture hall.[86] But from the early Greeks and Romans through Burton, Darwin, and Freud, authorities have regarded situations such as speaking in public, meeting new people, talking with people in authority, or talking with strangers as generative of anxiousness. Treating them as anxiety disorders pathologizes extensive domains of social and personal life; in the case of social anxiety disorder these are precisely the kinds of domains that are most likely to lead naturally to anxiousness.

The boundaries between responses to realistic external threats and anxiety disorders can never be precise. Psychiatric thought, however, has always recognized that the contexts in which symptoms develop is one crucial way to differentiate natural from pathological symptoms. The arbitrary figures that result from the failure to distinguish pathological from natural worries render highly suspect the rates of GAD and SAD (and the other anxiety disorders) that the NCS uncovers. The use of the *DSM* categories in community surveys has not solved the problem of how to define a psychiatric case; it has only swept it under the rug. "By simply altering slightly the wording of a criterion," Herb Kutchins and Stuart Kirk note, "the duration for which a symptom must be experienced in order to satisfy a criterion, or the number of criteria used to establish a diagnosis, the prevalence rates in the United States will rise and fall as erratically as the stock market."[87] Kutchins and Kirk are only half-correct. Prevalence rates in recent epidemiological studies go in only one direction: upward.

DISASTERS

For thousands of years, observers have realized that threatening events naturally lead to fears and worries. The very definition of normal fear and worry is that they occur when people have something to be afraid of or worried about. Normal anxiousness in the context of highly threatening events has traditionally never been viewed as disordered. Indeed, the *DSM* takes great pains to distinguish anxiety disorders from natural responses to realistic threats. Even the highly flawed NCS makes some attempts to separate non-excessive fears from disordered conditions.

Recent studies of the mental health impact of disasters, however, have overcome any restraints that common sense and millennia of medical thought provide.

Empirical studies of mental health after natural disasters have always shown that enormous proportions of affected populations develop symptoms of distress. Immediately after catastrophes such as hurricanes, floods, or earthquakes, almost everyone reports some distress.[88] One review notes that soon after natural disasters, "incidence rates of post-disaster symptomatology approach 100 per cent."[89] Rates of normal anxiety are directly related to factors such as the loss of property, displacement from homes, threats to physical integrity, disintegration of the community, loss of employment, and similar stressors that lead the future to be uncertain. Such normal worries continue as long as the highly stressful situation remains but subside as soon as living conditions normalize. For example, very high proportions of people were anxious soon after the terrorist attacks of September 11, 2001. Several months after the attacks, however, their levels of anxiety returned to normal, indicating that their initial fears were natural and not signs of anxiety disorders.[90] Disasters, however, can also lead to mental disorders in a small proportion of affected individuals whose symptoms endure well after the disaster-related social adversities have gone away.

Studies of the mental health of community members who have suffered disasters face a constraint that is not present in most community studies: they must be conducted very soon after the disaster occurs. Moreover, because respondents face many exigencies, few are willing to spend a great deal of time dealing with lengthy interviews. Therefore, researchers must not only get into the field to begin their interviews quickly, they must also use quite brief measures of psychological conditions.

The K6 scale is one of the spin-offs from the NCS. The scale consists of just six questions that are a combination of items that measure anxiety and depression: "During the past 30 days, how often did you feel so sad (nervous, restless or fidgety, hopeless, that everything was an effort, worthless) that nothing could cheer you up?" Scores of all the time (4 points), most of the time (3 points), some of the time (2 points), a little of the time (1 point), and none of the time (0 points) are summed for a possible score ranging from 0 to 24. Someone who scores 13 or more is considered to have a "serious mental illness." Someone who scores just 8 or more is thought to have a "probable mental illness."

The K6 was not designed to measure responses to highly stressful situations such as disasters. The NCS researchers originally developed the K6 as a way to identify community members who should undergo a second-stage interview to see if they have a psychiatric disorder. That is, its items were not themselves interpreted as indicators of mental disorder but as first-stage screens that might identify people who a later clinical interview might diagnose as having a serious disorder.

This aspect of the K6 questions is similar to the function of the gate questions of the NCS that were reviewed above: to indicate what proportion of people might benefit from a second-stage diagnostic interview, in order to eliminate those who need not be further interviewed. The items are completely a-contextual and make no attempt to establish whether the anxious and depressive feelings are a natural response to a life situation. Their nature is such that they will identify people who will screen positively in a second-stage interview, but they will also capture many false positives that the diagnostic measure will, in theory, negate. Nevertheless, the K6 has become a common stand-alone instrument that is itself used to assess rates of mental disorder after disasters *without* a subsequent diagnostic interview.[91]

The lack of contextual grounding in the K6 questions means that it is particularly unsuitable for use in highly stressful contexts such as the aftermath of disasters. Not only are its questions insensitive to context, but its use in disaster research is precisely the sort of situation that expectably produces findings of huge levels of anxiety and distress. In the absence of a second-stage interview, enormous numbers of people who have suffered realistic losses and have realistic worries will be wrongly treated as though they have anxiety-depression disorders. The disastrous situation itself would produce most of the symptoms, impairment, and distress that arise in its aftermath.

All the same, the K6 is now applied to populations that are undergoing the consequences of serious disasters that will naturally produce fears, worries, and depression. Worse, the instrument is not used as a screening measure that is preliminary to a second-stage clinical interview, but as a direct measure of mental disorder. The result has been a massive pathologization of normal emotions.

Hurricane Katrina, one of the worst natural disasters in American history, is a case in point. It resulted in the deaths of over a thousand people, led to a massive relocation of over half a million people, and resulted in over $100 billion of property damage. Moreover, a slow and ineffective governmental post-disaster response led stressors to endure long after the initial damage they created. It created a situation where millions of people lost their homes, jobs, and communities and faced unexpected threats to their future well-being.

Studies of the mental health effects of Hurricane Katrina have unsurprisingly found that the population in the affected area was under massive amounts of stress. The largest study of over a thousand residents of New Orleans and other areas that were directly exposed to Hurricane Katrina asked respondents to rate their hurricane-related stress exposure on a scale from 0 to 10, where 0 meant no stress at all and 10 meant the most stress you can imagine a person having.[92] The study also asked respondents about their experiences with ten hurricane-related stressors, including risk of death to themselves or a loved one, criminal victimization, physical illnesses or injuries, extreme physical adversity, housing difficulties, and property and income loss. The median level of exposure was an 8, indicating an extraordinary amount of stress in this population. Over 90% of respondents in the New Orleans area and over 80% outside New Orleans reported experiencing some hurricane-related stressor. In New Orleans, over 70% reported property loss and housing adversity. Nearly 30% of this group reported experiencing five or more serious stressors.

The study found that about 20% of the entire sample scored between 8 and 12 on the K6. A third of the New Orleans sample fell in this range. People who said they experienced any four of the K6 items "some of the time" during the past month would score in this range. An additional 17% of the New Orleans sample and 10% of the remainder of the sample had scores ranging from 13 to 24 on the scale. Overall, half of the New Orleans sample and a quarter of the rest of the sample had scores of 8 or above on the K6. Experiencing stressors—especially physical illness and injury, physical adversities due to the storm, or financial loss—was especially related to higher scores on the K6.

Remarkably, the authors of this study conclude that they have found a *"high prevalence of DSM-IV anxiety-mood disorders."*[93] Indeed, they equate K6 scores from 8 to 12 with "probable mild/moderate mental illness" and scores from 13 to 24 as "probable serious mental illness." In their eyes, Hurricane Katrina caused half of New Orleans residents and a quarter of residents in the other affected areas to become "mentally ill."

Although the authors claim to have uncovered the presence of an enormous amount of *DSM* disorder, their findings are not remotely related to what the *DSM* would call "mental disorder." The K6 was developed as a screen for mental disorder; it was not intended to be a stand-alone measure. Moreover, it was meant to be a screen only in the general population, not in a population that had undergone extreme stressors. To be a valid measure of mental disorder in a highly stressed population, it would have to contain numerous safeguards that could distinguish realistic threats and losses from disorders. In fact, it lacked a single constraint when applied to a population where even high levels of anxiousness and depression would not be "excessive," "unreasonable," or "disproportionate." Studies that use measures such as the K6 show the naturalness of distress in disaster-related situations but reveal nothing about the extent to which disasters cause mental disorder.

Scales such as the K6 impose no boundaries between natural and pathological responses but treat all positive symptoms as signs of disorder. Moreover, such studies are conducted during the extreme uncertainty of a post-disaster period when people have no idea whether and how their lives will be put back together. People who have had their house ruined in a flood or hurricane, been relocated outside of their community, and lost their job and subsequently report feelings of nervousness, restlessness, sadness, and the like are considered to have a "serious mental illness." The boundaries of pathology have spread so broadly that they incorporate completely natural responses to highly distressing events, hopelessly confounding normal and pathological responses in the aftermath of a disaster. The result has been an enormous broadening of what is considered to be a pathological result of a traumatic situation.

The utter confusion of disorder and natural distress that this study illustrates would have been incomprehensible during most of psychiatric history. Recall the admonition of the Present State Examination in the 1970s: "Do not, *of course*, include anxiety appropriate to the situation, e.g. going into battle, narrowly avoiding a traffic accident, realistic fear of punishment, anxiety during an examination, etc."[94] Likewise, it is hardly imaginable that a clinician would consider "mentally ill" a patient who has recently survived a major disaster that destroyed her home, ruined her possessions, forced the relocation of her family, and bankrupted her finances and then affirmed that she is feeling anxious and depressed. Calling half the population of a major metropolitan area "mentally disordered" after a natural disaster based on such feelings is inconsistent with any sensible concept of mental disorder. Consider, then, that the most respected investigators in the field conducted this study, the major funding agency in the field of mental health financed it, and the most prestigious psychiatric journal published its results. It is plain that in the attempt to create a scientific approach to psychiatric disorder, psychiatry is instead coming perilously close to transforming itself into a pseudoscience that has rendered its own domain of mental disorder meaninglessly broad and its assertions about mental disorder vacuous.

Such confusions have practical human consequences. The most pressing need of most disaster victims is social services that can restore their homes, livelihoods, and communities. "What people need during the first few days," counsels British psychiatrist Simon Wessely, "is the support of their family and friends and assistance with information, finances, travel, and the planning of funerals. The most appropriate immediate mental health interventions are practical, not emotional."[95] Most people are resilient and can deal with their negative emotions by turning to their lay social support networks.[96] They rarely require or can benefit from professional mental health counseling that calling them "mentally ill" implies they require. The danger of using expansive conceptions that classify even the most obviously natural emotions as mental disorders is that the results of the social devastation of natural disasters are transformed into individual pathologies in need of mental health treatment.

The community studies of the 1950s and 1960s that uncovered extraordinarily high rates of mental disorder were widely mocked. The use of scales such as the K6 recreates the same problems that led to the discrediting of these earlier scales. Disaster researchers that measure generalized distress using instruments that do not distinguish disorder from responses to real contextual threats risk the same fate.

If the results of such studies get more credibility now than in the past, it is not because they use more valid methods. Instead, the cultural climate in the early twenty-first century seems more amenable to labeling as mental disorders even the most natural emotions resulting from life circumstances.

CONCLUSION

Epidemiologists have not solved the problem of how to define a psychiatric case in community populations. In fact, definitions of psychiatric disturbance intrinsically involve ambiguity and uncertainty. In the absence of any conclusive gold standard for a valid concept of mental disorder, they can uncover as much seeming psychopathology as they desire by altering the parameters of what experienced symptoms are required, how long they must last, and how severe they must be. When they abandon contextual constraints altogether, as in the case of the K6 scale used with Katrina victims, enormous numbers of non-disordered people can be made to seem as if they have mental disorders.

The only valid way to ensure that studies measure mental disorders rather than realistic worries and fears is to relate the measurement of symptoms to the actual contexts in which they develop and to natural human tendencies to experience distress due to our species-typical biologically designed emotions. The *DSM* itself suggests the basis for such measurements and makes good-faith efforts to focus on disordered anxiety conditions. Many epidemiologists, however, have chosen to minimize the study of context and of natural human emotional dispositions, and thus to maximize the amount of disorder their studies generate.[97]

CHAPTER 7
PTSD

Post-traumatic stress disorder (PTSD) has become an emblematic diagnosis of our time. "At the beginning of the twenty-first century," write historians Paul Lerner and Marc Micale, "PTSD is perhaps the fastest growing and most influential diagnosis in American psychiatry."[1] Although PTSD is a young diagnosis, only entering psychiatric nosology in 1980, it has already generated a gigantic industry of consumers, therapists, and researchers.

Individuals suffering the often extreme emotional effects of confronting extraordinary traumas deserve social support and any therapeutic help that may be beneficial. However, the psychiatric diagnosis of PTSD, which classifies some individuals' struggles with traumatic experiences as psychiatric disorders, raises a number of difficult questions about the boundaries between normality and pathology. One is the fundamental question of how humans are naturally designed, if at all, to respond to what we now consider traumatic events, some of which were presumably not all that rare in the challenging and unforgiving environments in which humans evolved. What does a "normal" response to traumas look like?

Horrific and shocking experiences challenge people's basic senses of values and reality and uproot fundamental assumptions regarding personal safety, mortality, and a just world. Such disturbing events lead to the difficult and lengthy challenge of reconstructing meaning systems to suit new circumstances, and human belief systems are clearly designed to be capable of such adaptation over time to changing circumstances. Extreme distress and extended grappling with the significance and consequences of such events are expectable results of traumas as one engages in such meaning reconstruction. Moreover, we are clearly not designed to leave behind traumatic memories forever. Because of the need to learn from experience and to avoid reentering situations where traumas can reoccur, evolution is unlikely to select responses that obliterate memories of traumatic events.[2] Given the possible intensity and prolonged nature of normal-range responses to extreme events, diagnosticians face a daunting challenge in sorting out what divides natural and disordered responses to such events.

Another particular characteristic of PTSD lies in the fact that, unlike other diagnoses, it requires not only a particular set of symptoms but also a particular type of cause for its existence. PTSD by definition arises as a consequence of some horrific experience; symptoms that would otherwise justify a PTSD diagnosis but that emerge in the absence of a traumatic precipitant cannot, by definition, indicate this disorder. This requirement raises the issue of what constitutes a trauma in the first place.

PTSD also raises complicated questions about the *uniqueness* of responses to traumatic events. No need exists for a special diagnosis if extremely disturbing events result in anxiety, depression, panic, and the like. Diagnosticians can classify such symptoms within existing categories of disorder; they do not require a particular trauma-related diagnosis. A special category is warranted only if the psychic results of traumatic events have singular characteristics that other diagnoses cannot capture. The symptom criteria for PTSD attempt to capture such a distinctive syndrome, but the question remains whether this syndrome is really distinctive to responses to traumas.

A further issue involves the intensely *moral* nature of the implications of many PTSD diagnoses. Perhaps more than any other *DSM* category, PTSD diagnoses involve questions of right and wrong in addition to dispassionate issues of fact. On one side, patients are viewed as victimized and in need of help; people who question sufferers' disordered status are seen as uncaring or immoral. On the other side, skeptics have regarded patients claiming PTSD diagnosis as cowards, malingerers, or fortune hunters. PTSD diagnoses, then, often create morally charged boundaries.

A final concern arises from the possibly iatrogenic nature of PTSD diagnoses. Normal responses to trauma involve memories of the disturbing event that often last well after the experience itself is over. But, like all memories, most will naturally fade over time, albeit often lengthy periods of time. Instead of facilitating natural healing processes, PTSD labels can sometimes perpetuate suffering by maintaining a focus on, and even creating identities around, memories of the traumatic event. Symptoms that might disappear over time if they were left alone can become protracted when they are organized around a PTSD diagnosis.

PTSD thus raises perhaps the most difficult diagnostic decisions of any anxiety disorder. This chapter first considers the issues involved in drawing the lines between normal and pathological reactions to horrific experiences. It then discusses the vast expansion of PTSD diagnoses since the late 1980s. Finally, it turns to some of the moral issues and controversies that this diagnosis has generated.

DIAGNOSING PTSD

While all anxious conditions have intrinsically fuzzy boundaries, it is usually easy to identify a considerable range of clear cases of normal fears and anxiety disorders. In contrast, it is difficult to know what even obviously natural and pathological responses to trauma are, because extreme stressors naturally entail intensely alarming memories and other disturbing consequences. From an evolutionary point of view, remembering traumatic events can help people learn from experience and avoid situations that led to the initial trauma; forgetting such events can hamper chances of survival.[3] It is particularly hard to establish the point at which natural recollections of traumatic experiences become pathological.

The criteria for PTSD, considered in more detail below, vary considerably across the *DSM-III*, *DSM-III-R*, and *DSM-IV*.[4] All of the manuals, however, make an intrinsic connection between traumas and particular symptoms tied to the patient's active memory of the event that are assumed to be pathological. These include intrusive memories and disturbing dreams about the traumatic event, feeling upset about reminders of the event, re-experiencing the event, unpleasant somatic sensations and heightened arousal, irritability, difficulty concentrating, sleep problems, and a feeling of danger when reminded of the event. A major problem, however, arises because these symptoms can be products of the inherent cognitive bias of fear mechanisms to promote reinforcement and recollection— rather than forgetting—of past traumatic experiences.[5] Moreover, symptoms of intrusion, avoidance, and hyperarousal that trauma researchers assume are intrinsically connected to *traumatic* events also characterize responses to non-traumatic stressors and even to other events that aren't traumatic at all.

Separating Normal from Pathological Symptoms

There is a central question to consider when evaluating whether PTSD criteria identify only mental disorders or encompass normal responses as well: Do these symptoms occur only in the case of extreme traumas, or do they also arise as a more general reaction to a range of stressors? The evidence suggests the answer is that these symptoms constitute a common way that people respond to a broad span of disturbing events.

Consider a study that asked college students questions about how often they relived or avoided thinking about, and insulated themselves in reference to, *the worst movie (or worst television program)* they had seen in the last few months.[6] The study used a common scale of PTSD symptoms that asked respondents about their reactions to traumatic events using such responses as "I thought about it when I didn't mean to" or "I tried to remove it from memory." It found that 41% of respondents scored in the high range, 31% in the medium range, and 28% in the low range of scores obtained from victims of events that are commonly viewed as traumatic. These results were only slightly lower than those found among survivors of an airplane crash. A number of other studies also find that levels of symptoms presumed to indicate PTSD are at least as high among people who have a variety of common interpersonal, academic, and occupational problems as those who have suffered from traumas.[7] For example, responses to a romantic partner's unfaithfulness typically involve intrusive and recurrent thoughts of sexual activities, avoidance of reminders of the affair, and symptoms of sleep difficulties, anger, and hyper-vigilance.[8]

Donna Brazile was a campaign aide to presidential candidate Albert Gore. Her feelings after Gore lost the presidency in 2000 provide a particular illustration:

> Campaigns are not for the fainthearted. They are tough—mentally, physically and spiritually. Once a campaign ends, an emptiness comes over you. You find yourself struggling to figure out how to become human again. . . . you're in a state of emotional disrepair . . . No matter how hard you try to contain it, you're both angry and sad. . . . I remember feeling lost and disillusioned. I was empty inside. . . . I had no idea what to do with my life. . . . I had no energy to start looking for work. I was obsessed with those chads: hanging, swinging and, my favorite, pregnant. Above all else, I did not want to quit fighting. . . . It will take you weeks to readjust and for the world to appear normal."[9]

Keep in mind that this reaction stems from a *political* campaign, not a military campaign. Brazile's comments remind us how difficult re-entry to usual roles can be after immersion in a different sort of life, but the condition she describes does not represent a mental disorder.

These examples indicate how typical symptoms used to measure traumas do not necessarily capture *disordered* responses but can indicate intrusive thoughts, feelings, and images that apply equally well to any disturbing occurrence, including recollections of such obviously non-traumatic experiences as watching a bad movie. Indeed, anyone who has tried to stop thinking about a song she cannot get out of her head could receive a substantial score on a checklist of "trauma" symptoms. It is not necessarily pathological to try to avoid thinking about stressful experiences (whether traumatic or not), minimize exposure to them, and become physiologically aroused when thinking about them.[10] No less than traumatic events, ordinary stressors such as the death of a loved one, interpersonal problems, or embarrassing and humiliating events can lead to rumination, re-experiencing, pondering, avoidance of reminders of the stressor, and selective attention.[11] Such events happen to most people at some point in their lives, creating the potential for a massive pathologization of natural responses to recollections of disturbing experiences.

The difficulties of separating normal and pathological responses to trauma perhaps stem from the lack of knowledge about how evolution designed people to react after they have been traumatized. Presumably, our ability eventually to adapt after such painful experiences was crucial to our survival. Symptoms of numbing and reduced awareness of the environment that are commonly interpreted as disordered symptoms of dissociation might be adaptive forms of natural responses to stressful occurrences. In the immediate aftermath of a trauma, people normally experience a short period of emotional numbness, followed by a longer period characterized by sleep difficulties, nightmares, intrusive images of the terrible events, and an avoidance of reminders associated with the trauma.[12] Without outside interventions, these disturbing symptoms often slowly go away, although they might occasionally reoccur. Such intrusive recollections may be involved in major adjustments of long-term memory for what is safe and what is dangerous, and may make people more likely to avoid the kind of experiences that led to their symptoms in the first place. Even if such speculations are accepted, our lack of an adequate theory of what natural responses to traumas entail creates a wide range of possibilities for setting the boundaries between natural and pathological traumatic responses. Because the processing of traumas involves so much suffering, it is tempting in such an evidential void to establish very broad definitions of trauma-related mental disorders.

What Is a Trauma?

PTSD is a stark exception to the *DSM*'s most basic classificatory principle: symptoms, rather than etiology, should establish different diagnostic categories. This principle is often necessary at this point in psychiatry's history because the causes of mental disorders remain largely unknown, so, unlike in the rest of medicine, causes cannot be the basis for distinguishing different disorders.[13] Yet PTSD symptoms such as intrusive, avoidant, and hypervigilant recollections of some trauma, *by definition*, result from traumatic situations; if they were not consequences of a trauma, logically they cannot indicate PTSD.[14] The trauma may not be the sufficient cause because not everyone who experiences a trauma develops symptoms; features of the person's history and personality, for example, no doubt play a role in whether the trauma causes enduring symptoms. However, it is a necessary part of the cause.

This causal assumption of the PTSD diagnosis sharply contrasts with the other anxiety disorders, as well as with the other mental disorders in the *DSM* more generally. For example, anyone who fulfills the symptomatic criteria for any other anxiety or mood disorder *ipso facto* has this condition. In contrast, people who meet all of the PTSD criteria cannot receive a diagnosis when their symptoms are not the result of an event that falls under the criteria for what a trauma is.

This causal link means that a singular aspect of PTSD among the major *DSM* diagnoses is that the boundaries of pathology depend not only on the types of symptoms that are considered to indicate disorder but also on what counts as a trauma in the first place. The same symptoms that would constitute a disorder if provoked by a trauma cannot indicate PTSD in the absence of a traumatic stressor. Because sharp boundaries between traumatic and non-traumatic stressors do not exist in nature, demarcations can be drawn in many places.

One problem involved in defining what constitutes a trauma is that different individuals have highly variable thresholds of what they perceive as horrific or upsetting. Since the time of Charcot, many clinicians have emphasized that the intensity and persistence of post-traumatic symptoms do not correspond with the nature and severity of the traumatic event itself.[15] Instead, personal vulnerabilities and meanings enter into what people define as traumatic. This raises the challenging issue of whether individual meanings should be taken into account in definitions of traumatic events. As we will see below, the answer to this question makes a vast difference in rates of PTSD.

Another problem regards the role of culture in defining what constitutes a trauma. Philosopher Mikkel Borch-Jacobsen discusses the case of the Quechua Indians of Peru, who commonly develop symptoms (which closely resemble PTSD symptoms) of what they call *Susto* after becoming frightened by stimuli including thunder, the sight of a bull or snake, or sightings of old Incan ruins.[16] Experiences that are traumatic for the Quechua would not be culturally appropriate reasons for developing PTSD symptoms among Westerners. Conversely, Borch-Jacobsen reports, a Quechua wouldn't develop symptoms of *Susto* after exposure to events such as natural disasters or accidents that can provoke PTSD among Westerners.

Cultural definitions of trauma can have powerful effects on who develops or is considered to have PTSD. For example, one reason for the vastly higher rates of

PTSD among soldiers in recent wars compared to earlier ones lies in changing expectations about what leads to trauma. Before the Vietnam War, combat was more likely to be associated with tests of manhood to be met through stoicism and resolve; after this war, combat came to be viewed as a source of terrible and long-lasting psychic wounds.[17] The consequences of transformed definitions of the nature and extent of traumatic experiences can have profound influences on the emergence of PTSD.

Are the Symptoms of PTSD Unique?

The symptoms of PTSD and those of other disorders are highly permeable. Traumatic events are associated with numerous pathological conditions including GAD, panic, depression, and increased substance use. Unlike PTSD, these other conditions need not entail a traumatic cause to be diagnosable. It is difficult to distinguish what *unique* symptoms are related to traumatic exposure. For example, studies of psychiatric outpatients show that levels of PTSD symptoms are equivalent among those who have and have not experienced traumatic events.[18] Moreover, the same people who develop PTSD typically also experience a range of other conditions, including mood and other anxiety disorders, after traumatic events; therefore, the distinctiveness of the PTSD diagnosis is questionable.[19] The term "PTSD" can easily be elided with numerous other conditions that result from traumatic experiences. Indeed, "PTSD" has recently become a shorthand notation for any disturbing psychic consequence of trauma.

The linkage of traumas with distinctive symptoms is quite new. Although psychiatrists and physicians have recognized and debated the psychic results of trauma since the latter part of the nineteenth century, psychiatric classifications before the *DSM-III* in 1980 never recognized any particular collection of symptoms that *specifically* resulted from a trauma. Instead, trauma victims in the nineteenth century developed symptoms of neurasthenia and other well-recognized categories. Likewise, shell-shocked soldiers in World War I developed paralysis of limbs, gait disorders, tremors, blindness, and other hysterical conditions that were not distinct from those of non-military neurological, medical, and psychiatric patients.[20] Soldiers who suffered from combat neuroses in World War II displayed symptoms of anxiety, depression, and psychosomatic illness that were comparable to those of many psychiatric outpatients at the time.[21] The psychological results of traumatic situations were encompassed within extant diagnoses, so no specific category of symptoms that was exclusively related to traumatic exposure was thought to be necessary. The extent to which PTSD involves a distinct collection of symptoms is still a debatable issue. Indeed, some psychiatrists claim that PTSD has no reality as a separate diagnosis; they consider it a natural form of distress stemming from the need to readjust to changing circumstances.[22]

So, what constitutes a trauma is hard to define, the responses to these events may or may not be pathological, and the symptoms that result need not be unique to PTSD. It is no wonder that the potential range of what constitutes PTSD is extremely variable. Given what we have seen in similar situations regarding other diagnoses, it is not surprising that the scope of PTSD has undergone a huge extension in recent years.

THE EXPANSION OF PTSD

PTSD has become, in anthropologist Allan Young's terms, "the Esperanto of global suffering."[23] The term "PTSD" pervades both media discussions and lay descriptions of responses to trauma, generally referring to unpleasant memories of horrible events. A large trauma industry has become widely institutionalized in schools, hospitals, police and fire departments, government, and industry as well as in mental health facilities.[24] Grief and trauma counselors, who did not exist twenty years ago, now flock to the scene of every catastrophe. The PTSD diagnosis has generated far more research than any other anxiety disorder. Articles about PTSD in the medical literature doubled between 1985 and 1995 and then doubled again between 1995 and 2005.[25] By 1999 more than 16,000 overall publications concerned PTSD.[26] If current trends continue, by 2015 it will spawn more than twice as many articles as the next most studied anxiety disorder.[27] The PTSD diagnosis has expanded extremely rapidly, become firmly institutionalized, and generated considerable controversy in a very short period of time.

Diagnoses before the *DSM-III*

The current range and scope of PTSD contrasts with traditional conceptions of the limited range of traumatic situations and the small number of people who were likely to become psychologically disturbed after traumatic exposure. Although it was known since the latter part of the nineteenth century that profound shocks stemming from horrific events such as train wrecks could have direct effects on the nervous system, no major psychiatric diagnosis captured the specific impact of traumatic experiences until after World War II. The epidemic of war neuroses that arose during this war demonstrated the inadequacies of extant psychiatric manuals, which had been developed for institutionalized patients. The diagnostic system embodied in the *Statistical Manual for the Use of Hospitals for Mental Disorder* could not adequately classify the vast majority of symptoms that psychically impaired soldiers displayed.[28] In particular, it could not classify chronic yet non-psychotic conditions that stemmed from exposure to traumatic events.

The insufficiencies of the *Statistical Manual* led the Veterans Administration to develop its own diagnostic system, which in turn spurred the American Psychiatric Association to create its first classification manual, the *Diagnostic and Statistical Manual of Mental Disorders (DSM)*, in 1952.[29] None of the major categories in the *DSM-I*—brain disorders, mental deficiency, psychotic disorders, psychoneurotic disorders, or personality pattern disturbance—could encompass long-lasting symptoms that arose after an environmental trauma among people with no previous histories of psychological problems. The *DSM-I* created a category of "Transient Situational Personality Disorders" for people with normal personalities who developed transient symptoms as a way of adjusting to an overwhelming situation.[30] These disorders were distinguished from psychoneuroses, which were assumed to arise from unconscious conflicts stemming from childhood experiences, and from personality disorders, which were developmental defects that had minimal anxiety. Among these transient situational reactions was "Gross Stress Reaction." This diagnosis was to be applied only for "previously more or less 'normal' persons who have experienced intolerable stress."[31] The *DSM-I* specified wartime combat and catastrophic events in civilian life as the two traumatic conditions leading to this reaction. Because gross stress reactions arose in normal individuals who had undergone unusually stressful experiences, the *DSM-I* states that GSR will "clear rapidly" once the individual is removed from the stressful situation.[32] The consequences of traumatic stress were assumed to be self-limiting unless some preexisting individual susceptibility was present. If symptoms were persistent, a different diagnosis, usually some psychoneurosis, was indicated.

By the time the *DSM-II* appeared in 1968, the influence of the military experience in World War II had receded, and no organized group had an interest in trauma-related diagnoses. This manual dropped the category of Gross Stress Reaction. It did include a general diagnosis of "Transient Situational Disturbances" that stated, "If the patient has good adaptive capacity his symptoms usually recede as the stress diminishes. If, however, the symptoms persist after the stress is removed, the diagnosis of another mental disorder is indicated."[33] In other words, any persistent condition would not be classified in this category but must be a psychoneurosis, personality disorder, or psychosis. Chronic symptoms, therefore, must be due to individual predispositions and not to exposure to a traumatic stressor.

Within the general category of Transient Situational Disturbances was a diagnosis of "adjustment reaction of adult life." Among its brief descriptions was the example of "Fear associated with military combat and manifested by trembling, running and hiding," virtually synonymous with a description of cowardice.[34]

The absence of a suitable diagnostic category for chronic combat-related stress in the *DSM-II* was to become highly significant during the development of the *DSM-III*. The existing literature had little resonance with the distinctive pathology of Vietnam veterans, whose memories compulsively intruded into their lives many years after their traumas had occurred. Indeed, major psychiatric textbooks published not long before the *DSM-III* did not even mention any similar condition.[35]

PTSD in the *DSM-III*

The aftermath of the Vietnam War completely transformed traumatic diagnoses. A highly politicized anti-war atmosphere pervaded much of the country, including many returning Vietnam veterans who had turned against the war. A vocal and well-organized subculture of anti-war veterans emerged, centered on Vietnam Veterans Against the War (VVAW). Within VVAW, a subgroup developed that consisted of anti-war psychiatrists (most notably Robert Jay Lifton and Chaim Shatan), disillusioned Veterans Administration therapists, and psychologically disturbed veterans.[36] They created a network of therapeutic "rap groups" where veterans could discuss their problems in the company of sympathetic peers. Based on their experiences in dealing with these groups, Lifton, Shatan, and others became convinced that massive numbers of veterans were experiencing a "post-Vietnam syndrome" marked by survivor guilt, flashbacks, rage, psychic numbing, alienation, and feelings of being scapegoated.[37] They emphasized both that veterans who did not receive appropriate treatment would become chronically disabled and that symptoms could have a delayed onset that began well after their wartime experiences had ended. The existing *DSM*, however, couldn't encompass veterans who displayed chronic pathology where traumatic memories compulsively intruded into their present lives.

Pre-*DSM-III* research about traumatized persons studied conditions such as "general nervousness," "anxiety neurosis," "depression," or "delirium," which could also occur among persons who had not suffered any traumatic event.[38] Studies occasionally noted symptoms that were intrinsically connected to the trauma, such as horrifying recollections of events, nightmares, and guilt for not having saved companions who died, but such symptoms were viewed as aspects of existing types of neuroses and not of a separate diagnostic category.[39] No psychological syndrome existed that captured chronic and specific effects of a trauma.

Coincidentally, around the same time the veteran's group was mobilizing against the absence of a suitable diagnosis for the psychic impacts of combat, the American Psychiatric Association created a task force in 1974 to revise the *DSM-II*. Under the overall direction of Robert Spitzer, it consisted of a number of subgroups that were charged with evaluating existing data and developing specific criteria for each of the disorders that would appear in the *DSM-III*. The anti-war psychiatrists took advantage of the revision process and aggressively tried to remedy the absence of a diagnostic category that covered the enduring psychological impacts of traumatic conditions. Lifton and Shatan operated within an ideological climate that was still hostile to the war effort and sympathetic to veterans' claims. They were able to persuade Spitzer to appoint them and a Vietnam veteran, Jack Smith (the sole member of the roughly 150 persons on the various *DSM* task forces to have no graduate degree), to the six-member advisory committee working on the Reactive Disorders section of the manual (the others were psychiatrists Nancy Andreasen, Lyman Wynne, and Spitzer himself).[40]

The development of the new PTSD diagnosis in the *DSM-III* had none of the trappings of other conditions such as field trials of criteria, tests of reliability, and statistical analyses of data. The veterans' advocates relied on the moral argument that failing to include a PTSD diagnosis in the new manual would be tantamount to blaming victims for their misfortunes.[41] In a highly charged cultural climate still reeling from the aftermath of the war, their ethical position prevailed over the data-driven arguments that succeeded in the creation of other diagnoses. The result was that the *DSM-III* incorporated a PTSD diagnosis that almost completely followed the recommendations of the anti-war psychiatric group.

The new event criterion required the "[e]xistence of a recognizable stressor that would evoke significant distress in almost everyone."[42] It was based on a model that assumed traumas of a sufficiently extreme severity were likely to produce chronic symptoms in otherwise normal individuals. The horrific quality of the events themselves, not personal definitions of trauma, were responsible for the resulting problems. This limited the range of applicability of the PTSD diagnosis to such extreme situations as combat, sexual violence, civilian disasters, or concentration camp survival.[43]

The anti-war psychiatrists' assumptions about the duration of PTSD symptoms sharply diverged from previous assumptions that most soldiers were resilient and over time would gradually adjust to their wartime experiences. To overcome the absence of any stressor-related diagnosis for chronic symptoms in the previous manual, *DSM-III* symptoms could emerge at any time subsequent to the experience of the trauma and did not need to coincide with the traumatic event. This incorporated both prolonged psychological disturbances and repressed symptoms that appeared long after the period of combat was over. The *DSM-III* criteria thus allowed for not only conditions that had acute onset and limited duration but also those that lasted for six months or more and those that had delayed onset of at least six months after the trauma.

The *DSM-III* criteria were silent about the distinction between normal and pathological responses to trauma. This omission, however, was not a serious issue thanks to the inherent constraints of the stressor criterion, which imposed the requirement of the "[e]xistence of a recognizable stressor that would evoke significant symptoms of distress in almost everyone." Extraordinary traumas marked by wartime combat, rape, or fires that led to severe burns framed the context of the subsequent symptoms. Therefore, it was the stressor criterion rather than the subsequent symptoms that limited the scope the PTSD diagnosis. Because this criterion clearly limited the diagnosis to people who had undergone extraordinary stressors, there would be little point in considering its potential to over-pathologize symptoms. The understandable failure of the *DSM-III* task force to consider what were natural reactions to trauma only became consequential after future manuals diluted the stressor criterion and applied it to wider and wider populations. These manuals, not the *DSM-III*, are responsible for the expansion of the PTSD diagnosis to virtually the entire population from its delineated origin in the conditions of combat veterans and a small number of other traumatized groups.

PTSD after the *DSM-III*

Most *DSM-III* diagnoses have remained basically intact or have undergone only minor changes. In contrast, each subsequent revision of the *DSM* substantially transformed the PTSD diagnosis. The first revision of the *DSM-III*, the *DSM-III-R* (1987), made minimal changes in the exposure criterion. It altered "[e]xistence of a recognizable stressor that would evoke significant distress in almost everyone" to require "an event that is outside the range of normal human experience and that would be markedly distressing to almost anyone."[44] This definition maintained the traumatic quality of events as an aspect of the severity of the event itself and not the individual's response to it. It also provided a list of examples that could be of lesser intensity than wartime combat, sexual assault, or severe burning: "serious threat or harm to one's children, spouse, or other close relatives and friends, sudden destruction of one's home or community; or seeing another person who has recently been or is being seriously injured or killed as the result of an accident of physical violence."[45]

The major extension of PTSD in the *DSM-III-R* came through changes in the symptom criteria. During the 1980s, a prominent social movement had developed that emphasized the widespread prevalence of repressed and then recovered memories of childhood sexual abuse. "The ordinary response to atrocities," according to a leading figure in this movement, psychiatrist Judith Herman, "is to banish them from consciousness."[46] The repression of traumatic experiences had little connection to the intense memories of veterans, who were all too able to recall their symptoms. However, a large cadre of therapists had developed who were committed to using techniques that would bring memories into consciousness after many years of repression.[47] This group required symptom criteria that recognized that traumatic experiences could be repressed as well as intrusive.

Primarily in response to the recovered memory movement, the revised criteria changed the category of numbed responsiveness to the external world to include the "inability to recall an important aspect of the trauma." Traumatic symptoms now encompassed recurrent and intrusive memories as well as the inability to remember some trauma. The *DSM-III-R* also significantly lowered the duration requirement of symptoms from six months to one month: long-lasting symptoms were no longer necessary for a PTSD diagnosis.[48] Symptoms of relatively brief duration, which would be especially common in natural responses to traumas, were now treated as pathological.

The *DSM-IV* (1994) brought about the major expansion of the PTSD diagnosis. The new criteria dropped the requirement that events be "outside the range of normal human experience" and must "cause distress in almost everyone." It replaced them with the requirement that "the person experienced, witnessed, or was confronted with events that involved actual or threatened death or serious injury, or a threat to the physical integrity of self or others" and that "the person's response involved intense fear, helplessness, or horror."[49] These changes immensely widened the boundaries of traumatic events.

The initial PTSD diagnosis in the *DSM-III* focused on extreme traumas. The revised stressor criteria of *DSM-IV* included all cases that the earlier definitions had captured but added many other experiences that the previous diagnosis did not encompass. The "confronted with" criterion extended the notion of exposure so widely that persons who were not even present at a traumatic event could potentially meet the diagnostic criteria. For example, someone who learns of the sudden and unexpected death of a close relative, or that a friend has died from natural causes, would meet the new stressor criterion. Even people who watched a disaster unfolding thousands of miles away on television could potentially become diagnosable under the new criteria.

The *DSM-IV* changed the nature of traumatic exposure in a second way. The requirement that the person's response involve "fear, helplessness, or horror" shifted the definitional criteria from the nature of the stressor itself to the subjective experience of the victim.[50] Individual temperament, personality, and reactivity now entered into what defined an event as "traumatic." This introduced a subjective element into the nature of the stressor itself, because only people who have a certain emotional reaction to the stressor are considered to have experienced a traumatic event in the first place. The *DSM-IV* thus radically changed definitions of trauma both to include a great heterogeneity of experiences and to partially locate the nature of trauma within the individual rather than the environment. These changes helped to create a vast array of pathology far beyond previous conceptions of PTSD. (However, it should be noted that the PTSD work group for the *DSM-5* is considering elimination of the required subjective emotional response and is also proposing some subtle limitations in the kinds of allowable traumas that need not be directly experienced.[51])

Community Studies of Trauma

The Epidemiologic Catchment Area Study (ECA), which was conducted shortly after the *DSM-III* was published in 1980, was the first major study to examine rates of PTSD among community members. Using the initial *DSM-III* criteria that required extraordinary stressors and extended duration, it found modest rates of the disorder. Data from the St. Louis site found that only 5 men and 13 women per 1000 met PTSD criteria at any time during their lives.[52] Only Vietnam veterans who had been wounded in combat reported high levels of PTSD. Another study using data from the North Carolina site of the ECA found a similarly low PTSD lifetime prevalence of 1.30% and a six-month prevalence of just 0.44%.[53] PTSD, as defined by the *DSM-III* criteria, rarely occurred in the general population.

Subsequent studies that used the *DSM-III-R* criteria, which required only one-month instead of six-month duration and which used broader stressor and symptom criteria, yielded far higher rates. In the early 1990s, the National Comorbidity Study (NCS) found that slightly over 60% of men and 50% of women in a large, national population reported some traumatic event—most commonly, witnessing someone being injured or killed, a natural disaster, or a life-threatening accident. These studies also reported considerably higher PTSD rates than studies that had used the initial *DSM-III* criteria. Nearly 8% of the population, including over 10% of women and 5% of men, had enough symptoms to receive a PTSD diagnosis at some point in their lives.[54] One study of Detroit-area residents during the 1980s found that about 40% reported exposure to events fitting the *DSM-III-R* definition of trauma. About a quarter of persons who were exposed to a traumatic event also developed PTSD: 11% of women and 6% of men reported PTSD, with an overall lifetime prevalence rate of over 9%.[55] The lifetime prevalence for women in the Detroit study was nine times higher than in the ECA study, and 35 times higher for men![56]

The *DSM-IV* revision drove rates of traumatic exposure even higher, to the extent that virtually the entire population had some "traumatic" experience.[57] One large community study found that 92.2% of males and 87.1% of females met the *DSM-IV* criteria for having encountered traumatic stressors.[58] Learning about the sudden, unexpected death of a loved one, reported by 60% of the population, was the event most responsible for the increase of traumatic stressors. Rising rates of PTSD did not stem from the presence of a more traumatized population or from the greater ability of researchers to identify traumatic disorders. Instead, they were the product of definitional changes that broadened the criteria for traumatic events and lowered the required duration of symptoms. Where boundaries are placed between natural and pathological experiences has an enormous impact on rates of PTSD. Trauma had moved from battlefield, blaze, or rape situations into the realm of everyday life.

9/11

The terrorist attack of 9/11 provides a prime example of how researchers and the trauma community used the expanded stressor criteria of the *DSM-IV* on a vast scale. Nonstop news coverage of the attacks meant that the whole population of the nation (indeed much of the world)—not just those who were directly exposed to the terrorist attacks—was "confronted with" a potentially traumatic event.

An early study of 9/11, published in the *New England Journal of Medicine*, was conducted within three to five days after the attack. Researchers asked 560 respondents from across the country whether they experienced five symptoms of PTSD: "Feeling very upset when something reminds you of what happened? Repeated, disturbing memories, thoughts, or dreams about what happened? Having difficulty concentrating? Trouble falling or staying asleep? Feeling irritable or having angry outbursts?" Forty-four percent of those surveyed reported at least one "substantial" symptom, and virtually everyone (90%) experienced at least "a little bit" of a symptom.[59]

Other research indicated that during the second month after the attack, 11.2% of persons in the New York City area and 4.3% nationwide suffered from PTSD, and 11.6% experienced clinically significant distress.[60] Another study found higher rates: 17% of the U.S. population reported post-traumatic stress two months after the attacks.[61] Other surveys taken during the first week after 9/11 took affirmative responses to such ordinary emotions as "fears of future terrorism," "fear of future harm to family as a result of terrorism," or reporting "quite a bit" of anger at Osama bin Laden as indicators of PTSD.[62] Such criteria indicated that nearly half of the U.S. population experienced some "symptom" of PTSD.[63] Likewise, over half of respondents said that at least one child was upset by the attacks.[64]

Such research treats any distressing recollection of a horrific event as pathological. Feeling upset or irritable and repeatedly remembering the events are treated as a sign of disorder despite the fact that such "symptoms" can be normal responses to catastrophic occurrences. The likely normality of such symptoms is indicated by the fact that, despite dire predictions that 9/11 would result in an enormous amount of psychological disorder, especially PTSD, symptom levels dropped precipitously soon after the attacks. While about 7.7% of Manhattan residents reported full-blown PTSD a month after the attacks, by six months after the attacks a negligible 0.7% had PTSD.[65] The almost immediate "recovery" of most people who were not directly affected by the attacks calls into question whether they ever had a disorder in the first place. Certainly, the precipitous decline in symptoms cannot be attributed to successful treatment efforts: despite predictions to the contrary, no rise in treatment rates occurred after 9/11.[66] Most people who received an initial diagnosis seem to have experienced natural, but transitory, responses to a highly disturbing experience.

Research about the psychological consequences of 9/11 not only fails to distinguish natural from pathological responses to traumas but also raises the issue of what it means to be "exposed" to a trauma. The *DSM-IV* exposure criteria encompass watching a traumatic event on television (as long as one had a horrified reaction) as well as actually experiencing the terrible event. As a result, people who were scrambling for their lives in the World Trade Center and seeing their colleagues die are equated with those who were in no danger while watching the towers collapse on their television screen from thousands of miles away. Indeed, the number of hours of television viewing was an especially good predictor of who reported a greater number of PTSD-related symptoms.[67]

The Military

Combat has historically been linked with psychological trauma, whether through "shell shock" in WWI, "combat neuroses" in WWII, or "PTSD" after Vietnam. In all of these conflicts, military authorities commonly refused to acknowledge the often dire psychic consequences of war. As the battle to insert PTSD into the *DSM-III* illustrates, psychologically wounded veterans had to make extensive efforts against strong opposition to have their conditions recognized.

Mental health professions have undergone a vast change in their assumptions about the extent to which PTSD will emerge as a result of combat experiences. Unlike military psychiatrists in previous conflicts, who believed that the vast majority of soldiers were resilient and could even develop greater emotional strength from participating in combat, mental health personnel expected that PTSD would be a common result of the Iraq and Afghanistan wars.[68] Like the broader mental health culture at the time, they embraced the view that PTSD was a widespread condition in wartime, that all soldiers could be potential victims, and that as many affected soldiers as possible should be treated for it. Indeed, in one study, a quarter of over 100,000 veterans who had come home from the Iraq and Afghanistan wars received some mental health diagnosis; 13% were diagnosed with PTSD.[69] Studies indicate higher rates of PTSD in close to 20% of members of combat units after returning from deployment in Iraq.[70]

The increased recognition and understanding of the psychic consequences of combat is a welcome development. Questions remain, however, about the extent to which aggressive efforts to identify and treat soldiers who are presumed to have PTSD actually identify disordered conditions and actually help the individuals so labeled. It is hardly surprising that a high proportion of soldiers who have just experienced long periods in a hostile environment, been threatened with sudden death or injury, and witnessed comrades blown up would experience many distressing feelings and re-experience the traumas they have witnessed. It is not clear, however, that these are psychiatric disorders as opposed to normal processing of such events. Yet, instead of distinguishing the truly traumatized from the normally distressed, current criteria appear to leave natural and pathological responses intertwined.

Such labeling could have substantial effects on subsequent behavior and self-identification. The intensity of the painful psychic impacts of traumatic events often naturally remits over time, especially when people have supportive resources that help them adjust to their experiences. For example, a recent Army report notes that the high rates of apparent mental disorder present in those returning from combat assignments decrease almost to baseline rates of those garrisoned at U.S. military bases after about 24 months, and fully to baseline by 30–36 months, suggesting that most symptoms classified as PTSD do remit on their own with time.[71] "Just as with a course of grief," psychiatrist Paul McHugh notes, "the most disturbing psychological symptoms gradually fade away, leaving the subject with some enduring sense of loss, the occasional bad dream, and perhaps some reluctance to revisit locations or arenas where the shock was experienced."[72] Telling individuals suffering from normal but painful emotions that they have a "post-traumatic stress disorder" can send a message that their emotions are actually pathologies in need of lengthy treatment. This message can unwittingly focus attention on, and stabilize, symptoms that might otherwise have dissipated with time. Moreover, it can divert attention from natural tendencies to resilience, self-healing, and, occasionally, even personal growth in the wake of tragedies.[73]

While not proof of iatrogenic effects, a striking increase of PTSD diagnoses has accompanied the growing attention given to this diagnosis. For example, despite the fact that risk of PTSD from a traumatic event drops as time passes, the number of Vietnam veterans who applied for PTSD disability almost doubled between 1999 and 2004.[74] Perhaps such increases represent a pool of genuinely disordered individuals who earlier were reluctant to seek help and were not recognized as disordered. However, the journalist Malcolm Gladwell notes how the dominant belief systems after World War II emphasized veterans' psychological resilience after even gruesome combat experiences.[75] Few veterans of this war suffered enduring disorders. In contrast, Gladwell observes that more recent therapeutic beliefs stress that traumas will have persisting psychic consequences unless they are treated. Indeed, rates of PTSD during the Iraq and Afghanistan wars have increased exponentially along with the acceptance of the notion that soldiers will not naturally get over the traumatizing impacts of combat. Paradoxically, in some individuals this expectation can create the very condition that it claims to describe—and hopes to relieve.[76]

While catastrophic events undoubtedly cause much psychic devastation, defining the problems of returning veterans in mental health terms might not be the optimum way of providing the support and resources that they require for successful reintegration. Findings that as many as 20% of returning veterans have PTSD lead to calls for increased identification of mental health problems and provision of mental health services.[77] While soldiers who have suffered from the emotional consequences of trauma warrant the best available treatment if they desire it, an overemphasis on the emotional impact of wartime experiences can turn attention away from other salient aspects of post-war adjustment. Returning veterans deserve help with negotiating complicated bureaucracies, finding employment and social services, reintegrating with families and friends, and coping with naturally distressing memories. Those who are understandably anxious and depressed about their war experiences and the difficulties they encounter when they re-enter civilian life might find monetary, occupational, educational, and interpersonal resources more useful than psychological treatment. An overemphasis on recollecting traumatic memories can deflect considerations of meeting the challenges of reintegration into civilian life while at the same time focusing on disturbing images that could otherwise gradually dissipate.[78]

It is of course crucially important to recognize PTSD as a disorder among our military personnel when it does in fact exist and where the natural human response to extreme stress has broken down in some way, blocking gradual adaptation to changed meanings and circumstances. Perhaps it is even helpful to err to some extent on the side of judging that there is possible disorder in order to avoid missing potentially serious cases. However, the gross pathologizing of an enormous amount of the likely normal suffering by military personnel, as is arguably occurring at present, has several downsides. It may misdirect therapy toward painful normal responses that would have naturally healed over time, encourage lengthy self-identified patient status that delays recovery, and provide incentives for remaining disabled.

However, at its core, the problem with expansive diagnosis of PTSD among veterans is that it does not represent an accurate and respectful portrayal of the nature of the very human responses such individuals have to the extreme stresses they are forced to undergo for their country. For example, military psychiatrist Charles Hoge notes that the normal physiological acclimation to the combat environment includes adjustment to prolonged extreme stress accompanied by chronic sleep restriction and reversal of circadian cycles, arguing that the expectation that such changes "will reset easily upon return home is unrealistic."[79] Military personnel, Hoge argues, understand that after they re-enter civilian life their symptoms are often extensions of the adaptive behaviors they learned in order to survive combat, not pathologies. The lengthy adjustment period upon returning home is likely partially due to the thoroughgoing need to undo the responses to combat that veterans have previously gone through.

Hoge also observes that veterans are frequently dissatisfied with the care they get for psychiatric symptoms because they perceive a "disconnect between their experiences as warriors and perspectives they encounter trying to obtain the help they need."[80] Appropriately normalizing some PTSD symptoms might actually benefit veterans, who tend to perceive that their condition is not a disorder and thus resist obtaining help for a pathologized condition. Hoge suggests conceptualizing PTSD within an occupational context:

> Military personnel are members of professional workgroups, similar to police and other first responders, trained to respond to multiple traumatic events; they do not normally perceive themselves as victims, nor their reactions as pathological. The paradox of war-related PTSD is that reactions labeled "symptoms" upon return home can be highly adaptive in combat, fostered through rigorous training and experience. For example, hyperarousal; hypervigilance; and the ability to channel anger, shut down (numb) other emotions even in the face of casualties, replay or rehearse responses to dangerous scenarios, and function on limited sleep are adaptive in war.[81]

This sort of partially normalizing perspective, which broadens the concern with PTSD beyond a narrowly defined clinical pathology to encompass how soldiers must be retrained for combat and then retrained once more to return to civilian life, corresponds better both to reality and to how military personnel see their symptoms. This would be a beneficial adjustment to the inflated pathologizing of post-traumatic suffering that currently appears to be occurring.

MORAL BOUNDARY SETTING

The boundaries between disordered and natural conditions are not simply conceptual or diagnostic issues. In addition, they can often become *morally* charged. Conflicts over diagnoses, illustrated most sharply in the case of schizophrenia, usually involve patients who reject psychiatric labels that are imposed on them. In contrast, conflicts over PTSD labels usually pit sufferers and their advocates who embrace this diagnosis against those who dispute whether or not they are truly disordered. Seemingly mundane issues involving decisions over statistical techniques, categorization rules, and symptom definition become intensely charged clashes between forces of good and evil. On one side, proponents demonize cynics who question the validity of PTSD diagnoses. On the other side, opponents decry the extension of victimized statuses to ever-widening groups of people.

This conflict stems from the unique status of the PTSD diagnosis, which displaces blame for psychological distress from victims to circumstances or people that are held responsible for the traumatic event. By rooting symptoms in a cause external to sufferers, PTSD can deflect blame from the individual, lead to therapeutic help, and (often) bring monetary compensation and other rewards. "It is rare," notes psychiatrist Nancy Andreasen, "to find a psychiatric diagnosis that anyone likes to have, but PTSD seems to be one of them."[82] Other psychiatric diagnoses rarely involve issues where the drawing of boundaries is not just a matter of diagnostic convenience but also an issue of justice and injustice.

Initial Conflicts

Moral contestation over psychological injuries arising from traumas emerged simultaneously with traumatic diagnoses themselves. Foreshadowing future controversies, victims of railway accidents sued railroad companies in efforts to gain monetary rewards for psychic conditions, which they called "railway spine," that they attributed to train crashes; the railroad companies in turn denied that crash victims could experience purely psychological effects of traumas unless they were already predisposed to develop them. In 1866 the eminent British surgeon John Erichsen wrote the first text on railway spine, claiming that nervous shocks deserved compensation no less than more precisely demonstrable physical symptoms.[83] In the same year, a cynical reviewer of Erichsen's text noted:

> The only differences which . . . are to be found between railway and other injuries are purely incidental and relate to their legal aspects. A man, whose spine is concussed on a railway, brings an action against the company, and does or does not get heavy damages. A man, who falls from an apple-tree and concussed his spine, has—worse luck for him— no railway to bring an action against.[84]

Others claimed that the distinctiveness of diagnoses of railway spine was "due, not to the specific peculiarities of train accidents, but to the annoying litigation and exorbitant claims for pecuniary damage that are constantly the grave result of their existence."[85] The unique aspect of railway spine, according to skeptics, was that unlike other diagnoses it led to monetary rewards.

Moral contestations continued during the world wars of the twentieth century in struggles between mentally damaged soldiers and military officers who accused them of cowardice. Shell shock and combat neuroses affected millions of men and had major impacts on armies' ability to conduct warfare. Most military officers and politicians as well as many psychiatrists felt that psychological damage from combat was a product of cowardice and malingering, which could be overcome only through harsh discipline. In a famous incident in 1943, General George S. Patton visited a military hospital in Sicily. Responding to a young soldier who identified himself as a psychiatric casualty, Patton slapped the soldier across the face, proclaiming "You're just a goddamned coward."[86]

Skeptics believed that normal individuals would naturally recover from traumas without long-term effects, while the minority of men who developed chronic disorders likely had constitutional predispositions to become mentally ill and used their premorbid weaknesses to exploit the availability of public pensions.[87] Other psychiatrists, however, found no evidence of pre-existing personal weaknesses and attributed breakdowns to war experiences themselves.[88] Because these debates occurred in the highly charged context of what actions constituted bravery, cowardice, and manliness as well as what sorts of wartime injuries entitled soldiers to receive compensation, they aroused deep moral passions.

Moral conflicts over the PTSD diagnosis began almost as soon as it was introduced into the *DSM* in 1980. As noted above, the initial large study of PTSD rates in the community uncovered quite low rates. The relative rarity of the condition was immediately equated with unsympathetic and hostile attitudes toward trauma sufferers. Veterans Administration psychologists Terence Keane and Walter Penk assailed the authors of the study, psychiatrist John Helzer and sociologist Lee Robins, for estimating that only 1% of the population displayed PTSD:

> We believe that post-traumatic stress disorder . . . is a serious psychiatric condition affecting many men and women who have survived life-threatening events, including combat, rape, political torture, and other disasters that often occur in the course of world events. Its effects should not be minimized.[89]

Findings about the rarity of PTSD are equated with disregard for human misery. Low prevalence rates are taken out of the realm of scientific discourse and placed into the moral sphere, where they are seen as indicating indifference to the victims of horrendous experiences. This initial salvo was a herald of a number of controversies that have accompanied the spread of trauma-related diagnosis.

The amount of PTSD among veterans of military conflict has been a perennial source of controversy. As we have seen, the PTSD diagnosis resulted from advocacy efforts that placed a chronic condition resulting from wartime stressors into the *DSM-III*. In 1983 the U.S. Congress mandated a large, retrospective study, the National Vietnam Veterans' Readjustment Study (NVVRS), which would ascertain the prevalence of PTSD among Vietnam veterans. Launched in the late 1980s, the NVVRS randomly sampled 1,200 male veterans, with additional control samples of non-veterans and women. Because the study used a population sample rather than a sample of veterans who were seeking compensation for PTSD, respondents did not have any obvious incentives to fabricate either traumatic exposures or resulting symptoms from their wartime experiences. Nevertheless, the NVVRS reported extraordinarily high rates of PTSD: 30.9% of veterans had developed PTSD at some point in their life, and an additional 22.5% had developed partial PTSD, so that over half of Vietnam veterans reported signs of PTSD. The study also found an extremely high current (in the late 1980s) PTSD prevalence rate of 15.2%, with an additional 11.1% of veterans reporting current partial PTSD. These figures were especially striking because they stemmed from interviews conducted about twenty years after most respondents would have served in Vietnam.

The rates of PTSD found in the NVVRS seem anomalous in several respects. First, psychiatric casualty rates during the Vietnam War itself were remarkably low compared to previous conflicts. Psychological reasons accounted for fewer than 5% of evacuations of soldiers out of Vietnam from 1965 through 1967, the period of most intense combat.[90] Overall rates of breakdowns during the war were only about 5 per 1000 troops.[91] One study of veterans in the immediate months after their return to the U.S. found that 4.1% had encountered emotional difficulties, a rate no higher than non-veteran controls.[92] These rates compared favorably to previous conflicts: 37 per 1,000 soldiers experienced psychological breakdowns in the Korean War; 70 per 1,000 during World War II.[93] Indeed, some psychiatrists reported that psychiatric casualties in Vietnam were as much as ten times lower than those during World War II.[94] Although the reasons for the rarity of psychopathology during the Vietnam War are not clear, possible factors include improved treatment in combat zones, expectations of quick recovery, and the ready availability of alcohol and illegal drugs as ways of coping with the stresses of war; however, the underreporting of psychiatric casualties may also have played a role.[95]

Nevertheless, enduring rates of chronic PTSD among Vietnam veterans decades later were strikingly higher than those found in veterans of previous wars. One long-term follow-up study found that only 1 of 107 World War II veterans met the

DSM-III criteria for PTSD in 1988.[96] Other long-term studies found that less than 1% of a sample of several hundred male veterans of World War II and the Korean War had a current PTSD diagnosis, and only 1.5% met PTSD lifetime diagnostic criteria.[97] The rates in the NVVRS were far higher than rates during and in the immediate aftermath of the Vietnam War as well as far higher than recorded rates in past wars.

Another anomalous finding in the NVVRS was that rates of PTSD had actually risen with the passage of time since the end of the Vietnam War. Virtually all other studies of traumatic symptoms showed that they develop almost immediately after the trauma and then rapidly decline.[98] No other study showed such high rates of delayed emergence of symptoms. There was no precedent for such elevated amounts of long-term and chronic conditions.

An additional anomaly was that only about 15% of Vietnam veterans had served in combat units whose members should be especially prone to develop PTSD; an additional 15% served in combat support roles. Thus, the number of soldiers stricken with PTSD appeared to be far higher than the number who actually faced combat. The NVVRS rates, if consistent with the notion that PTSD must result from some direct or indirect exposure to combat, required that virtually every veteran who served in a combat or combat support role developed PTSD. Finally, the NVVRS figures were much higher than those found in previous studies of Vietnam veterans. One study by the Center for Disease Control, the Vietnam Experience Study (VES), reported a current prevalence rate of only 2.2%, about seven times lower than the NVVRS.[99] For many reasons, the amount of PTSD in the NVVRS study seemed to be implausibly high.

In 2006 social psychologist Bruce Dohrenwend and colleagues published a reanalysis of the NVVRS data that used more rigorous methods.[100] This reanalysis found rates of PTSD that were 40% less than the NVVRS estimates. Lifetime estimates dropped from 30.9% to 18.7%, and current prevalence (meaning prevalence in the late 1980s) fell from 15.2% to 9.1%. These figures, although considerably lower than those of the NVVRS, still indicated substantial rates of PTSD among Vietnam veterans. They also confirmed that higher exposure to combat situations was the most important predictor of PTSD, so dissimulation of symptoms was unlikely to account for the initial NVVRS results.

The extreme range of prevalence estimates in studies of Vietnam veterans, varying from 2.5% to 9.1% to 15.2%, comes from setting different cut points for the boundaries between natural and pathological symptoms. When researchers apply the same cut points to the VES and the NVVRS data, they find very similar estimates. For example, the VES mandated that all symptoms had to be connected to the traumatic event, whereas the NVVRS required that only intrusive symptoms needed to have such a connection.[101] A second source of variance depends on whether recall of symptoms is based on a one-month or six-month framework. When comparable scoring procedures are used, prevalence rates from both studies produce similar results: strict cut points produce estimates of 2.9% and 2.5% and broad cut-point estimates of 15.8% and 12.2% in the NVVRS and VES, respectively.[102]

Another major source of the varying results stems from decisions about how much impairment PTSD symptoms must cause to be considered pathological. The NVVRS, following *DSM-III* criteria, did not require any impairment to be present for a diagnosis to be made. Symptoms could be pathological even if they were not impairing. The Dohrenwend et al. re-estimation required that symptoms were more than slightly impairing, such that pathological symptoms involved "[s]ome difficulty in social, occupational, or school functioning, but generally functioning pretty well, has some meaningful interpersonal relationship OR some mild symptoms (e.g., depressed mood and mild insomnia, occasional truancy, or theft with the household)."[103] When researchers adjusted for the degree of impairment and documentation of combat exposure, lifetime rates of PTSD fell from 22.5% to 18.7% and current rates declined from 12.2% to 9.1%. This represented a 40% drop in current PTSD from the initial estimates.

Psychologist Richard McNally, a commentator on the Dohrenwend et al. reanalysis, noted that even this drop meant that veterans who were "functioning pretty well" were considered to be suffering from the disorder of PTSD.[104] He showed how if the boundary for impairment is moved one more step on the scale to be "[m]oderate difficulty in social occupational, or school functioning OR moderate symptoms (e.g., few friends and conflicts with peers, flat affect and circumstantial speech, occasional panic attacks),"[105] then the original 15.8% rate, which dropped to 9.1% in the Dohrenwend reanalysis, falls to just 5.4%, a 65% drop from the original estimate.

This seemingly esoteric debate over methodological decision rules became embroiled in passionate moral struggles. Placing a cut point at "moderate" rather than at "some" impairment was viewed as denying the suffering of deserving victims. The defenders of the NVVRS analysis accused the critics of "reliance solely on anecdotal evidence," while their own analysis involved "careful consideration of multiple well-validated measures that involved multiple assessment methods."[106] Traumatologists scorned McNally's analysis and questioned his truthfulness.[107] In fact, each party simply used a different decision rule for how much impairment a diagnosis of PTSD should require. Behind the employment of scientific rhetoric was a deeply moralistic intent to show that critics of the NVVRS found PTSD to be a "minor problem" where the "real problem is veterans faking combat exposure and PTSD symptoms to qualify for service-connected disability."[108]

Is the prevalence of PTSD among Vietnam veterans 15.2%, 9.1%, 5.4%, or 2.5%? The answer is that, first, many of these reactions almost certainly represent the normal suffering and challenges of re-adaptation to civilian life that go along with military service and deserve our attention and support but are not disorders. But, second, we have insufficient knowledge of the nature of our minds to establish precisely which if any of these represents the *true* prevalence of PTSD, and it may be that no such identifiable true prevalence can be confidently established without much greater understanding.

In any case, it seems certain that the boundaries of PTSD are inherently fuzzy. There is no correct general answer to whether moderate, mild, or no impairment should be required for a diagnosis, because normal and pathological conditions can be impairing, and the degree of impairment must be considered in context to discern what it suggests about the condition. The results of decisions about whether to link all or just some symptoms to stressors, the length of time that symptoms must endure, and how impairing they must be are attempts to formulate indicators of some theorized internal dysfunction that we know little about, that may not even exist, and that, if it does exist, is surely not sharply delineated. While some of these rules might be more or less defensible than others, each rests on theoretical assumptions about the nature of normal behavior under stress and on diagnosticians' preferences for certain kinds of rules. Nevertheless, in the context of diagnosing PTSD, they become infused with morally charged questions about right and wrong ways to help suffering people.

9/11

The response of traumatologists to questions about the extent of PTSD after the terrorism of 9/11 echoes Keane and Penk's attacks that questioned the apparent rarity of PTSD in the initial studies of this condition. In one study, psychologist Richard McNally and epidemiologist Naomi Breslau cited the evidence mentioned above that showed a drastic decline in rates of mental disorder in the wake of 9/11 such that less than 1% of Manhattan residents reported PTSD six months after the attack.[109] Moreover, most people in this small group already had diagnosed mental disorders before the attack. The vast majority who reported possible symptoms of PTSD soon after 9/11 were in all likelihood undergoing normal, transient distress responses.

Psychiatrist Randall Marshall, an editor of the volume in which Breslau and McNally's chapter appeared, was incredulous, asking, "Where does one begin to respond to Breslau and McNally's assertion that there 'was no mental health epidemic after 9/11'?" He compares their claims to "conspiracy theorists who believed the moon landings had actually been elaborately staged." Marshall goes on to accuse these scholars of not just scientific but also moral failure:

> It is unfortunate, but this chapter abandons the basic principle that mental health scientists should concern themselves with recognizing and responding to public health needs. The ethical consequences of minimization or outright denial of human suffering after large scale traumatic events are profound. (It) was perhaps inevitable that an event with profound political consequences from the start would become politicized.[110]

For Marshall, the issue that 9/11 was responsible for high rates of PTSD is settled for most scientists. "If we are committed to the scientific process," he notes, "our definition of trauma should derive from empirical findings and aim to maximize recognition of treatable psychiatric disorders."[111] Marshall equates a high prevalence of PTSD with "science" while at the same time counting such common problems as sleep difficulties, worries about future terrorist attacks, and reluctance to fly on airplanes as indicators of "PTSD." Worse, he accuses people who question such loose boundaries of being "non-scientific."

In fact, Marshall and other traumatologists use "science" as a *moral* boundary to accuse those who do not agree with cut points that establish high prevalence rates of being indifferent to suffering. Yet, in the absence of any sound definition of disorder, there is no "scientific" way to demarcate the boundaries between disordered and natural responses to trauma. Marshall's values lead him to desire to "maximize recognition of treatable psychiatric disorders," which he justifies as being committed to "the scientific process." He invokes science to justify his value commitment. His use of science, however, is not as a commitment to objective inquiry but as a moral bludgeon to discredit those who disagree with him.

Child Sexual Abuse

Controversies over the traumatic effects of sexual abuse also display the intensely moral conflicts that can arise over the boundaries of psychological disturbance. Child sexual abuse, in particular, has such high moral valence that it might seem to lead inevitably to traumatic consequences. A study that attempted to show that this morally loaded trauma was in fact a quite heterogeneous type of stressor with a variety of psychological consequences turned out to be the most notorious study in the history of the American Psychological Association (APA).[112]

Psychologists Bruce Rind, Philip Tromovitch, and Robert Bauserman conducted an analysis, published in the APA journal *Psychological Bulletin*, that examined all 59 studies that looked at the psychological consequences of reported child sexual abuse among students who were currently in college. Their goal was to show how a seemingly unitary category, child sexual abuse (CSA), was actually extremely varied. For example, most researchers used legal definitions of CSA that encompassed both the rape of a 5-year-old girl by her father and the willing sexual involvement of a 15-year-old boy with an 18-year-old girl. While some events defined as CSA would undoubtedly be traumatic, many others would not necessarily be so. The authors expected that the very broad range of CSA experiences should lead to a wide variety of psychological consequences among students who reported them. They predicted that violent and/or unwanted abuse experiences would have long-lasting effects but that consensual actions, which were legally but not subjectively defined as abusive, would have no enduring negative impacts.

The review found that college students reporting CSA events were only slightly more psychologically maladjusted than those who had not experienced them. Two-thirds of males, although only about a quarter of women, actually reported neutral or positive reactions to their "abuse" experiences. Indeed, over a third of men found that their experiences were *positive* at the time they occurred. The authors concluded that definitions of traumatic stressors should not rely on heterogeneous legal categories but should be limited to those with harmful and unwanted occurrences.

Several months after the study was published, radio talk show host Dr. Laura Schlessinger condemned it on several broadcasts. Her attacks mushroomed, and a number of conservative groups denounced not only the study but also the APA itself for advocating child sexual abuse. Then-Majority Whip Tom DeLay of the House of Representatives called for formal action against the APA because of its advocacy for "normalizing pedophilia." The panicked CEO of the APA, Raymond Fowler, commended DeLay for his "strong personal and professional commitment to the serious problem of child abuse" and continued, "the sexual abuse of children is a criminal act that is reprehensible in any context. . . . It is the position of the Association that sexual activity between children and adults should never be considered or labeled as harmless or acceptable."[113] Among other concessions, Fowler guaranteed Delay that in the future APA journal editors would "fully consider the social policy implications of articles on controversial topics." The House unanimously voted 355 to 0 to condemn the article, followed by a unanimous voice vote in the Senate. "We know of no other prior instance," wrote two officers of the APA, "in which a specific scientific article has been singled out for censure in a congressional resolution or a scientific organization chastised for publishing it."[114]

Boundary-setting for traumatic events thus can become an ethical issue that involves right and wrong positions. Traumas are morally charged categories that are incompatible with notions of fuzzy boundaries and ambiguous psychic impacts. In the past, skeptics who considered sufferers of trauma to be malingerers or cowards predominated. At present, advocates of widespread trauma occupy the moral high ground. They associate narrow boundaries with victim-blaming and broad ones with support for the traumatized. At the extreme, scholars who question the broad boundaries of PTSD diagnoses, such as psychologist Elizabeth Loftus and literary critic Elaine Showalter, have received death threats.[115] While the moral valence of PTSD has shifted away from its skeptics toward its advocates, the ongoing controversies it creates have deep roots that go well beyond any narrow scientific dispute.

CONCLUSION

In one sense, PTSD exemplifies the general expansion of perceived psychopathology in recent decades. Its spread, however, results from unique factors that mark it as an especially characteristic condition of late twentieth and early twenty-first century life in Western societies. It is difficult to connect growing rates of PTSD to any actual rise in the symptoms connected to the diagnosis. Overall, wars, natural disasters, violent crime, accidents, sexual abuse, and other widespread causes of PTSD have been no more common during this period compared to most of human history. Nor is it plausible to connect growing knowledge about the psychopathological impact of such traumas to rising rates of PTSD diagnoses: knowledge about natural and disordered responses to traumas has not increased in recent years. "There is," notes psychiatrist Simon Wessely, "probably little we could now teach either the Regimental Medical Officers of the First World War, or the psychiatrists of the Second, about the psychological effects of war."[116] It remains extraordinarily difficult to separate normal from pathological reactions because severe distress expectably accompanies extreme stressors.

Instead, changes in diagnostic criteria and in the surrounding culture, including the formation of advocacy movements, account for expanding rates of PTSD. The PTSD diagnosis originated in a particular historical situation to meet the needs of Vietnam-era veterans and other victims of extraordinarily stressful situations. It subsequently came to embrace a far broader range of traumatic situations, to incorporate subjective responses, and to expand the types of symptoms indicative of traumatic effects. These changes resulted primarily from efforts of clinicians and researchers who seek to broaden the range of people who should receive mental health services and secondarily from the greater willingness of trauma victims to define themselves as needing such services. The rhetoric surrounding PTSD, which links the diagnosis to suffering, victimhood, and service need, is especially conducive to promoting its growth. In the current cultural climate, these moral claims have been easily expanded to a growing number of groups. Unfortunately, advances in treating the suffering that stems from life's terrors have not matched the increasing numbers of people who are seen as in need of mental health services to help them cope with an ever-increasing range of negative circumstances classified as traumas.

CHAPTER 8

The Transformation of Anxiety into Depression[1]

Earlier chapters have used an evolutionary perspective to distinguish normal from disordered anxiety conditions. We argued that the separation of genuine anxiety disorders from natural anxiety that no longer fits current social conditions can help prevent the widespread pathologization of anxiety. However, conceptual adequacy is hardly the only—or even the primary—determinant of how diagnoses are actually formulated. In fact, conceptions of mental disorders are collective cultural entities whose meanings, practices, and importance fluctuate over time and with changing social circumstances.[2] Their social significance waxes and wanes depending on such factors as professional norms, economic incentives, media portrayals, scientific and diagnostic fashions, and interest group pressures. In addition, the emphasis placed on any particular type of mental illness depends on its relative significance compared to the attention that other types of mental health problems receive.

Anxiety conditions were at the forefront of medical and psychiatric, as well as cultural, attention in the United States during the post-World War II era. The poet W. H. Auden's phrase "Age of Anxiety" famously captured the dominant aspect of the fear and malaise afflicting the population at the time. The most recent community surveys show that anxiety is still the most widespread mental health problem and that treatment for anxiety conditions is growing.[3] Nevertheless, since the 1970s, depression—considered to be a rare disease in the post-World War II period—has supplanted anxiety as the focus of mental health treatment, research, and public attention.[4] This chapter considers the oscillating importance of anxiety and, in particular, the puzzle of why depression rather than anxiety became the emblematic mental health condition of our age after the publication of the *DSM-III* in 1980. It also briefly addresses the possibility that there will soon be a swing back to an emphasis on anxiety disorders.

ANXIETY AND THE STRESS TRADITION

The stress tradition encompasses a diffuse and multifaceted array of psychic, somatic, and interpersonal problems that often arise as responses to the strains of everyday life.[5] The common psychological features of these problems include a mélange of symptoms involving nervousness, sadness, and malaise. The typical physical symptoms consist of headaches, fatigue, back pain, gastrointestinal complaints, and sleep and appetite difficulties, often accompanying struggles with interpersonal, financial, occupational, and health concerns. These complaints account for a large proportion of cases found in outpatient psychiatric and, especially, in general medical treatment.

Since the discovery around the late 1700s of fibers composing the nervous system, professionals and laypeople alike were likely to call this varied combination of symptoms problems of "nerves," emphasizing the somatic side of complaints.[6] General physicians were typically the frontline responders to anxiety conditions that involved somatic components, using alcohol, opiates, and a variety of patent medications to palliate the array of nervous symptoms.[7] Primary responses to psychic problems without somatic components often included prayer or talking with friends, clergy, or physicians.[8]

For much of the twentieth century, the equally amorphous term "stress" captured the same heterogeneous range of psychic and somatic conditions.[9] During this era, anxiety and its siblings "nervous disease" or "neuroses" became the central themes of what came to be called the "stress" tradition.[10] In the first half of this century, two general views reflected how stress operated, both of which focused upon anxiety. One school, reflecting a strong Freudian influence, identified "stress" with "neuroses" that were considered psychosocial as opposed to medical problems.[11] The second school, rooted in the work of biologist Walter Cannon and physiologist Hans Selye, emphasized the biological roots of stress reactions.[12] Selye termed the multitudinous consequences of stress the "General Adaptation Syndrome," indicating the wide array of conditions that fell into this domain. Both stress traditions focused on anxiety as their central component, although they also featured relatively mild forms of unhappiness and low mood.

In contrast to this focus on anxiety, before the 1970s depression was usually considered a relatively rare condition involving feelings of intense meaninglessness and worthlessness, often accompanied by vegetative and psychotic symptoms and preoccupations with death and dying.[13] Moreover, depression was more likely to be associated with hospitalized patients than with the clients of general physicians or outpatient psychiatrists. But beginning in the 1970s and continuing into the present, "depression" rather than "anxiety" has become the common term used to indicate the set of common psychic and somatic complaints associated with the stress tradition. Depression now dominates clinical practice, treatment, and research as well as images of mental health problems in the broader culture.[14]

Why did depression replace anxiety as the featured condition in outpatient diagnosis and treatment—as well as in the public consciousness—during the last part of the twentieth century? It is difficult to even imagine any "real" cause—whether biological, psychological, or social—that would explain why the actual prevalence of one condition has risen at the same time as the other has fallen during this time period. Instead, several factors, including changing norms of psychiatric classification, professional and political advantage, and economic organization and marketing, came together toward the end of the twentieth century to transform an "age of anxiety" into an "age of depression."

THE TRANSFORMATION OF ANXIETY INTO DEPRESSION

Before the 1970s, "anxiety" was the common term used to capture the nonspecific nature of the most common mental health problems seen in outpatient psychiatry and general medical practices.[15] During this period, the cultural conception of anxiety was not so much a particular type of psychiatric illness as a general psychic consequence of the demands and pace of modern conditions of life. Dominant theories emphasized how a variety of psychosocial stressors, especially family- and work-related problems, caused "stress," "nerves," and "tension," which were all manifestations of anxiety. The ubiquitous nature of anxiety made it the most symbolic condition of American society, as well as of psychiatry, in the post-World War II era.

Anxious patients were especially likely to be found in the offices of general physicians. As Karl Rickels, a leading expert on the treatment of psychiatric problems in primary medical care, noted in 1968, "An abundance of tensions, fears, worries and anxieties confront mankind today, and, in fact, anxiety is seen in the majority of patients visiting the physician"[16] One overview of the kinds of problems found in general medical practice asked the question "What illnesses are being treated?" and answered, "Most of what primary care physicians see, they label 'anxiety.'"[17]

Anxiety conditions also dominated the presentation of problems in outpatient psychiatric practices. Psychiatric diagnoses in the *DSM-I* (1952) and *DSM-II* (1968) reflected the centrality of the "psychoneuroses," which were grounded in anxiety. In 1962, for example, anxiety was the most prevalent psychoneurotic condition: according to the *National Disease and Therapeutic Index*, about 12 million patients received diagnoses of anxiety reactions compared to just 4 million with diagnoses of neurotic depression.[18] One large study at the time indicated that three-quarters of neurotic patients received some anxiety diagnoses, whereas most of the rest were simply considered "neurotic." In contrast, depression was "absent from the diagnostic summaries."[19]

The global conception of stress-related problems in the 1950s and 1960s affected mental health research as well as treatment, so the most prevalent categories of research in the major psychiatric journals explored both general topics (e.g., behavioral science) and policy issues (e.g., mental health services).[20] Particularly during the last half of the 1960s, these journals featured publications using a psychosocial framework. Research on mental problems in the community also relied on measures that reflected a nonspecific view of psychic disturbance, although they emphasized symptoms of anxiety.[21] But because depression was associated with psychotic symptoms, epidemiological surveys rarely featured questions about this condition.

In addition, the prevailing drug treatments during the 1950s and 1960s were also directed at conditions that were considered to reflect problems of "anxiety." A revolution in the treatment of mental health problems had begun in the 1950s when the development of meprobamate (Miltown) created the first mass market for the treatment of generalized stress.[22] Miltown was called a "tranquilizer" and was marketed for the relief of anxiety, tension, and stress associated with anxiousness and its accompanying somatic symptoms.

Miltown became the most popular prescription drug in U.S. history. By 1965 physicians and psychiatrists had written 500 million prescriptions for it, and as early as 1960 about three-quarters of all American physicians were prescribing Miltown.[23] By the late 1960s, the spectacular success of the benzodiazepine Librium, which was introduced in 1960, displaced Miltown. In turn, Valium succeeded Librium as a blockbuster anti-anxiety drug, becoming the single most prescribed drug of any sort. By 1973, 20% of all women and 8% of all men reported using a minor tranquilizer each year.[24]

During the 1950s and much of the 1960s, the concept of "depression" barely existed for submelancholic conditions, and "antidepressant" medications were reserved mainly for serious depressive conditions found among hospitalized patients.[25] In the *DSM-I* and *DSM-II*, non-psychotic forms of depression were conceived of as a defense mechanism that allayed underlying feelings of anxiety. In contrast, these manuals prominently featured depressive psychoses. "Thus, in these years," according to epidemiologist Jane Murphy and psychiatrist Alexander Leighton, "depression was usually thought of as a psychotic rather than a neurotic disorder."[26] General physicians rarely prescribed antidepressants, which were far overshadowed by tranquilizers in the public consciousness. Because physicians and psychiatrists treated less severe forms of depression with the minor tranquilizers, no market existed for antidepressant drugs aimed at depressive conditions that were not very serious. Depression was also of relatively minor importance in American popular magazines. "In the 1960s," reports historian Laura Hirshbein, "there were three times as many articles about anxiety as there were about depression."[27]

Then, in the 1960s, clinicians and researchers started to pay more attention to depression, particularly emphasizing its prevalence among patients in primary medical care.[28] This led advertisers to begin to place ads for the antidepressant tricyclics and monoamine oxidase inhibitors (MAOIs) in medical and psychiatric journals. By the end of the decade, the disparity between anxiety and depressive diagnoses had narrowed, although anxiety was still far more common than depression. Depressive diagnoses in outpatient treatment grew to 8 million, whereas those of anxiety remained at around 12 million.[29]

Treatment statistics during the 1970s reflected a growing interest in depression. In the decade's first half, the management of depression became as common as that of anxiety, and by 1975 the 18 million diagnoses of depression surpassed the 13 million diagnoses of anxiety.[30] From 1980 to the present, the upward trajectory of depressive diagnoses has been especially apparent. Between 1987 and 1997, the proportion of the U.S. population receiving outpatient treatment for conditions that were called "depression" increased by more than 300%.[31] In 1987, 0.73 persons per 100 adults in the U.S. were treated for depression, but by 1997, these rates had leaped to 2.33 per 100. Twenty percent of patients in outpatient treatment in 1987 had a diagnosis of some kind of mood disorder, mostly major depressive disorder (MDD); depressive diagnoses nearly doubled by 1997 to account for 39% of all patients in this setting.

In contrast, the rates of any anxiety diagnosis among treated patients rose much more slowly, from 10.5% in 1987 to 12.5% in 1997.[32] By 1996–1997, diagnoses of mood disorders were more than three times as common as anxiety diagnoses in office-based psychiatry.[33] A large study of psychiatric practice conducted in 1997 by the American Psychiatric Association is illustrative, finding that over half of patients had mood disorders and about a third had a principal diagnosis of MDD, whereas just 10% had received a diagnosis of some anxiety disorder.[34]

Recent figures present a mirror image of the overwhelming dominance of anxiety in general medicine and psychiatry during the 1950s and 1960s. In 2002, 51.7 million outpatient visits were for mental health care. Depression accounted for 21 million of these, compared to only 6.2 million for anxiety.[35] Likewise, by the early part of the twenty-first century, general physicians were more than twice as likely to make diagnoses of depression as anxiety.[36] In sharp contrast to depressive diagnoses' much faster growth than anxiety diagnoses, epidemiological studies indicate that rates of anxiety actually grew faster than rates of depression from the early 1990s through the early 2000s. Whereas the lifetime prevalence of depression was basically stable during this period and actually declined slightly from 17.3% to 16.6%, the comparable prevalence of anxiety rose from 22.8% to 28.8%.[37] Whatever actual problems people sought mental health care for, the treatment system and, in all likelihood, the patients themselves were calling them "depression." For example, depression is the single most common topic of online searches for pharmaceutical and medical products, attracting nearly 3 million unique visitors over a three-month period in 2006.[38]

The takeover of the stress marketplace by the "antidepressant" class of selective serotonin reuptake inhibitor (SSRI) medications strengthened the association between common mental health problems and depression. When the SSRIs came on the market in the late 1980s, anti-anxiety drugs were about twice as likely to be prescribed in outpatient visits as were antidepressants.[39] But at that point, the trends changed abruptly. Between 1985 and 1993–1994, prescriptions for anti-anxiety drugs plunged from 52% to 33% of all psychopharmacological visits; the number of users of anti-anxiety drugs grew very slowly after that, rising from 5.5 million to 6.4 million in 2001.[40]

Conversely, from 1996 to 2001, the number of users of SSRIs increased rapidly, from 7.9 million to 15.4 million. By 2000, antidepressants were the best-selling category of drugs of any sort in the United States; fully 10% of the U.S. population was using an antidepressant.[41] In fact, these drugs were used so widely in general medical practice that in 2003–2004, 310 of every 1000 female patients received a prescription for an antidepressant.[42] Prescriptions for SSRIs continued to grow: by 2006, Americans had received over 227 million antidepressant prescriptions, an increase of more than 30 million since 2002.[43] Antidepressants were prescribed for mood and anxiety disorders alike, gaining unchallenged control of the market once held by the anxiolytic drugs.[44]

The conditions and treatments of the stress tradition thus underwent a widespread transformation between 1955 and the present. The heyday of anxiety during the 1950s and 1960s was followed by its steep decline beginning in the 1970s, a decline that accelerated during the 1980s and 1990s and increased more gradually in the early 2000s. Over the past half-century, those mental health conditions in physicians' offices, psychiatric clinics, research, and popular culture that were seen as problems of "anxiety" came to be called "depression." Likewise, antidepressants replaced anxiolytics for their treatment. What factors account for this major relabeling of mental health problems?

HOW DEPRESSION CAPTURED THE STRESS MARKETPLACE

Diagnostic Specificity

Diagnostic specificity has been the master trend in the recent history of psychiatric classification. For most of history, only a few imprecise categories such as mania, melancholia, and hysteria were used to describe severe psychiatric conditions. No distinct diagnoses or treatments were given for common mental conditions that did not feature serious symptoms. But during the twentieth century, scientific norms increasingly demanded that medicine and psychiatry treat specific diseases. "This modern history of diagnosis," according to historian Charles Rosenberg, "is inextricably related to disease specificity, to the notion that diseases can and should be thought of as entities existing outside the unique manifestations of illness in particular men and women: during the past century especially, diagnosis, prognosis, and treatment have been linked ever more tightly to specific, agreed-upon disease categories."[45]

The stress tradition's variable and fluctuating mixture of psychic distress, somatic problems, and life difficulties lacked the diagnostic specificity needed to give disease entities medical legitimacy. Although pure forms of anxiety and depression do exist, they are the exceptions rather than the rule. Indeed, the co-presence of symptoms of anxiety and depression is far more common than isolated forms of each condition; for example, more than two-thirds of people with major depression also report an anxiety disorder.[46] Nevertheless, beginning in the 1970s, intense pressures were placed on the psychiatric profession to embrace as the standard for definitions of their subject matter the norms of diagnostic specificity accepted in the rest of medicine.

Before the 1970s, the ill-defined, amorphous, and protean conditions that patients brought to general physicians and mental health specialists did not pose a major problem for the psychiatric profession. The supremacy of psychodynamic perspectives meant that diagnostic norms did not dictate sharply bounded, discrete categories of disorder. Instead, explanations emphasized unconscious mechanisms that were not specific to particular symptoms.[47] For example, the *DSM-II* definition of the psychoneuroses stated, "Anxiety is the chief characteristic of the neuroses. It may be felt and expressed directly, or it may be controlled unconsciously and automatically by conversion, displacement and various other psychological mechanisms."[48] In addition, although analysts distinguished a variety of disorders, their treatments were not specific to particular conditions. Moreover, at the time, most clients paid directly for their therapy, so there were no third-party payers to require specific diagnoses. Neither theoretical nor financial concerns forced psychiatry to differentiate among various types of disorders.

During the 1970s, however, this situation began to change rapidly as demands for specificity placed tremendous pressure on psychiatry to alter its diagnostic system. Generalized conceptions—whether "psychoneuroses," "stress," or "nerves"—became a millstone around the neck of the psychiatric profession (although they remained common in popular discourse). The unreliability of the *DSM-II*'s cursory diagnoses subjected psychiatry to much criticism and ridicule, and even questions about its legitimacy. Prominent critics such as Thomas Szasz mocked psychiatry because it could not even define its central domain of "mental illness." Others, like D. L. Rosenhan, conducted highly publicized studies purporting to show that psychiatric labeling worked to hospitalize people who were not sick at all.[49] Psychiatry was under attack from many fronts, including the libertarian right, the Marxist left, and feminists, all of whom focused on its perceived suppression of individual freedom.

Discontent was growing as well among members of the psychiatric establishment as stinging critiques from its own ranks questioned its knowledge base. Many academic studies, most prominently the U.S.–U.K. Diagnostic Project that systematically compared the diagnostic practices of American and British psychiatrists, indicated that even the most basic psychiatric categories had an appalling lack of reliability.[50] Moreover, the reigning psychosocial model did not provide a solid grounding for why psychiatrists—as opposed to many other professionals, including clinical psychologists, counselors, social workers, or nurses—should have professional dominance over the treatment of mental illnesses.[51] Psychiatry, which in the twentieth century had always had a shaky position within the prestige hierarchy in medicine, was in danger of losing its legitimacy as a scientific discipline and its authority in the broader culture. It became clear that the maintenance of psychiatric authority depended on replacing the conceptions of "psychoneuroses" and "stress," which were at the heart of the *DSM-II* classificatory system.

The National Institute of Mental Health (NIMH) also faced a serious crisis in the 1970s. During the 1950s and 1960s, the agency had emphasized the study of general personality, developmental, and social issues, which were more closely related to the stress tradition than to specific types of mental illness. It awarded 60% of its grant funding to psychologists and social scientists and less than 40% to psychiatrists and other medical and biological scientists.[52] After Richard Nixon ascended to the presidency in 1969, his administration and Congress began to attack the NIMH for sponsoring research on social problems such as poverty, racism, and violence. Although this type of research accounted for only about a fifth of the institute's portfolio, it was a lightning rod for attacks on its overall mission. Psychosocial research thus had become a political liability in the institute's efforts to secure funding from Congress and the executive branch.[53]

By the late 1970s, biologically oriented researchers had joined the fight against psychosocial research by the NIMH. They were deeply concerned that research on social problems would damage the institute's reputation and subject it to a backlash against all its research programs.[54] These researchers argued that a narrower focus on the study of specific mental disorders would both enhance the quality of scientific research and justify the institute's mission in the face of political opposition.

Around the same time, family advocacy groups became a major lobbying force concerned with the NIMH. These groups, such as the National Alliance for the Mentally Ill, were primarily composed of family members with children suffering from severe mental illnesses. They lobbied the NIMH to shift its focus from broad social research to the study of the biological underpinnings of specific mental disorders and treatments for them. These efforts culminated in a 1982 directive from Congress that ordered the NIMH to stop its support of social research.[55] The transformation from research on general psychosocial problems to specific biologically based diseases was a great success, and beginning in the early 1980s funding for the institute sharply increased.

Another spur toward specificity of diagnosis was the mandate from the Food and Drug Administration (FDA) to the pharmaceutical industry to target psychoactive drugs to specific biomedical conditions.[56] During the 1950s and 1960s, the popularity of the benzodiazepines stemmed from their effectiveness as remedies for general life stresses and protean conditions of anxiety, with little consideration of whether or not they treated explicit disease states. Studies of this period found that only about a third of the minor tranquilizers were prescribed for specific mental disorders, while the rest were given as a response to more diffuse complaints and psychosocial problems.[57] For example, a review of psychoactive medications at the time concluded that "only about 30 percent of use is in identified mental disorders and the remainder covers the rest of medicine."[58] The vocabulary of the era dictated that these drugs would be called "anti-anxiety" or "tranquilizing" drugs, and the problems they treated were considered problems of generalized "anxiety," although they often involved co-occurring depression.

Pharmaceutical companies presented the tranquilizers to physicians and psychiatrists as drugs that treated a variety of nonspecific complaints including anxiety, tension, depression, and mental stress. Advertisements (which at the time were directed at physicians, not consumers) emphasized that these drugs provided relief for such common problems as dealing with unruly children, traffic jams, demanding bosses, and housekeeping.[59] In the 1970s, however, government regula-tors began to enforce more stringently the legislative requirement dating from 1962 that drug companies target the marketing of their products to particular biomedical conditions.[60] In addition, growing coverage by private and public insurance meant that few patients paid the bulk of their insurance costs, and third-party payers reimbursed clinicians only for treating a specific disease. These factors placed pressure on mental health providers to call the conditions they treated "diseases" or "disorders" rather than more amorphous problems of living.

The emphasis on generalized conditions and treatments had been suitable for an era when psychodynamic explanations that emphasized unconscious mechanisms were dominant; the most seriously ill patients, with more specific conditions such as schizophrenia and manic depression, were concentrated in inpatient institutions and so were rarely found in outpatient settings; clients paid for treatment out of their own pockets; and therapies were nonspecific. By 1980, though, it was appar-ent that classifications focusing on specific disease entities were needed to increase psychiatry's professional legitimacy, obtain reimbursement, and meet regulatory standards for prescriptions. For psychiatry, however, the re-categorization of the nebulous conditions in the stress tradition as specific diagnostic entities had to maintain the specialty's ascendant position in the huge market of stress-related con-ditions. The question is why depression rather than anxiety took center stage in psychiatry's reinvention of its classificatory system.

THE RISE OF BIOLOGICAL PSYCHIATRY

Professional competition within psychiatry is one reason for the rise of depression and decline of anxiety as the discipline's central point of reference. Psychodynamically oriented psychiatrists emphasized anxiety-related conditions but paid relatively little attention to depression. During the 1970s, however, a group of biological psychiatrists became intensely concerned with the unscientific nature of psycho-analysis and the damage it was doing to efforts at developing psychiatry as a branch of medicine. Research-oriented psychiatrists who generally favored biological perspectives regarding mental illness led the opposition against the *DSM-II* and its etiologically based and unreliable categories.[61] They were far more interested in studying specific diseases than amorphous stress conditions, and at that time— because of the close connection of anxiety to the psychodynamic tradition— depression was a more effective vehicle than anxiety for biological psychiatrists in realizing their scientific aspirations.[62] "Depression," asserts historian Laura Hirschbein, "became a phenomenon around which professionals in the latter part of the twentieth century made claims about psychiatry."[63]

Depression fit the professionally desirable conception of a severe and specific disease that could be associated with biological causes. Indeed, depression was considered to be a very serious condition connected to suicide and psychosis and thus, for the most part, was outside of the stress tradition.[64] In addition, far more than anxiety, depression was theoretically grounded in brain chemistry and conceptions of chemical imbalances. The two most significant biological articles during the 1960s both explored the relationship between low levels of biogenic amines in the brain and depressive illness.[65] These early breakthroughs cemented the coupling of biological approaches and depressive conditions. The biological grounding of depression heightened its appeal for the research-oriented psychiatrists who were in charge of revising the *DSM* classification system. "Major depression," summarizes historian Edward Shorter, "served the then-nascent field of biological psychiatry in the way that psychoneurosis had once served psychoanalysis."[66]

THE *DSM-III*

Although biological psychiatry and its central vehicle of depression were gaining ground during the 1970s, the implementation of the *DSM-III*, which the American Psychiatric Association issued in 1980 and which we discussed in Chapter 4, was the central turning point leading to the transition from anxiety to depression. The manual radically changed the nature of psychiatric diagnoses, based on the foundational principle that diagnostic criteria should not assume any particular etiology of symptoms. This strategy allowed its advocates to claim theoretical neutrality and so mitigate the opposition of clinicians who did not adhere to the core group's biological orientation.[67] The goal of purging etiological assumptions was especially consequential for the anxiety disorders.

The unifying concept of *DSM-I* and *DSM-II* was that the symptoms of all of the psychoneuroses were defenses against underlying anxiety. A successful attack on this etiological concept required the wholesale destruction of the global concept of anxiety neurosis. As an alternative, the *DSM-III* developed definitions of various specific conditions that emphasized how each was a discrete and qualitatively distinct disease.[68] Unlike the *DSM-I* and *DSM-II*, which had placed both depression and anxiety within the same psychoneurotic category, the *DSM-III* formulated anxious and depressive conditions as completely distinct. It also carved away conditions such as hysteria and hypochondriasis that had previously been core aspects of anxiety-related states, putting them into separate groups. The psychoneuroses were split into four distinct general categories: anxiety disorders, affective disorders, dissociative disorders, and somatoform disorders.

Four particular aspects of the differential definitions of the affective and mood disorders in the *DSM-III* facilitated the desirability of using major depressive disorder (MDD) rather than any single anxiety condition as a diagnosis for what had been considered to be general stress conditions. The first was the very different ways in which the manual differentiated the various conditions of anxiety and depression. As discussed earlier, no single category of anxiety was preeminent. The anxiety classification was divided into phobic, anxiety states, and post-traumatic stress disorder (PTSD), as well as numerous subtypes of each.[69] For example, there were several types of phobias including simple phobia, social phobia, and agoraphobia, which itself was split into conditions that did or did not display panic disorder. Generalized anxiety disorder, which on its face might be viewed as the core anxiety condition, was instead made a residual category to be diagnosed only when symptoms of phobic, panic, or obsessive-compulsive disorders were not present.

Subsequent research on anxiety disorders illustrates the impact of the differentiation of anxiety into a number of disorders without a focus on any particular condition. After 1980, the vast majority (83%) of studies published in psychiatry, psychology, and related fields focused on a single anxiety disorder. These journals featured panic disorder/agoraphobia (36%), PTSD (28%), and OCD (27%) to an almost equal degree. Less than 10% of articles focused on GAD, which had been the central anxiety condition in psychodynamic theory.[70] Current studies of anxiety remain balkanized and without a central focus.[71]

The *DSM-III*'s treatment of depression sharply contrasted with the division of the anxiety disorders into many distinct conditions. Major depressive disorder (MDD) was the only significant category of non-psychotic depression among the affective disorders. Psychotic forms of mood disorders were identified with bipolar disorder, which was the sole psychotic state of any note within the larger affective disorders category. Unipolar states of psychotic depression were virtually indistinguishable from MDD. Melancholic depression—the central depressive condition before the *DSM-III*—became a subcategory of MDD.[72] People could qualify for a diagnosis of melancholy, which required symptoms of greater severity in the morning, early-morning awakening, marked psychomotor retardation, weight loss, and excessive guilt, only if they had already met the MDD criteria. The submersion of melancholia into the broader MDD category ensured its fall into obscurity.[73]

The condition of dysthymia supposedly was created to be a form of minor depression that would contrast with the state of major depression represented by MDD.[74] While the three necessary symptoms of dysthymia (raised to four symptoms in subsequent editions of the manual) might have been a suitable diagnosis for many people with conditions linked to the stress tradition, the diagnosis was given only to those adults whose symptoms had lasted for at least two *years*.[75] This precluded anyone except those with the most long-standing conditions from receiving a diagnosis of dysthymia.

MDD was clearly the singular non-psychotic diagnosis in the affective disorders category, encompassing conditions ranging from melancholia through the depressive neuroses to short, reactive depressions. The MDD symptoms captured both the amorphous and short-lived consequences of psychosocial problems that marked the stress tradition and the serious and chronic conditions that in the past had been associated with melancholic depression.

Research on depression subsequently reflected the overwhelming dominance of the MDD category. Beginning in 1981, MDD began a steep upward trajectory and by 2000 had a citation rate about five times higher than all other depressive labels combined.[76] Citations for conditions of "melancholic," "endogenous," or "psychotic" depression fell dramatically beginning in the early 1980s and had almost disappeared by 2000.[77] Unlike anxiety, with its multiple centers of research and publication, depression was almost completely identified with MDD. Major depressive disorder was unquestionably the core non-psychotic affective disorder, which helped it to replace anxiety as the heir to the stress tradition.

A second reason why depressive diagnoses took over the stress tradition from anxiety had to do with the *DSM-III*'s allocation of the most general symptoms of distress to the different major diagnostic categories. The definition of MDD included such global symptoms as sadness, sleep and appetite difficulties, fatigue, and lack of concentration, which afflicted many people with mental health problems that fell into the stress tradition.[78] The capacious MDD criteria thus could cover a heterogeneous group of people, ranging from irritable adolescents who constantly sleep, overeat, and are uninterested in school to morose elderly people who cannot sleep, eat little, and feel worthless.[79] In contrast, the diagnostic criteria for the various anxiety disorders were far more specific and centered on narrower manifestations such as intense fears of specific objects or situations, obsessions and compulsions, and post-traumatic stress.

The anxiety diagnosis that potentially could have encompassed the generalized aspect of symptoms—generalized anxiety disorder (GAD)—became a mere phantom in the *DSM-III*. The hierarchical system of diagnosis in the *DSM-III* privileged diagnoses of depression over those of anxiety: anxiety diagnoses would not be made in the presence of coexisting depressive disorders. Because of the extensive co-occurrence of depressive and anxious symptoms, this increased the likelihood of making depressive rather than anxiety diagnoses. Moreover, GAD could not be diagnosed in the presence of other anxiety conditions.[80] Because GAD almost always was found together with these conditions, it was rarely diagnosed at all. Finally, the criteria for diagnosing GAD bewildered clinicians. "In fact," psychologist David Barlow summarized, "the category of GAD in *DSM-III* produced so much confusion that few clinicians or investigators could agree on individuals who would meet this definition."[81] The new diagnostic criteria therefore made MDD a more appropriate label than anxiety for the ubiquitous symptoms of stress that so many patients displayed.

Third, the duration criteria for the anxiety conditions were considerably longer than for MDD. Most anxiety conditions required "persistent" symptoms, usually of at least six months duration, which ruled out diagnoses of short-lived responses to stressful conditions.[82] In contrast, symptoms that endured for a mere two weeks met the MDD qualifications.[83] Transient responses to stress, therefore, could meet diagnostic criteria for depression but not anxiety.

Finally, and perhaps most important, the disparate treatment of the contextual basis of anxiety and depression favored diagnoses of depression over those of anxiety. A very high proportion of patients enter mental health and, especially, primary medical care settings with psychosocial problems that are often the proximate reasons for their symptoms. Yet, as we noted, the diagnostic criteria for all of the anxiety diagnoses were hedged with many qualifiers that distinguished them from contextually appropriate symptoms. For example, only "irrational" or "unreasonable" fears qualified for diagnoses of phobia, thus ruling out proportionate and reasonable fears.[84] Or, panic disorders had to occur "unpredictably" and could not be responses to life-threatening situations.[85] The treatment of anxiety according to the *DSM-III*, therefore, ruled out proportionate responses to dangerous situations as possible diagnoses.

In contrast, many patients who were reacting to stressful psychosocial contexts could meet the MDD criteria. Bereavement was the sole relevant exclusionary criterion for depression: people grieving the death of an intimate who otherwise met the MDD criteria would not be so diagnosed as long as their symptoms were not especially severe or long-lasting. But no comparable exclusions were made for those who met the criteria after they were laid off from jobs, rejected by romantic partners, or informed of a serious medical diagnosis for themselves or an intimate. Unlike the diagnostic criteria for the anxiety disorders, the MDD criteria did not preclude diagnoses even when symptoms were proportionate responses to the losses that provoked them. The range of conditions in the stress tradition that featured mixed depressive and anxious symptoms thus became more amenable to depressive than anxiety diagnoses.

Whether the problems that people bring to therapy have changed much over the past half-century is questionable,[86] although their labels have dramatically altered. The *DSM-III* unintentionally created the conditions for depression, rather than anxiety, to incorporate the disparate manifestations of stress and thus become the central diagnosis of the mental health professions. "One of the more irritating consequences of *DSM-III*," complained psychiatrist Donald Klein, a specialist in anxiety disorders, "has been the plague of affective disorders that have descended upon us."[87]

FROM ANXIOLYTICS TO ANTIDEPRESSANTS

A major consequence of the *DSM-III*'s new categorizations was to make depression a more promising target for the new class of antidepressants—the selective serotonin reuptake inhibitors (SSRIs)—that came on the market in the late 1980s. The SSRIs now dominate the treatment of non-psychotic mental disorders, including MDD and the various anxiety disorders as well as many other conditions. In practice, there is little evidence that the SSRIs' efficacy has any relationship to the diagnostic categories in the *DSM*. They act very generally to increase levels of serotonin in the brain that both raise low mood states and lower levels of anxiety, and thus could just as easily have been marketed as anti-anxiety medications.[88]

By the late 1980s, however, it made more sense for companies to market products aimed at a wide array of stress conditions as "antidepressants" rather than as "anti-anxiety" drugs. A backlash against the anxiolytic drugs had developed in the early 1970s when the media turned sharply against their use, showing in many stories their addictive potential, use in suicide attempts, and other negative side effects. In response, patients, with backing by organized advocacy groups, filed numerous lawsuits against the manufacturers of these drugs.[89] In addition, the rise of the feminist movement, which harshly assailed these drugs because of their assumed role in upholding patriarchal norms and keeping women confined in oppressive social roles, was another nail in the tranquilizers' coffin.[90]

The result was, according to historian Edward Shorter, a "general hysteria about addiction from pharmaceuticals that swept American society in the 1970s."[91] Stimulated by hostile congressional hearings, government agencies including the FDA and Drug Enforcement Agency (DEA) confronted the pharmaceutical industry and attempted to restrict the use of the benzodiazepines.[92] This backlash resulted in their classification in 1975 by the DEA as Schedule 4 drugs, which required physicians to report all prescriptions written for them and limited the number of refills a patient could obtain.

Although most psychopharmacologists insisted that the tranquilizing drugs were rarely abused or sources of addiction, the regulatory actions and attendant media publicity destroyed their legitimacy and led to a sharp decline in their use.[93] After twenty years of steadily rising sales since their introduction in the mid-1950s, consumption of the anxiolytic drugs plunged. From a peak of 104.5 million prescriptions in 1973, the number dropped to 71.4 million by 1980 and continued to plummet throughout the 1980s.[94] Pharmaceutical companies had difficulty marketing anti-anxiety drugs. "By the mid-1980s," writes psychopharmacologist David Healy, "it had become impossible to write good news stories about the benzodiazepines."[95] Moreover, because their patents had expired, pharmaceutical companies had no interest in either promoting the anxiolytic drugs or conducting new trials that could show their safety and efficacy.

Despite the growing interest in depression in the 1960s and 1970s, antidepressants did not gain any traction in the general marketplace of drugs and were rarely prescribed in general medical practice, instead usually being reserved for the most seriously ill patients.[96] Despite their relative invisibility compared with tranquilizers, antidepressants had several marketing advantages over the anxiolytic drugs. Unlike the tranquilizers, which became popular because they could be used to treat a wide array of common psychosocial problems of people in the community, the early antidepressant drugs—the tricyclics and MAOIs—were prescribed for the problems of severely depressed populations. This connected them with the newly desirable notions of specificity, in contrast to the tranquilizing drugs' ubiquitous range of effects. In addition, the antidepressants were not linked to the problems of addiction and dependency associated with tranquilizers.[97]

Because the FDA required manufacturers to prove a drug's efficacy for some biomedical condition, the SSRIs could not be marketed for generalized distress, only for specific diseases.[98] In contrast to the many particular anxiety disorders of the *DSM-III*, the unification of depression around the MDD criteria put depression in the best position to encompass the amorphous symptoms of the stress tradition. Given the hostile cultural and regulatory climate toward anti-anxiety drugs when the SSRIs came onto the market in the late 1980s, it made much more marketing sense for manufacturers to promote them as antidepressants than as anti-anxiety agents.

As had so often happened in psychiatric history, the development of a treatment shaped the nature of the illness that it was supposedly meant to treat. Network television shows, national newsmagazines, and best-selling books widely featured the SSRIs as antidepressant medications. In particular, the publication in 1993 of Peter Kramer's wildly popular *Listening to Prozac: A Psychiatrist Explores Antidepressant Drugs and the Remaking of the Self* cemented the coupling of the SSRIs with the treatment of depression.[99] Advertisements for Prozac soon began using the imagery depicted in Kramer's book, using slogans such as "better than well" and showing women cheerfully fulfilling both work and family roles. This imagery differentiated the SSRIs from the clientele of the older antidepressants and positioned this class of drugs as the direct heir of the tranquilizers. Because a drug was called an "antidepressant," depression seemed to be the condition that was being treated. Much as "anxiety" had during the 1950s and 1960s, "depression" came to refer to the disparate experiences of suffering connected to the stress tradition during the 1990s and early 2000s.

The FDA's loosening of restrictions on direct-to-consumer (DTC) drug advertisements in the late 1990s both enhanced the popularity of the SSRIs and reinforced their link to depressive illness. Many of these ads were aimed at selling the disease of depression itself, rather than a particular type of antidepressant.[100] They relentlessly pushed the view that "depression is a disease" linked to deficiencies of serotonin in the brain. Advertisements typically connected the most common symptoms of depression from the *DSM*'s diagnosis—sadness, fatigue, sleeplessness, and the like—with common situations involving interpersonal problems, workplace difficulties, or overwhelming demands, themes similar to the messages of ads in the 1950s and 1960s. What was different is that the psychic consequences of these problems were now being called "depression" instead of "anxiety," "tension," "nerves," or "stress."

THE RETURN OF ANXIETY?

The transition of the age of anxiety into the age of depression demonstrates that diagnoses are contingent upon the impact of changing social circumstances. The emphasis placed on any particular type of mental illness also may be influenced by the relative amount of attention other types of mental health problems receive. If so, the rise (or decline) of one type of diagnosis may lead another type to fall (or increase). There are some signs, in fact, that anxiety could displace depression and recapture its hold on the stress tradition.

Many of the patents for the use of SSRIs to treat depressive conditions have expired, so far cheaper generic drugs are now threatening to take market share and drastically lower the profits derived from the trademarked brands.[101] In addition, the rapid rise of diagnoses of bipolar conditions that are treated with second-generation antipsychotic drugs is fracturing the market for depression treatments. Some mood states that would have been diagnosed as MDD are now called "bipolar" conditions that can be treated with lucrative patent-protected medications.[102] Indeed, by 2008 sales of antipsychotic medication had surpassed those of antidepressants, and they were the most profitable class of any kind of drug.[103] Economic considerations seem likely to drive the pharmaceutical market away from depression as the condition to be treated.

Anxiety should become a particularly attractive target for trademarked SSRIs.[104] As shown in Chapter 6, more than a quarter of the population experiences enough symptoms of anxiety disorders to meet *DSM* criteria, making the group of anxiety disorders the most prevalent of any general category of mental health conditions.[105] As one marketing report points out,

> ...anxiety disorders are considered the most prevalent of psychiatric disorders. However, poor diagnostic rates and treatment outcomes mean there is still considerable scope for manufacturers to move into the anxiety market.... Despite a fifth of the total population across the seven major markets suffering from an anxiety disorder only a quarter of these individuals are diagnosed and therefore treated. As a result, drug manufacturers are failing to maximize revenues from the anxiety disorders market. Investment in awareness campaigns is essential.[106]

The boundaries between depression and anxiety are permeable enough that the same drugs can easily be marketed as responses to anxiety rather than to depression.

While the differentiation of the many forms of anxiety in the *DSM-III* initially enhanced the appeal of the unitary condition of MDD, each form of anxiety now can become a segmented market. For example, in 1999 the FDA approved Paxil for the treatment of social anxiety disorder (SAD) and Zoloft for PTSD; two years later Paxil and Effexor gained approval for the treatment of GAD. Old drugs can seem innovative and up-to-date when they are prescribed for new indications. Different brands can target a variety of specific types of anxiety conditions and capture distinct niches. The extraordinary success of GlaxoSmithKline's efforts to promote Paxil as a treatment for SAD indicates the huge potential of anxiety conditions as pharmaceutical targets. A vast advertising campaign blitzed the media in 1999, shortly after Paxil was approved for treating SAD, which previously had been viewed as a rare disorder. Paxil became the largest selling antidepressant at the time, with sales of $3 billion a year, and consumers now widely recognize social anxiety as a reason to seek drug treatment.

Transformations also may move from the class of antidepressants to that of anxiolytic drugs. The same sort of counter-reaction to the anxiolytic drugs that occurred in the 1970s shows signs of reemerging against the SSRIs, with questions being raised about their efficacy, side effects, potential addictiveness, and safety.[107] If this backlash against the SSRIs grows, drug companies could develop a marketing strategy that will once again emphasize the anxiolytic drugs as first-line treatments for problems of stress. Indeed, while still dwarfed by the antidepressant market, prescriptions for benzodiazepines grew from 69.4 million in 2002 to 80.1 million in 2006.[108]

The diagnosis of depression is also no longer as useful to psychiatry as it was over the past quarter-century. The profession's scientific credibility is now far greater than it was in the 1970s, its diagnostic system is generally regarded as reliable, and its biological models are widely accepted. The reasons for psychiatry's turn away from anxiety—its association with the indefinable category of psychoneurosis, with psychodynamic treatments, and with the presumed addictive nature of the tranquilizers—have long been forgotten, leaving few traces in cultural memory. But anxiety has never gone away, and it will be surprising if such a ubiquitous and universal condition does not once again come to the forefront of the stress tradition.

CONCLUSION

This chapter has addressed an apparent paradox. On the one hand, epidemiological studies consistently show that, taken as a class, anxiety disorders are the most common form of disorder. Moreover, they indicate a sharp rise in the prevalence of this condition since 1980. One would thus expect anxiety to be the most medically treated mental problem, as was markedly the case in the decades before the *DSM-III* appeared. But, on the other hand, over the past few decades, depression has become by far the most treated and discussed condition.

We have suggested that part of the explanation for the paradox lies in the logical structure of the *DSM-III*'s categorization of disorders and the details of its diagnostic criteria. While the manual split anxiety into many distinct conditions, major depression was clearly the central category of mood disorders. Whereas anxiety diagnostic criteria demanded persistent and excessive or unreasonable reactions as a requirement for disorder, major depression's lack of such contextual grounding and its minimal duration requirement rendered it a more suitable diagnosis than anxiety for brief responses to stress. Moreover, depression is given some hierarchical dominance over anxiety disorder diagnosis in the criteria's exclusion clauses. In sum, a major unplanned consequence of the *DSM-III* was a paving of the way for the emergence of depression as the central diagnosis of the psychiatric profession after 1980.

Physicians traditionally described anxiety and depression as commonly occurring together in a matrix of distress symptoms—which makes perfect sense, for sadness about what is happening or has happened is likely to go along with anxiety about what might happen as a result. In a quest for diagnostic purity, the *DSM-III* separated anxiety from depression, but in such a way that depression became the more favored diagnosis for distress responses. Paradoxically, having artificially separated what had always before been recognized as commonly going together, psychiatry now finds itself grappling with the "puzzle" it has created for itself of why these supposedly pure conditions should so frequently be found together, and the developers of the *DSM-5* are considering adding mixed depression-anxiety conditions to the manual.[109]

But the nuances of the *DSM*'s diagnostic criteria cannot solely account for the dramatic and rapid changes we documented in the turn of psychiatry's focus from anxiety to depression. Although psychiatric science strives in the long run to identify natural kinds of etiological processes that form coherent categories that "carve nature at its joints," a variety of social factors influence the precise way these categories are formulated, the boundaries that are drawn in fuzzy areas, and the way the categories are deployed socially. In the case of the shifting emphasis between anxiety and depressive disorders, a variety of professional, economic, regulatory, and cultural factors also helped to shape these changes.

From the latter part of the nineteenth century until the mid-twentieth century, under the influence of psychoanalysis, physicians and psychiatrists often formulated mental health problems as problems grounded in stress, nerves, and anxiety. They rarely saw such conditions as specific disease entities because there was no point to detailed classificatory conceptions in an era where dominant paradigms emphasized nonspecific etiological mechanisms and undifferentiated forms of treatment, and third-party reimbursement was rare. The sociohistorical underpinnings of diagnosis began to change drastically during the 1970s when the unreliability of its undifferentiated conditions threatened the basic legitimacy of the psychiatric profession. Research psychiatrists and government funders of research began to turn their attention to the study of specific disease entities, while the rise of third-party reimbursement reinforced the need to formulate mental health problems into discrete disorders. Moreover, regulatory agencies forced drug manufacturers to prove the efficacy of their products with recognized disease conditions rather than generalized problems of living. At the same time, the attacks on the anxiolytics associated tranquilizers with addiction and negative side effects. When the SSRIs were developed in the 1980s, their consequent marketing as antidepressants meant that physicians and psychiatrists became more likely to call the conditions they treated "depression" as opposed to "anxiety." Depression and antidepressant drugs had captured the vast market of stress-related conditions.

Psychiatric classifications inevitably reflect not only the attempt to identify real and distinct underlying dysfunctions but also the social forces prevailing in any particular historical era.[110] Which conditions are diagnosed and how they are treated will depend not only on the symptoms that patients display but also on factors that include professional fashions in diagnoses, the financial rewards from various treatments, the activities of various interest and regulatory groups, cultural images of disorder, and the concerns of funding agencies. The amorphous psychic, somatic, and interpersonal problems that bedeviled humans long before the emergence of standardized diagnoses will continue to underlie whatever specific labels are used to classify them. However much we strive to make psychiatric classifications reflect natural kinds, given our ignorance of the mechanisms and evolutionary histories underlying these conditions, the deployment of psychiatric categories will inevitably reflect prevailing social and cultural forces.

CHAPTER 9

Setting Boundaries between Natural Fears and Anxiety Disorders

W hen are our fears normal and when do they reveal that something has "gone wrong" with our minds? There is no *precise* answer to this question. In this regard, anxiety is no different from most other mental conditions because the boundaries between mental disorders and normal conditions are usually ambiguous. No sharp lines, for example, divide natural sadness from depressive disorder, attention deficit disorder from boisterousness, or bipolar disorder from ordinary mood swings.

It is, however, especially difficult to distinguish normal anxiety from disordered anxiety conditions. Other normal negative emotional reactions—such as depression that is a proportionate reaction to a loss, restlessness that is a natural response to an overly constraining school environment, or mood swings that are anchored in changing romantic circumstances—tend to appear sensible when understood in context. One might want to medically treat such reactions for practical reasons, but they are not psychiatric disorders. For several reasons, normal anxiety, even when placed in context, does not always make sense as a reasonable response to danger.

First, our fears arise not only to currently real threats but also to genetically programmed situational triggers representing ancient dangers that may no longer pose risks at all in our current circumstances. Fears of wild animals, darkness, or strangers—fears that humans appropriately developed in prehistory—linger within us, although they rarely if ever have much adaptive value under modern conditions, and they often are seriously maladaptive. Second, seemingly unreasonable fears emerge in response to situations or objects that are generally not dangerous but that occasionally pose serious threats to which it is best to rapidly respond (as in the "smoke detector principle") and thus are advantageously feared in general despite their usually benign nature. These fears, too, are often preprogrammed and insensitive to our knowledge, as when we become anxious about being in a high place even when we know that in this instance there is no danger of falling, or we have a pronounced startle response to a harmless shadow.

Third, we respond with fear to situations that posed idiosyncratic threats earlier in our lives and then stuck in our minds, even if they pose no current danger. Fear is biologically designed as a protective mechanism and is highly sensitive to past dangers that people have encountered, so that only in the light of their past history will some of their fears make sense. Finally, the combination of great normal variation in individual anxiety tendencies with the low threshold for the emergence of anxious emotions means that many people have anxious personality dispositions. Such high-end but normal-range personality variation in anxiety responses may seem to those who are calmer to be overly reactive and can readily be confused with anxiety disorder.

Such natural yet seemingly irrational fears may be problematic for us in our current social environments, but they are nevertheless not dysfunctions of psychological mechanisms. They represent how our fear mechanisms were designed to function; nothing has "gone wrong" with our minds. Consequently, understanding the distinction between normal and disordered anxiety requires that we go beyond immediate context to understand both our individual and our species-typical evolutionary history.

When natural anxieties are problematic and unreasonable, it has proven very tempting to characterize them as mental disorders in order to bring medical treatment to bear on the problem. The imprecise borders between natural fears, evolutionary mismatches, nervous personalities, and anxiety disorders have facilitated the drawing of broad boundaries for anxiety disorder because the great degree of fuzziness means that plausible lines between normality and pathology can be drawn in many places. Social institutions, moreover, greatly prize clarity of boundaries and so attempt to draw clear lines among these conditions even where our ignorance makes a precise boundary difficult to justify.[1]

We have argued for five theses regarding the drawing of such boundaries:

1. Despite explicit symptom-based criteria, the boundaries between disorder and non-disorder remain quite ambiguous in diagnostic manuals because natural and pathological anxieties often share the same anxiety symptoms.

2. Considerable normal individual variation in anxiety levels creates difficulties in making any general statements about when the intensity of anxiety must indicate disorder versus high-end personality differences.
3. Even the most meaningful and real distinctions can possess fuzziness at the borders of contrary categories. Just as there is no sharp line between day and night, though they are genuinely different, so the distinction between normal and disordered anxiety can be real even if the boundary is indefinite.
4. Especially when a lack of conceptual clarity exists about a distinction, social values (e.g., the pressure to speak in public) tend to implicitly determine what is seen as the "real" boundary between categories, and these social values may come to be mistaken for a naturally given dividing line. Thus, the inherent ambiguities of drawing boundaries can be exploited to yield expansive disorder categories.
5. Such social pressures and influences can occasionally go beyond simply influencing where an arbitrary boundary is drawn and can sometimes lead to the misclassification of substantial domains of clearly normal cases of fear as mental disorders. Such cases do not just exploit the vagueness of the lines between normal and disordered anxiety but also get the classification grossly wrong and thus mislead patients and the public.

There is nothing wrong with using therapy to help people adjust to social demands. Indeed, this may be a desirable form of what one of us has labeled "psychological justice."[2] However, misrepresenting normal fears as mental disorders is incorrect, undermines informed consent, and erodes an important distinction between social control and treatment of disorder.

The most plausible explanation for the rise in presumed anxiety disorders in recent decades lies in changes in how and where psychiatry decided to draw the line between disorder and non-disorder, encompassing much of what had formerly been the terrain of normal distress. Although psychiatry occasionally demedicalizes a condition, as it did with homosexuality in 1973, it has not generally been responsive to concerns about the dangers of the expanding boundaries of pathology. "Researchers," psychiatrist Robert Spitzer shrewdly notes, "always give maximal prevalence for the disorders that they have a particular interest in. In other words, if you're really interested in panic disorder, you're going to tend to say it's very common. You never hear an expert say, 'My disorder is very rare.' Never. They always tend to see it as more common."[3] In addition, because of the seemingly technical nature of the *DSM* diagnostic criteria, other institutions generally take psychiatry's expansive diagnostic criteria as unchallengeable "givens." Moreover, expanded boundaries of pathology were carried into the community population via epidemiological studies rather than being limited to clearly disordered treated populations. It is unlikely that the revisions planned for the forthcoming *DSM-5* will do much to remedy this situation.

THE *DSM-5*

Why won't the *DSM-5* help matters? The work group on anxiety disorders for *DSM-5* has made a good-faith attempt to improve the anxiety disorders criteria and has made many modest improvements. However, it has approached the revision of these criteria sets without an adequate conceptual compass and without a critical look that would rein in the explosive increase in diagnosable anxiety disorders. The rationales and literature reviews that it uses to justify various proposals make little or no mention of problems with over-diagnosis and false positives—this just does not seem to have been prominently on the radar of the work group, despite the enormous expansion in anxiety disorder prevalence estimates in recent years. In the end, their clarifications serve to reveal rather than eliminate the weaknesses in the *DSM*'s approach to diagnosing anxiety disorders.

Consider again, for example, the *DSM-5* proposal for the criteria for specific phobia, the most common anxiety disorder according to epidemiological surveys. The work group recommends that disordered versus normal fear should be distinguished by whether the fear or anxiety is out of proportion to the actual danger posed by the specific object or situation.[4] As we argued in Chapter 5, this proposal entirely ignores what we know about human nature when it comes to fear—as well as other emotions, such as love and optimism. Humans are not biologically designed to always be reasonable in this way. This criterion would, for example, classify Seligman's refusal to eat Béarnaise sauce after getting sick the evening he ate it as a disorder, because he knew that it was not the cause of his illness and so his aversion was irrational. However, this type of abhorrence is a prototype for the biologically designed normal development of many fears.

The proposed criteria pathologize many such irrational fears of circumstances that are generally harmless in current environments but are species-typical prepared fears. There is nothing necessarily disordered about such fears. At some high threshold, where the fear is so intense and insensitive to reassurance that it impairs major areas of natural functioning, one could properly label such anxieties as disordered. This would, however, be a radically different and more demanding criterion than the one proposed for *DSM-5*.

The current *DSM-IV* and the prospective *DSM-5* approaches to diagnosis both ignore species-typical evolutionary shaping of anxiety and pathologize human irrationality. We have suggested that the harmful dysfunction (HD) approach provides a better alternative. The HD view of disorder requires that there be harm in the form of severe anxiety and its consequences, but it also requires that the harm must be due to a mental dysfunction where something has gone wrong with the way anxiety mechanisms are designed to function. Thus, there are two dimensions that together determine disorder: degree of harm and degree of dysfunction. These two dimensions need not go together, because mild anxieties can be dysfunctions and severe anxieties can be normal. The *DSM* runs together these two requirements and tends to see severity of anxiety, with its associated discomfort and disruption of role performance, as determining disorder. In reducing a two-dimensional concept to one severity dimension, the *DSM* collapses the crucial distinction between intense normal anxiety and disordered anxiety. The resulting confusion undermines the integrity of research on the causes and treatment of anxiety disorders.

Moreover, the result of the *DSM*'s inflation of natural fear into psychiatric disorder is that we ignore the social roots of much of our anxiety. When we choose lives and careers that naturally fill us with anxiety, we and those close to us then question whether we are mentally disordered, and we feel guilty that our anxieties preclude us from operating at peak efficiency. We also reduce our acceptance of those who are naturally higher in anxiety. Turning away from our biologically designed nature as a baseline for classification encourages a social control orientation in which inefficient emotions are addressed as problems within the individual rather than as results of demands for conformity to social norms interacting with normal human nature. If we instead recognize the true nature of the situation, other options for responding become apparent.

The special ambiguities of anxiety have allowed psychiatry to deploy the concept of anxiety disorder in ways that may seem plausible but do not in fact match our concept of disorder, which requires that something must have gone wrong with mental functioning. Consequently, it is not the concept of disorder but rather a complex configuration of interest groups as well as more general cultural trends and social values that has determined the range of conditions that are actually defined as disorders in need of treatment.

THE BATTLE OVER THE COMMODIFICATION OF CALMNESS

While we have focused on how psychiatric classifications influence the extent of pathology, psychiatry is not the only social force responsible for the expansion of anxiety disorders. The ubiquity of anxiousness and of anxiety-causing situations in our society, combined with the improvement of medicines that reduce anxiety, transformed anxiety into a particularly attractive target for social interests that strive to profit from distressing emotions. The pharmaceutical industry has been an especially powerful force in exploiting the flawed diagnoses of the psychiatric profession. In particular, the development of meprobamate (Miltown) in the mid-1950s created a huge potential market for anxiolytic drugs. As Chapter 8 indicated, the tranquilizers were initially marketed as treatments for general states of "anxiousness," "nerves," "tension," and "stress" more than for anxiety disorders.[5] During this period, advertisements, which were directed at physicians rather than consumers, not only emphasized the normality of anxiousness but also touted the value of tranquilizers (the "mother's little helpers" of which the Rolling Stones would later famously sing) in dealing with everyday stressors.[6]

Occasionally, the ads even explicitly grounded anxiety in the mismatch between evolutionary fears and modern environments—which should have suggested that the anxieties were normal parts of modern life rather than medical disorders. For example, an ad for Librium that appeared in the September 15, 1969 issue of JAMA juxtaposed a caveman and a businessman. In contrast to the caveman's "appropriate" responses to the short-term physical threats that he faced in his ancient situation, the businessman brought the same strategies to bear on modern circumstances, where they are "inappropriate."[7]

Before the 1980s, however, a number of forces constrained the industry's efforts to enlarge markets for psychoactive drugs. From the 1950s onward, congressional committees regularly criticized pharmaceutical company efforts to promote pills as

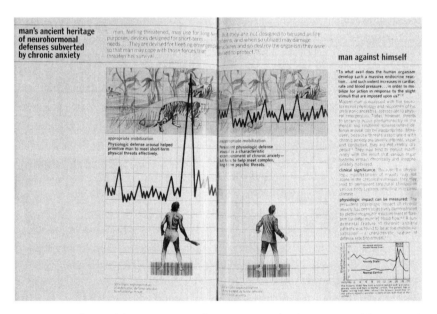

Figure 9.1: Librium ad from JAMA September 15, 1969. Used with permission of the New York Academy of Medicine Library.

remedies for the anxieties of everyday life.[8] The Food and Drug Administration (FDA), the major federal agency regulating the use of psychoactive medication, also often counterbalanced the drug industry's attempts to enlarge the boundaries of disorder. Beginning in 1962, the FDA required that drugs be efficacious for some established disease.[9] Although the agency did not rigorously implement its mandate at the time, this regulation created a powerful incentive for drug companies to seek ways to market their products as remedies for specific disorders rather than problems of living.

Prodded by Congress, the FDA confronted the pharmaceutical industry's widespread promotion of anxiolytic drugs for relieving psychosocial problems. The adversarial relationship between the FDA and the pharmaceutical companies became especially sharp in the early 1970s, when the agency began enforcing its mandate to control the promotion of anxiolytic drugs.[10] Its commissioner, Charles Edwards, explicitly distinguished the frustrations of daily living from mental disorders, noting in testimony before a congressional committee in 1971 that the tranquilizers were not intended for use with the "ordinary frustrations of daily living" but only for patients suffering from anxiety conditions that were psychiatric disorders.[11] "What has happened," he asserted, "is the advertisers, the promoters of these drugs, have taken these symptoms out of context and applied them to the day-to-day situations that we are all confronted with. As a result they have developed this totally misleading advertising."[12]

The FDA opposed what was clearly the promotion of tranquilizers for psychosocial problems. For example, advertisements for Sandoz Pharmaceutical's drug Serentil proclaimed:

> For the anxiety that comes from not fitting in. The newcomer in town who *can't* make friends. The organization man who *can't* adjust to altered status within his company. The woman who *can't* get along with her new daughter-in-law. The executive who *can't* accept retirement.... Serentil is suggested for *this* type of patient.[13]

The FDA demanded that Sandoz publish corrective advertisements that stated: "The FDA considers the advertisement misleading in several respects. For example: the FDA states that the principal theme of the ad suggests unapproved uses of Serentil for relatively minor or everyday anxiety situations encountered often in the normal course of living."[14] The agency went further, sending a letter to all sponsors of new drug applications for psychotropic prescription drugs, telling them "to cancel promptly all advertising and promotion of such drugs which recommend or suggest their use for everyday or minor life stresses...."[15] In 1980, the FDA began to require that labeling for the benzodiazepines state, "(drug name) is indicated for the management of anxiety disorders or for the short-term relief of the symptoms of anxiety. Anxiety or tension associated with the stress of everyday life usually does not require treatment with an anxiolytic."[16]

The National Institute of Mental Health (NIMH) is the primary federal agency responsible for research and policy regarding mental illness. In the first two decades after it was established in 1949, the NIMH generally supported psychosocial treatments for psychic conditions that were not serious mental disorders and took an active stance against the use of tranquilizers for problems of living. In 1963 Dr. Fritz Freyhan, then in charge of clinical studies at the National Institutes of Health, testified before a Senate hearing regarding drug research and regulation. He expressed concerns about the "overuse, if not abuse" of the minor tranquilizers and questioned the usefulness of these drugs.[17] Critiquing an ad that appeared in an issue of *Time* magazine sent to physicians, which claimed Librium could prevent nervous breakdowns and other disorders, Freyhan indicated that there was "no shred of evidence to lend substance to such claims."[18] Likewise, the director of the NIMH, Stanley Yolles, expressed his concerns to a Senate hearing in 1967:

> To what extent would Western culture be altered by widespread use of tranquilizers? Would Yankee initiative disappear? Is the chemical deadening of anxiety harmful? . . . I feel that myself and my colleagues—or so it seems to be evident from the sales statistics—are so easily seduced by the clever advertisement.[19]

Like the FDA, the NIMH asserted that drug treatments should be reserved for responding to genuine disorders and not used for psychosocial problems. This stance perhaps represents a streak of American Calvinism that itself warrants critique,[20] but it at least provided some counterforce to the pharmaceutical industry's attempts to promote the routine use of medication for problems of living.

Ironically, psychiatry's development of the symptom-based *DSM-III* criteria in the 1980s provided the pharmaceutical industry with the diagnostic entities it needed to market their products for recognized disease conditions. Because the criteria encompassed natural distress as well as genuine disorders, calling both "disorders," they provided the tools for anxieties to be treated medically without any attention to the earlier concerns of federal regulators. Moreover, since the early 1980s, the relationship between government agencies and the drug industry has changed. During the Reagan and G. H. W. Bush presidencies, the FDA moderated its adversarial stance toward the drug companies, and the NIMH promoted the use of the *DSM* categories despite their broad definitions.[21] The result was that no countervailing powers now question the use of drugs as treatments for widespread conditions that are not clearly disordered. During this period, drug company profits soared, with some of those profits used to support psychiatrists' research, education, and other activities in a way that created a controversially close relationship between pharmaceutical manufacturers and psychiatrists.[22] Consequently, in recent decades the drug industry has had an outsized effect over the psychiatric profession. The greatest influence of pharmaceutical companies, however, has stemmed from its enhanced ability to reach anxious people and cite the *DSM* criteria to convince them that they have anxiety disorders in need of chemical correction.

IDENTIFYING THE ANXIOUS

We have largely focused on the definitions of anxiety disorders found in the *DSM* and their application in epidemiological studies, but the diagnostic process is informally initiated before physicians or other mental health professionals apply diagnostic labels. Before the 1990s, individuals themselves typically decided whether to initiate treatment for anxiousness. Since then, commercial and public health strategies that encourage anxious individuals to enter treatment have become far more pervasive and aggressive. These strategies tend to use watered-down versions of the *DSM* criteria in ways that are geared to capture as many people as possible within the category of "disorder." The development of new ways of identifying anxious people, convincing them that they have anxiety disorders, and encouraging them to seek treatment is a further important reason behind the expansion of anxiety disorders.

Toward the end of the 1990s, a crucial change greatly extended the cultural boundaries of pathology. Until the end of the twentieth century, pharmaceutical ads targeted physicians rather than consumers.[23] In 1997 the Food and Drug Administration (FDA) loosened restrictions on drug makers so that they could advertise their products directly to the public. Since that time, the drug industry has spent huge sums to promote the most common disease entities of the *DSM*, capitalizing on the vague boundaries between normality and pathology to suggest that widespread symptoms of distress might signify the presence of a mental disorder. In addition, pharmaceutical companies have powerful incentives to sell products not just for treating existing diseases but also for creating new conditions and new populations in need of chemical management. Spending on direct-to-consumer (DTC) advertisements more than tripled after 1997, reaching nearly $5 billion by 2008.[24] The impact of DTC ads was so enormous that by 2007 drugs became the second most advertised type of product in the United States, behind only automobiles.[25]

When the *DSM* criteria filter into pharmaceutical advertisements, they lose the contextual constraints that limit the diagnoses of the various anxiety disorders.

Current DTC ads present situations that resemble the tranquilizer ads of the 1950s and 1960s, showing women (and occasionally men) trying to cope with conflicts between work and family obligations, demanding bosses, giving talks, and the like. Yet they differ from the earlier ads because they indicate that what is being corrected is a disease rather than the normal result of stressful conditions. Efforts to persuade people to define themselves as having anxiety disorders elide the *DSM* qualifiers and collapse natural fears, evolutionary mismatches, nervous personalities, and genuine anxiety disorders alike into disorders. Anxiety symptoms themselves become grounds for potential diagnosis, ensuring that many everyday worries and concerns will be seen as disorders that ought to receive medical treatment.

Generalized anxiety disorder (GAD) is potentially the most profitable anxiety condition because it involves the broadest and most frequently occurring symptoms of anxiousness (such as restlessness, fatigue, difficulty concentrating, irritability, muscle tension, and sleep disturbance). However, the *DSM* constraints over this condition tie its symptoms to a number of events or activities rather than a single context, require at least six-month duration (in the *DSM-IV*), and explicitly distinguish GAD from realistic worries. When these constraints are applied, this condition has a moderate prevalence rate; when they are removed, the prevalence of GAD skyrockets.[26]

Drug ads for GAD embody messages that symptoms themselves can be signs of disorder and grounds for seeking medications. For example, an ad touting Lexapro as a treatment for GAD shows only the three symptoms of "nervous and edgy," "trouble sleeping," and "feeling sad," without indicating any of the qualifiers in the diagnostic criteria. By using only the most common possible symptoms of anxiousness and tying them to the most common symptoms of depression, it indicates that symptoms alone, regardless of context, can indicate the need for a drug that treats a disordered condition.

GlaxoSmithKline's advertising campaign that touted the use of Paxil for GAD just after the 9/11 terrorist attacks went even further in expanding the boundaries of this condition. In the weeks following the attack on the World Trade Center, Glaxo positioned Paxil as the antidote to post-9/11 anxiety. The background images for its ads showed the twin towers collapsing. "Your worst fears," agonized one woman, seated at a kitchen table, "the what-ifs . . . I can't control it." "I'm always thinking something terrible is going to happen," another woman fretted. "It's like a tape in my mind," a third confessed. "It just goes over and over and over."[27]

These ads present what is in many respects the *opposite* of a condition warranting a GAD diagnosis. They connect anxiety to a single event, the terrorist attacks of 9/11, which the *DSM* explicitly rules out as a cause of GAD. Moreover, the ad portrays anxiety as arising immediately after the event, not as the enduring worry the criteria require. It also shows reactions that seem reasonably proportionate to the anxiety-provoking situation and therefore again would not meet the *DSM* criteria. When anxiety was unchained from the *DSM* constraints, millions of people could connect the high anxiety they felt after 9/11 to the seeming anxiety disorder the Paxil ad portrays. Other Paxil ads for GAD don't just remove the *DSM* constraints, they also suggest that even natural worries, concerns, and fears are signs of disorder. "It's like I never get a chance to relax. At work I'm tense about stuff at home. At home I'm tense about stuff at work."[28] Such ubiquitous advertisements thoroughly blur the boundaries between disorders and natural anxiety, pushing the threshold for pathology lower and lower.

DTC ads strip GAD of its contextual constraints and can lead normally anxious people to define themselves as having a disorder that requires chemical correction. Some conscientious physicians might not heed consumer requests for drugs to control appropriate normal fears stemming from work and family conflict or a terrorist attack. Many others, however, either will be unaware of the GAD diagnostic criteria or will dispense medications in response to patient desires regardless of whether their conditions meet these criteria. Busy GPs spend an average of only 15 minutes per patient visit, and their training leads them to be action-oriented and to write prescriptions instead of using alternatives.[29]

The extraordinary success of GlaxoSmithKline's efforts to promote social anxiety disorder (SAD) indicates the vast potential of anxiety conditions as pharmaceutical targets. "Every marketer's dream," according to Paxil's product director, "is to find an unidentified or unknown market and develop it. That's what we were able to do with social anxiety disorder."[30] As noted in the previous chapter, SAD was viewed as a rare disorder until the late 1990s. Shortly after Paxil was approved for the specific treatment of social anxiety in 1999, GlaxoSmithKline mounted an extensive publicity effort, spending over $90 million dollars on a barrage of print and television ads with the message "imagine being allergic to other people." Another widely broadcast ad for Paxil asks, "Is she just shy or is it social anxiety disorder?" Given that as many as 90% of Americans report feeling shy at some point in their lives, such an ad is certain to raise concern among a huge range of potential customers.[31] Other Paxil ads feature very common situations, such as extreme nervousness when preparing to give an important talk at a business meeting, proposing a toast at a wedding, or entering a dating situation. These are exactly the kinds of situations where people naturally feel anxious, generating a potentially enormous market for Paxil. Equating common symptoms with a mental disorder has been a shrewd and effective marketing technique.

These ads were just the tip of the iceberg of a gigantic public relations effort by the firm Cohn & Wolfe aimed at fundamentally reshaping public perceptions of social anxiety from being shy and uneasy in social situations to having a mental disorder treatable with drugs.[32] Other aspects of the campaign involved placing stories in newspapers, mass-market magazines, and television talk shows, often using celebrities, psychiatric experts, and testimonies from members of consumer advocacy groups about the pervasiveness of social anxiety disorder and disabilities resulting from SAD. A prime example was the appearance on popular talk shows and in print stories of the football star Ricky Williams's purported experiences with SAD.[33] Viewers and readers had no way of knowing that Williams's story was part of an expensive and high-powered promotion orchestrated by drug companies and implemented by public relations firms to promote the use of Paxil for his putative condition. The campaign was highly successful—Paxil became the largest selling antidepressant at the time, with sales of $3 billion a year. Social anxiety is now a common and well-recognized mental illness.

People have always sought relief, often through chemicals, for the unpleasant emotional experience of anxiety. What has changed is that they are now urged to make self-diagnoses of a mental disorder and then seek medication for help with their condition on the basis of common and context-free symptoms, thus conceptually framing such decisions in a biased way. The tremendous acceptance of these drugs, their widespread promotion, and their easy accessibility have led to a new cultural model of self-understanding about the nature of anxiousness. Ubiquitous DTC advertisements exploit the nature of symptom-based criteria and at the same time abandon the *DSM* contextual qualifiers excluding proportionate anxiousness from diagnoses. They transform natural anxiousness into an anxiety disorder, shifting the always-blurry boundaries between normality and pathology further and further in the direction of disorder.

SELF-SCREENING

DTC ads have been the major, but not the only, vehicle for getting people to self-define as having an anxiety disorder. Other strategies supplement direct marketing techniques: producing public service messages, promoting anxiety screening days, and packaging stories for the news media.[34] The Internet is one of the most common sources of information about anxiety (and other) disorders. It offers a variety of screening tests, often developed and sponsored by pharmaceutical companies, which allow people to self-diagnose anxiety disorders.

A typical test is found on AllPsych Online, which calls itself "The Virtual Psychology Classroom."[35] The site is enormously popular, registering over 11 million visitors from 2002 to 2009. "This test," the site indicates, "is based on the predominant symptoms of anxiety disorder as listed in the DSM-IV." Yet, in contrast to the *DSM*, all except two of the ten items have no contextual qualifiers. Instead, they ask questions such as, "Do you worry about things such as work or school more days than not?"; "Is it difficult for you to fall asleep due to too many thoughts in your head?"; "Do you notice your muscles getting tense frequently or feel tension in the muscles of your lower back, neck, or eyes?" (The two exceptions that do mention context are: "Do you often feel restless or on edge even when nothing is going on around you to cause these feelings?" and "Do you often feel irritable or tense even when nothing is going on which would justify this feeling?")

Popular screening scales for other anxiety conditions similarly lack any concern for the naturalness of a "symptom." For example, a common test for social anxiety asks people whether they fear situations such as talking to someone in authority, going to a party, calling someone you don't know very well, meeting strangers, or trying to make someone's acquaintance for the purpose of a sexual or romantic relationship.[36] These situations can be of particular concern to adolescents because the teenage years are particularly likely to feature doubts about social skills and concerns over social embarrassment. The result is that contextually appropriate worries are equated with the presence of disorder that requires medical attention. Moreover, the questions focus on the kinds of evolutionary fears of social evaluation and interaction with strangers that would naturally afflict large proportions of the population. Thus, the translation of the *DSM* criteria into screening instruments and messages in the public sphere often involves the loss of their qualifiers and leads to even more encompassing criteria for identifying possible disorders.

PROACTIVE STRATEGIES FOR IDENTIFYING THE ANXIOUS

Individuals themselves choose whether to seek treatment after viewing a DTC ad, hearing a public service announcement, or taking an Internet screening test. Such strategies, however, cannot influence people who are not interested in obtaining or acting on this information. To reach this broader population, policies promoting early intervention and prevention must reach people who do not think that they have a mental disorder or who don't voluntarily respond to appeals urging them to seek treatment. Attempts to impose screening and subsequent diagnostic tests on those who have not self-defined as anxious raise difficult issues about the boundaries between legitimate medical care and the coercive surveillance of private emotions.

Fueled by the large numbers of individuals that epidemiological studies identify as having anxiety disorders but as not receiving treatment for their conditions, aggressive methods of detecting and treating anxiety have emerged. Yet, the respondents that these surveys identify as having untreated mental disorders do not themselves report that they want care but don't get it because of cost, lack of access to professionals, or ignorance about where to obtain treatment. Instead, their most important reasons are, "I wanted to solve the problem on my own," "I thought the problem would get better by itself," and "I don't have a problem."[37] Indeed, over 83% of people considered to have a less serious type of mental disorder reported that they didn't seek treatment because they don't believe they have a problem.[38]

Despite the denials of respondents that they require or want professional intervention, screening advocates nevertheless urge forceful action to get people to enter treatment. "NCS results," researchers note, "show that the psychological barriers to seeking treatment will require more than mere public relations management targeted to the uninformed."[39] Surely, screening advocates correctly assert that some people with serious mental disorders may need, but do not obtain, treatment and that professionals should be educated to recognize such instances. However, such concerns are also being used as a rationale for transforming common emotional states from personal matters to conditions warranting public monitoring. The assumption that people who experience intense anxiety that falls under *DSM* criteria must have disorders even when they do not think they do raises complex moral, social, and civil liberty issues that have yet to be addressed.

Screening for Anxiety Disorders in Primary Medical Care

During the past decade, mental health educators and advocates, policymakers, and the pharmaceutical industry have vigorously promoted outreach programs to try to ensure that people who don't self-define as mentally ill are nevertheless brought into contact with mental health treatment.[40] Screening programs in primary medical care settings seem especially appropriate because so many persons with the combination of somatic and psychological symptoms that characterize anxiety conditions visit general physicians instead of mental health specialists.[41] Although depression has been the major focus of screening efforts in primary care to date, the development and use of screening measures for anxiety has been growing.

The GAD-7 exemplifies such scales.[42] It asks patients seven questions about how often during the last two weeks they were bothered by:

1. Feeling nervous, anxious, or on edge
2. Not being able to stop or control worrying
3. Worrying too much about different things
4. Trouble relaxing
5. Being so restless that it is hard to sit still
6. Becoming easily annoyed or irritable
7. Feeling afraid, as if something awful might happen

An answer of "several days" gets a score of 1, "more than half the days" a score of 2, and "nearly every day" a score of 3. Nearly a quarter of primary care patients receive scores of 10 or greater, which the authors indicate "represents a reasonable cut point for identifying cases of GAD."[43]

Although the developers of this scale claim that it is "specifically linked to the *DSM-IV (Text Revision)* criteria," it actually deviates from these criteria in a number of ways. The *DSM* criteria require "excessive anxiety and worry," symptoms that persist "more days than not for at least 6 months," and symptoms that are "about a number of events or activities" rather than a single concern.[44] In addition, they require that "[t]he person finds it difficult to control the worry." The GAD-7 uses none of these qualifiers. A single concern (such as a fear of losing one's job) could satisfy the screening criteria, not to mention alarm about the medical condition that brought the person to seek medical care in the first place. Needless to say, such concerns are often normal responses to threatening contexts.

In addition, it is especially difficult to distinguish somatic symptoms associated with anxiety, such as restlessness or inability to relax, from similar symptoms that are associated with many common physical conditions or with the consequences of medications people take for these conditions. Moreover, GAD-7 symptoms need persist for only two weeks instead of the six months needed to satisfy the *DSM* criteria. Given the a-contextual nature of the screening items, it is unsurprising that about a quarter of patients in primary care meet criteria for GAD. Its widespread use could lead to a massive pathologization of anxiety in this setting.

The Consensus Statement on Social Anxiety Disorder goes even further than the GAD-7 in loosening the criteria for anxiety disorders.[45] The text of the statement indicates that situations such as fear of buying goods in a small shop or feeling anxious in a supermarket line because of anticipating having to talk to the checkout clerk are likely to indicate anxiety disorders. If these anxieties are adequately intense, these examples do reflect at least arguable cases of disorder, but the decontextualized questions the Consensus Statement develops for use in primary care settings encompass a much broader range of conditions as disorders. It recommends that physicians ask all patients who appear to be reticent or shy just two questions: (1) Are you uncomfortable or embarrassed at being the center of attention? and (2) Do you find it hard to interact with people? Such anxious feelings can be omnipresent among people with normal-range anxiousness, not to mention those with introverted personality dispositions. The Statement also notes, "Once diagnosed with social anxiety disorder, the patient must be reassured that he or she has a recognized medical condition for which there is effective treatment."[46]

Screening for anxiety disorders in primary medical care settings is especially likely to extend the boundaries of disorder into natural fears and worries. A mental health specialist who has ample time to interview the patient might distinguish normal reactions to negative life circumstances from an anxiety disorder. The instruments recommended for rapid application by time-pressured general physicians, however, do not allow for such distinctions. The result, especially in primary care settings where anxious symptoms abound, can be to pathologize enormous numbers of people, many of whom might be normally anxious or shy but not disordered.

Screening in Schools

Screening adolescents in the schools that they attend has been a preeminent concern of preventive efforts with anxiety, because screening advocates assume that anxiety disorders have both temporal and causal priority relative to other kinds of disorders. Anxiety typically arises during the teenage years or even earlier. "In general," report Kessler and Waters, "anxiety disorders were the most likely to be temporally primary, with 82.8% of NCS respondents having one or more anxiety disorders reporting that one of these was their first lifetime disorder."[47] The presumed early onset of anxiety disorders and lack of timely treatment for them lends particular urgency to uncovering untreated cases of anxiety among the young: "It is consequently of great importance to develop aggressive outreach and treatment programs for young people with mental disorders."[48]

If anxiety disorders can be prevented at an early age, the argument goes, it ought to be possible to prevent the subsequent onset of depression, substance abuse, and other disorders. Such early intervention and treatment programs might avert the growing severity of existing disorders, subsequent onsets of additional disorders, and dire social and psychological impairments that are consequences of early onset disorders.[49] For example, the authors of an NCS report estimate that early interventions to treat social phobia could also prevent about 20% of all drug dependence disorders and up to 25% of mood disorders.[50]

The Multidimensional Anxiety Scale for Children (MASC) is the most highly regarded screening scale for young people at present.[51] The scale asks adolescents if they have experienced physical symptoms such as tenseness, restlessness, dizziness, and stomach aches; social anxiety such as looking stupid in front of others, having others laugh at or make fun of them, and feeling embarrassed; separation anxiety under circumstances such as going to camp, being alone, or watching a scary movie; and harm avoidance leading to always obeying others, avoiding getting upset, and asking permission.

Its authors claim that the MASC measures "the core features of disorder that may be most responsive to specific prevention efforts."[52] Yet the vast majority of "symptoms"—such as tenseness, fear of looking stupid in front of others, feeling anxious when going away from home, or always obeying others—are often normal emotions, especially among adolescents. Because the scale does not provide any context for symptoms, it hopelessly confounds natural forms of anxiousness with possible anxiety disorders. The result is that the MASC indicates that a third or more of all students are at risk for an anxiety disorder and thus are candidates for pharmaceutical or psychotherapeutic interventions.[53]

Such scales are developed as first-stage screening instruments to be followed by clinical interviews, but diagnostic interviews using *DSM* criteria will themselves be prone to treat normal, intense anxiety among adolescents as pathological. In addition, in situations of mass screening where time-consuming clinical evaluations are often unfeasible, the initial results of the screening instrument themselves can be emphasized because of the sheer number of people being processed.[54]

Professionals should take particular care that the common emotional turmoil of adolescence is not mistaken for a mental disorder. Monitoring the varying emotions of adolescents—and especially the moodiness, irritability, nervousness, and worries to which normal adolescents are regularly subject—may or may not be a good idea. But it is surely an idea that deserves serious and honest discussion before it is wholeheartedly embraced. Because of the faulty assumption that screening uncovers a disordered condition, however, such discussions rarely occur regarding screening for anxiety. Some children and adolescents who report anxiety symptoms will develop more serious disorders later in life; however most anxiousness at early ages does not represent the early stages of a full-blown mental disorder but is a normal aspect of adolescence. Researchers don't know how to differentiate the first from the second group, so they treat both as pathological. This inevitably results in treating many people suffering from transitory conditions who will get better on their own. Such treatment also entails the costs of side effects of therapy, stigma, and a wasteful use of scarce resources.

Of course there may well be benefit—as yet scientifically unproven—in screening, identifying, and treating some cases of intense adolescent anxiety in genuinely disordered individuals. However, the possible offsetting costs in mass screening as the way of identifying such cases, with its likely associated false-positive diagnoses, are less frequently considered and can be considerable. The emergence of a self-fulfilling prophecy is always possible because labels of mental disorder can transform individual identity, mood, and perception and unintentionally create the disorder that the intervention was supposed to prevent.[55] Adolescents in particular can face stigma and ridicule from their peers when they are perceived as having a mental illness. "Not surprisingly," reports sociologist David Karp, "young people will often go to great lengths to keep secret their use of psychiatric medications."[56] Such medications in a sense directly influence who people *are* and thus have far more wide-ranging social and self-identity impacts than the treatment of specific bodily diseases.[57] Especially (although not exclusively) among adolescents, the problems associated with psychiatric labels are a cause for deep concern. This should seemingly indicate more caution in pushing people to seek treatment, especially through mechanisms that are not self-initiated, such as screening programs.

Current screening programs are—and ought to be truthfully labeled as—methods of identifying distress, both normal and pathological. Many identified anxiety conditions are most likely normal reactions to environmental stressors. Recognizing the normality of many identified "symptoms" encourages a policy of watchful waiting (with counseling or social support if requested) to see whether symptoms persist, rather than routine referrals for professional treatment. Such a framework allows a more optimistic and accurate prognosis and less potential for stigma for many teens, as well as adults, who do screen positively.

SOCIAL VALUES AND THE TREATMENT OF ANXIOUSNESS

The use of decontextualized criteria that encourage expansive definitions of anxiety disorders and screening programs for them does not mean that these efforts are without merit. There is nothing necessarily wrong with helping people to identify and seek help for natural anxiousness as well as anxiety disorders. Indeed, a good argument can be made that society ought to provide its members methods of relief from the high anxiety that is integral to many social roles and circumstances.[58] Decisions about the wisdom of promoting any particular type of treatment stem partly from its relative risks and benefits and partly from value-laden choices about what kinds of conditions ought to be treated and what sorts of treatments ought to be provided.

The weight of extant evidence does show that both pharmacological and psychological treatments can often effectively relieve symptoms of many anxiety conditions.[59] Certainly unresolved issues exist about the magnitude and durability of these effects, the degree of negative side effects, and how drug and psychotherapeutic therapies compare to alternatives such as, for example, beginning an exercise regime, starting meditation classes, getting informal social support, or changing jobs or relationships.[60] Overall, however, both antidepressant and anxiolytic drugs as well as psychological therapies can at least temporarily relieve anxiety conditions for a fairly large portion of people who receive them.

Because no studies compare the relative benefits of therapies for contextually appropriate anxieties, evolutionarily natural anxieties, and disordered anxieties, their differential effectiveness is unknown. However, the only way that people can obtain treatment—and that their clinicians can obtain reimbursement for providing it—is when conditions are defined as disorders.[61] So why shouldn't as many anxious people as possible be labeled and receive medication and other therapies?

Treating Normal Anxiousness

People ought to have full information about the nature of their conditions before they decide whether to engage in some treatment. They should be aware that symptoms of anxiety do not necessarily indicate the presence of an anxiety disorder. Calling the feelings associated with anxiety "symptoms," and a collection of such symptoms an "anxiety disorder," prejudges what response they ought to make. If patients and their doctors assume that anxiousness is a disorder, they are more likely to take for granted that medication is warranted.[62] This doesn't mean, however, that normal symptoms of "stress" never warrant medical relief.

Consider anthropologist Margaret Mead's testimony before a congressional committee investigating problems in the drug industry during the 1960s:

> But I do believe it is worthwhile to avoid the stress that comes when the plumbing breaks down and both cars are broken and you can't find your husband to telephone him, and the child in nursery school, three children in nursery school, you were going to pick up 15 miles somewhere else, if a pill will permit you not to burst into tears under these circumstances but go next door and borrow another car, I think it is a good idea . . .[63]

Anxiety conditions, even when they are not disorders, can create suffering that deserves clinical attention if people desire it.[64] Unlike current advocates, however, Mead did not pretend that many of the conditions medications were treating were anything other than the natural results of stressful circumstances.

Non-disordered conditions can warrant treatment when individuals believe it will help them and when effective and safe treatments are available. Helping such people to lower their anxiety, however, is not the same thing as treating a disorder. Labeling a non-disordered condition as a "disorder" skews the decision of whether and how to treat the condition. In some cases it can also mask real issues in how people live their lives and deflect attention from social critique and change.

Treating Mismatches

Another issue in the treatment of anxiety stems from the difference between the presence of a disorder and a mismatch between normal human nature and changing environments. Distinctive social values and environmental demands can create mismatches that place normal human variation at a disadvantage. Humanity's success in creating artificial environments that have little similarity to the ones in which our species developed its natural fears accounts for much of our anxiety about things that are no longer dangerous. The use of psychiatry to minimize the resulting difficulties can allow anxious individuals to participate fully in social roles. Drug and other treatments can help them overcome their fears and enhance their role performances just as, for example, people who work on night shifts and suffer from a mismatch between the hours their jobs demand and their natural circadian rhythms can benefit from drugs that minimize the consequences of this mismatch. Treating individuals whose occupations require them to give talks or travel long distances can be regarded as a matter of psychological justice.[65]

The use of psychiatry to minimize the psychological distress that stems from such mismatches, however, is also prone to abuse. If mismatches are mistaken for disorders in which something is wrong in the person, those who cannot conform to new values can be labeled as disordered if social values change. As the pace of environmental change grows, and as increasing numbers of people spend more time in artificially created environments, the potential for mismatches to generate conditions that are labeled as "anxiety disorders" is also likely to grow. The temptation to medically enforce conformity to novel social demands and values will also increase the likelihood of labeling such mismatches as defects in the person.

In the past, overcoming problematic anxiety arising from normal variation in human nature when that anxiety was mismatched with a new type of environment was in part a matter of cultivating strong character or "virtue"—not the treatment of mental disorder.[66] Exchanging the concept of "courage" for one of "mental health" might impoverish our moral discourse and exert pressure to conform to occupational and social demands that may not be to our liking, when what may be needed is a broader reexamination of our social structure and our own niche within that structure.

The "emotional time machine" places normal individuals with their biologically designed emotional reactions into a new environment for which they were not designed and in which their anxious feelings may be personally and socially problematic. We may want to adjust natural, but currently disadvantageous, human emotions to fit more comfortably into these novel environments, yet retaining the distinction between disorder and mismatches is crucial. Otherwise, changing social demands for efficiency, productivity, and conformity in novel social circumstances may be expressed as the relabeling of such mismatches as disorders and lead to relentless calls for the treatment of natural anxiousness.

CONCLUSION

Scientific progress in understanding anxiety disorders depends on our ability to study etiologically homogeneous conditions. The conditions that current diagnostic systems now label as anxiety disorders, however, are not at all homogeneous. Rather, they involve several quite distinguishable etiologies of intense fear. Disorders are failures of biologically designed functioning that cause harmful outcomes. They are distinct from normal anxieties that are contextually appropriate responses to immediate threats, from anciently prepared innate fears, and from intensely anxious personality dispositions.

Optimal scientific progress and proper informed consent when treating anxiety both depend on making these basic conceptual and etiological distinctions. When a condition is considered to be a disorder—and thus there is presumed to be some defect in the individual—medical treatment is generally considered the appropriate response. While treatment is not limited to medical disorders (think, for example, of cosmetic surgeries), disorder status almost invariably prompts treatment. Calling unreasonable but natural aspects of human nature "disorders" can lead psychiatry to cross the boundary of medicine into the realm of enforcing adherence to social norms.

Knowing that much of our anxiety is normal can itself relieve some of the anxiety. Accepting that we have constructed lives or are in environments where particular artificial triggers interact with our innate programming to produce anxiety can open up possibilities for finding better social niches or lifestyles. If we suffer "impairment" in some social role performance, then we have to decide whether that "impairment" represents a natural response to programmed dangers or instead is truly damaged functioning. If the former is the case, then we might think about changing our roles. When that strategy is impossible, we might want to think about using drugs or other therapies to cope with what is actually a natural emotion. But in general, although what we have argued does not change the fact that one is anxious, it can help dissipate the shame and social pressures we often feel when we are considered to have an anxiety disorder.

Treating individuals can be justifiable when they want help in mastering fears and anxieties that inhibit them from optimal social functioning, but this does not necessarily involve correcting a dysfunction. Many of our multitudes of fears are not products of brains that have gone wrong; instead, they are unfortunate aspects of our nature as humans. We retain both our humanity and our broadest range of therapeutic options when we recognize that much of our anxiousness is natural and not a sign of mental disorder.

NOTES

CHAPTER 1

1. Kessler et al., 2005a.
2. American Psychiatric Association, 1980, p. 225.
3. Regier et al., 1998, p 111.
4. Kessler et al., 2005a.
5. Moffitt et al., 2009.
6. Foderado, 2008.
7. Kendler, 2008.
8. Galea et al., 2003.
9. *New York Times*, May 3, 2003.
10. Kaiser, 2003.
11. Galea et al., 2007.
12. Sulzberger & Wald, 2009.
13. Weiss, Seifman, & Olshan, 2009.
14. Thirlwell, 2011.
15. Garbowsky, 1989.
16. Saul, 2001, p. 6.
17. Bell, 2008.
18. Freud, 1909, p. 158.
19. Montaigne, 1955, p. 53.
20. Jackson, 1986, p. 42.
21. Sareen et al., 2005.

22. Solomon, 2008, p. 515.
23. Gajilan, 2008.
24. Saul, 2001, p. 7.
25. Darwin, 1872/1998, p. 43.
26. http://www.kpho.com/health//19368709/detail.html.
27. Tooby & Cosmides, 1990.
28. Rachman, 1978, p. 255.
29. Turner, 2000.
30. E.g., Evans-Pritchard, 1937/1976.
31. Bourke, 2005, p. 33–36.
32. Scott, 2007.
33. In addition, the manual divides agoraphobia into the two types of with or without panic disorder, has a category of anxiety disorder that is caused by a medical condition or is substance-induced, and a category that is not otherwise specified. American Psychiatric Association, 2000, p. 433.
34. American Psychiatric Association, 2000, p. 449.
35. American Psychiatric Association, 2000, p. 456.
36. American Psychiatric Association, 2000, p. 433.
37. American Psychiatric Association, 2000, p. 432.
38. American Psychiatric Association, 2000, p. 467–468.
39. American Psychiatric Association, 2000, pp. 471–472.
40. American Psychiatric Association, 2000, pp. 462–463.
41. American Psychiatric Association, 2000, p. 476.
42. E.g., Aristotle, 1991, p. 153; Marks, 1987.
43. E.g., Bourke, 2005, pp. 189–192. LeDoux, 2002, pp. 289–90.
44. Freud, 1926//1989.
45. Plato, 1992.
46. Kierkegaard, 1844/1980.
47. May, 1977, p. 182.
48. Kierkegaard, 1844/1980, p. xiii.
49. Heidegger, 1977, p. 108.
50. Goldstein, 1963. Tien, 1979.
51. Quoted in Lewis, 1970, p. 72.

CHAPTER 2

1. Andreasen, 1984, p. 8.
2. Insel & Cuthbert, 2009.
3. Saul, 2001, p. 37.
4. Mayberg et al., 1999.

5. Watson & Raynor, 1920.
6. E.g., Bandura, 1977; Kazdin, 1978; Wolpe, 1969.
7. Poulton & Menzies, 2002; Poulton, Waldie, Thomson, & Locker, 2001; Poulton, Thomson, Davies, Kruger, Brown & Silva, 1997;
8. Bandura, 1977.
9. Grinker & Spiegel, 1945b.
10. John, 1941.
11. Lazarus, 1994.
12. Watson, 1924.
13. Ohman, 2001.
14. Mineka, Davidson, Cook, & Keir, 1984.
15. Seligman, 1971.
16. LeDoux, 2002.
17. LeDoux, 2002, p. 252.
18. Reznek, 1987, p. 212.
19. See especially Scheff, 1966; Sedgwick, 1973.
20. Sedgwick, 1973, pp. 30–31.
21. David, 2008, p. 24.
22. Gay, 2002.
23. E.g., Mirowsky & Ross, 1989; Bolton, 2008. Note that because courage or other desirable traits might be unusual and lie at an end of a dimension, the statistical-deviance account of disorder would generally limit disorders to traits that are at a negative end of the distribution, such as high fear.
24. Grinker & Spiegel, 1945b.
25. Dillon, 2008.
26. Kakutani, 2008.
27. Bolton, 2008.
28. E.g., Kessler et al., 2003.
29. Stein, Waler, & Forde, 1994, p. 408.
30. Buckley, McKinley, Tofler, & Bartrop, 2010.
31. E.g., Bourke, 2005, pp. 138–39.
32. Murphy, 2006. For a contrasting view see Klein, 1981.
33. Damasio, 1994, p. 255.
34. Nesse, 1990, p. 281.
35. James, 1900, p. 4.
36. Buller, 2005, p. 425.
37. Tooby & Cosmides, 1990, p. 419. See also Buller, 2005.
38. E.g., Tooby & Cosmides, 1990; Pinker, 1999; Buss, 1995.
39. Kessler, 2009.

40. Nesse & Jackson, 2006.
41. Aldrich et al., 2010.
42. Nesse, 1990; Buss, 1995.
43. Ohman, 1986.
44. E.g., LeDoux, 1996.
45. Saul, 2001, pp. 41–43. See also Kandel, 1998.
46. E.g., Cannon, 1932/1963.
47. Lee, Wadsworth, & Hotopf, 2006.
48. Griffiths, 1997.
49. Hobbes, 1651/2009, p. 110.
50. Kierkegaard, 1844/1980.
51. Ohman, 1986, p. 128.
52. Watson & Raynor, 1920.
53. Marks, 1987.
54. LeDoux, 1996, pp. 131–2.
55. Marks, 1987, p. 52.
56. Seligman, 1971.
57. Hebb, 1968; Cook & Mineka, 1989.
58. Mineka, 1992.
59. Darwin, 1872/1998, p. 365.
60. Darwin, 1872/1998, p. 294.
61. Darwin, 1872/1998, p. 309.
62. Davidson, 2003, p. 330.
63. Darwin, 1872/1998.
64. Quoted in Charlesworth & Kreutzer, 1973, p. 103.
65. Marks, 1987, p. 150.
66. Tien, 1979, p. 11.
67. Marks, 1987, p. 40.
68. Freud, 1926/1989; Bowlby, 1969.
69. Tien, 1979, p. 21.
70. Marks, 1987.
71. Valentine, 1930.
72. Darwin, 1872/1998, p. 297.
73. Ekman & Friesen, 1971.
74. Schweder & Haidt, 2000.
75. Job iv., 13.
76. Cited in Marks, 1987, p. 112.
77. Gibson & Walk, 1960.
78. Walk & Gibson, 1961.

79. Poulton & Menzies, 2002.

80. Gibson & Walk, 1960.

81. Menzies & Clarke, 1995, p. 41.

82. Routtenberg & Glickman, 1964.

83. E.g., Wierzbicka, 1999; Konstan, 2006; Gross, 2006.

84. Konstan, 2006, p. 260.

85. Okano, 1994.

86. Fisher, 2002.

87. Gay, 2002.

88. Benedict, 1934; Nance, 1976.

89. Huizinga, 1924; Tien, 1979, Chapter 7.

90. Horney, 1937.

91. Freud, 1926/1989, p. 136.

92. Kagan, 1976; Kagan et al., 1978.

93. Super & Harkness, 2011.

94. Lazarus, 1994.

95. Tien, 1979, p. 33.

96. Bowlby, 1970, p. 86.

97. Rachman, 2004.

98. Buss, 2009.

99. Nettle, 2006.

100. E.g., Gould & Lewontin, 1979.

101. Pinker, 1999, p. 386.

CHAPTER 3

1. Wakefield, 1992a, 1992b, 1999.

2. Lazarus, 1994.

3. Aristotle, in particular, emphasized how fear was tied not just to dangerous situations but to cognitive appraisals of dangerous situations. See Fortenbaugh, 2002.

4. Quoted in Graver, 2007, pp. 85–86.

5. See especially, LeDoux, 1996, 2002.

6. As LeDoux (1996, 2002) emphasizes, the amygdala is not the only part of the brain related to anxiety. Among other brain regions, the hippocampus and prefrontal cortex, as well as the monoamine system, are also involved in stimulating anxiety.

7. LeDoux, 1996, 2002.

8. Darwin, 1872/1998

9. Plato, 1974; Cates, 2009; Hume, 1740/1967.

10. LeDoux, 1996, p. 224.
11. William James, 1884. "What Is an Emotion?" *Mind*, 9, 188–205. Well before James, the Stoic philosophers had already grounded emotional feelings in corporeal bodily states. See Graver, 2007.
12. Ohman & Mineka, 2001.
13. Nesse, 2005.
14. In fact, however, the annoyance that constant alarms create often leads them to be disabled or ignored. This seems to be the case with the apparatus designed to alert personnel of oil leaks on off-shore drilling platforms, a facilitating factor in the disastrous BP oil spill in the summer of 2010. See Wald, 2010.
15. The smoke detector principle explains why critiques of the evolutionary perspective that emphasize how most spiders and snakes are not poisonous are misguided. E.g, Richardson, 2007, p. 16.
16. Bulmer, 2003, p. 149.
17. Mineka, 1992.
18. Davidson, 2003; Bowlby, 1970, p. 81.
19. Kagan, 2007.
20. Marks & Nesse, 1994.
21. Marks, 1987.
22. MacDonald, 1981, p. 41.
23. Finlay-Jones & Brown, 1981.
24. Tooby & Cosmides, 1990.
25. LeDoux, 1996, p. 174.
26. Kaufman, 1947.
27. Spiegel, 1943.
28. Quoted in Graver, 2007, p. 96.
29. Marks & Nesse, 1994.
30. Wing, Cooper, & Sartorius, 1974.
31. Galea et al., 2007.
32. Kandel, 1998.
33. Nesse & Jackson, 2006.
34. Nesse, 1998.
35. Stern, 1995, pp. 126–161.
36. Stern, 1995, p. 126.
37. Marks, 1987.
38. Sapolsky, 2004.
39. Nesse, 1998.
40. Szasz, 1974.

41. Damasio, 1994.
42. Poulton & Menzies, 2002.
43. Nesse, 1998.
44. Quoted in Bourke, 2005, p. 116.
45. Curtis et al., 1998.
46. Tien, 1979, p. 14.
47. Marks & Nesse, 1994; May, 1977, pp. 91–92.
48. Ohman & Mineka, 2001.
49. Gardner, 2008.
50. Tien, 1979, p. 8.
51. Black, 2011.
52. Ruscio et al., 2008.
53. Marks, 1987, p. 19.
54. Sapolsky, 2004, p. 323.
55. Bloom, 2010.
56. Tien, 1979, pp. 213.
57. Ruprecht, 2010.
58. Quoted in Graver, 2007, p. 96.
59. Although the nature of dominance hierarchies usually produces more anxiety among subordinates, weak or uncertain positions of power can lead dominants to become anxious about their ability to maintain their superior positions. See Sapolsky, 2004.
60. Goodall, 1990. See also Gilbert, 2001, p. 744.
61. Higley et al., 1996.
62. Trower & Gilbert, 1989; Stein & Bouwer, 1997.
63. Gilbert, 2001, p. 739.
64. Gilbert, 2001.
65. Ruscio et al., 2008, p. 18.
66. Andrews & Thomson, 2009.
67. Glassner, 1999, p. 61.
68. Wald, 2008.
69. Bourke, 2005, p. 332.
70. E.g., Campbell-Sills & Stein, 2005; Bolton, 2008.
71. E.g., Szasz, 1974; Cooper, 1967.
72. http://www.huffingtonpost.com/2009/05/01/miss-californias-breast-i_n_194385.html.
73. Aristotle, 2009, VIII.1155a5.
74. Bowlby, 1970.

CHAPTER 4

1. Burton, 1621/2001, p. 258.
2. Plato, 2005, 355a–357e.
3. Quoted in McReynolds, 1985, p. 137.
4. Quoted in McReynolds, 1985, p. 138.
5. Cicero, 1927, p. 355.
6. Simon, 1978, p. 229.
7. Quoted in Burton, 1621/2001, p. 387.
8. Roccatagliata, 1986, p. 135.
9. Simon, 1978, p. 228.
10. Roccatagliata, 1986.
11. Jackson, 1986.
12. Burton, 1621/2001, pp. 169–170.
13. Burton, 1621/2001, p. 381.
14. Burton, 1621/2001, part 3, p. 142.
15. Burton, 1621/2001, part 3, pp. 143–148.
16. Burton, 1621/2001, part 3, p. 148.
17. Burton, 1621/2001, pp. 423–424.
18. Burton, 1621/2001, p. 424.
19. Burton, 1621/2001, p. 261.
20. Burton, 1621/2001, p. 424.
21. Burton, 1621/2001, p. 258.
22. Burton, 1621/2001, pp. 431–432.
23. Burton, 1621/2001, p. 337.
24. Quoted in Jackson, 1986, p. 293.
25. Jackson, 1986, p. 295.
26. Shorter, 1994, pp. 127–128.
27. Glas, 1994.
28. Jackson, 1986, p. 296, 297.
29. Shorter, 1997, p. 22.
30. Micale, 1994.
31. Shorter, 1997, p. 129.
32. Beard, 1869, p. 218.
33. Mitchell, 1867.
34. Shorter, 1992, p. 230.
35. Shorter, 1992, p. 223.
36. Shorter, 1992; Lutz, 1991.
37. See especially Kleinman, 1986.
38. Quoted in Lewis, 1976, p. 21.

39. Westphal, 1871–72.

40. Heckelman & Schneier, 1995, p. 3.

41. Kraepelin, 1896.

42. Boyd et al., 1984.

43. Maudsley, 1879.

44. Janet, 1903/1976.

45. Lewis, 1970, p. 66.

46. Shorter, 1992.

47. E.g., Shorter, 1997; Crews, 1999.

48. Klerman, 1987; Breier, Charney, & Heninger, 1985; Michels, Frances, & Shear, 1985.

49. Freud, 1894/1953, pp. 45–61.

50. Freud, 1926/1989, p. 32.

51. E.g., Freud, 1916–17; Freud, 1933.

52. Freud, 1926/1989, p. 59.

53. Freud, 1926/1989, p. 107.

54. Freud, 1957, p. 80.

55. Freud, 1957, p. 136.

56. Freud, 1926/1989, p. 54.

57. Freud, 1926/1989, pp. 75–76.

58. Freud, 1926/1989, p. 37; Rycroft, 1988, p. 77.

59. Freud, 1930, p. 82.

60. E.g., Klerman, 1985.

61. Freud, 1926/1989, p. 104.

62. Freud, 1926/1989, p. 63.

63. Freud, 1926/1989, p. 103.

64. Rycroft, 1988, p. xii.

65. Michels, Frances, & Shear, 1985.

66. Freud, 1933/1965.

67. Freud, 1933/1965, p.83.

68. Quoted in Lane, 2007, p. 154.

69. Freud, 1926/1959, pp. 778–79.

70. Freud, 1926/1959, p. 777.

71. Freud 1957, p. 83

72. Freud, 1926/1959, p. 66.

73. Freud 1933/1965, pp. 88–89.

74. Freud, 1926/1959, p. 79.

75. Freud, 1926/1959, p. 25.

76. Freud, 1926/1959, p. 53.

77. Quoted in Michels, Frances, & Shear, 1985, p. 609.
78. Glas, 1994, p. 32.
79. Grob, 1991b, p. 96.
80. Grob, 1991a.
81. American Psychiatric Association, 1952, p. 31.
82. American Psychiatric Association, 1952, pp. 31–32.
83. American Psychiatric Association, 1952, p. 33.
84. American Psychiatric Association, 1952, p. 33.
85. American Psychiatric Association, 1952, pp. 33–34.
86. American Psychiatric Association, 1952, p. 32.
87. American Psychiatric Association, 1952.
88. American Psychiatric Association, 1968, p. 39; Horwitz, 2002; Kirk, 1999.
89. Cooper et al., 1972.
90. Kirk, 1999.
91. Healy, 1997.
92. Kirk & Kutchins, 1992; Horwitz, 2002.
93. Arnold, 1782, p. 20.
94. Spitzer, 1978; Spitzer, Williams, & Skodol, 1980; Wilson, 1993; Kirk & Kutchins, 1992; Horwitz, 2002.
95. Bayer & Spitzer, 1985.
96. Wing, Cooper, & Sartorius, 1974, p. 147.
97. Feighner et al., 1972.
98. Feighner et al. 1972, p. 59.
99. Feighner et al., 1972.
100. Klein & Fink, 1981.
101. Healy, 1997, p. 193.
102. American Psychiatric Association, 1980.
103. Lane, 2007, p. 43; Healy, 1997, p. 237.
104. Wakefield, 2001; Horwitz, 2002.
105. Horwitz, 2002, p. 239.
106. Tyrer, 1984, p. 79.
107. Spitzer et al., 1994.
108. Freud, 1926/1989, p. 107.
109. Freud, 1957.
110. Akiskal, 1998.
111. American Psychiatric Association, 1980, p. 232.
112. Cox et al., 1995. Pincus et al., 1993.
113. Tyrer, 1984, p. 79.
114. Blazer et al., 1996.

115. American Psychiatric Association, 1980, p. 225.
116. American Psychiatric Association, 1980, p. 228.
117. American Psychiatric Association, 1980, p. 231.
118. American Psychiatric Association, 1980, p. 234.
119. American Psychiatric Association, 1980, p. 236.
120. Indeed, the *DSM-5* work group distinguishes disorders on the "obsessive-compulsive spectrum" from anxiety disorders. See Phillips, 2009.
121. American Psychiatric Association, 1980, p 238.
122. The *DSM-III-R* changed the diagnostic criteria for generalized anxiety disorder to require "unrealistic or excessive anxiety or worry." American Psychiatric Association, 1986, p. 252.
123. American Psychiatric Association, 1986;, 1994;, 2000.
124. American Psychiatric Association, 1986, p. 252.
125. American Psychiatric Association, 2000, p. 473.
126. American Psychiatric Association, 2000, p. 462.
127. American Psychiatric Association, 1980, p. 228.
128. American Psychiatric Association, 1986, p. 243.
129. American Psychiatric Association, 1986, p. 243.
130. Oddly, the *DSM-III-R* also changed the requirement for simple phobia from persistent and irrational fears to only persistent fears. Yet, in contrast to social phobia, the *DSM-IV* changed the requirement back to "marked and persistent fear that is excessive or unreasonable." American Psychiatric Association, 2000, p. 449.
131. Horwitz and Wakefield, 2007.

CHAPTER 5
1. LeBeau et al., 2010, p. 164.
2. American Psychiatric Association, 2000, p. 432.
3. Wakefield, Pottick, & Kirk, 2002.
4. American Psychiatric Association, 2000, pp. 471–472.
5. American Psychiatric Association, 2000, pp. 440–441.
6. American Psychiatric Association, 2000, p. 462.
7. American Psychiatric Association, 2000, p. 449.
8. American Psychiatric Association, 2000, p. 462.
9. American Psychiatric Association, 2000, p. 433.
10. American Psychiatric Association, 2000, p. 667.
11. Wakefield, 2000.
12. Lewis, 1970, p. 77.
13. Taylor & Brown, 1988.
14. Quoted in Treffers & Silverman, 2001, p. 5.

15. E.g., Mineka, 1992.
16. Seligman & Hager, 1972.
17. Seligman, 1971, p. 312.
18. Seligman, 1971, p. 316.
19. American Psychiatric Association, 2000, p. 449.
20. LeBeau et al., 2010, p. 164.
21. American Psychiatric Association, 2000, p. 449. Reprinted with permission.
22. LeBeau et al., 2010, p. 163.
23. LeBeau et al., 2010, p. 163.
24. LeBeau et al., 2010, p. 163.
25. LeBeau et al., 2010, p. 163.
26. Horwitz & Wakefield, 2007.
27. http://articles.cnn.com/2009–09-09/us/meade.excerpt.hln_1_ew-ay-breath?_s=PM:US).
28. American Psychiatric Association, 2000, p. 456. Reprinted with permission.
29. Bogels et al., 2010.
30. Bogels et al., 2010, p. 183.
31. Bogels et al., 2010, p. 182.
32. Bogels et al., 2010, p. 182.
33. Freud, 1957, p. 80.
34. American Psychiatric Association, 2000, p. 476. Reprinted with permission.
35. Andrews et al., 2010, p. 134.
36. Andrews et al., p. 134.
37. Andrews et al., p. 143.
38. Krueger, 1999.
39. Andrews et al., 2010, p. 139.
40. Andrews et al., 2010, p. 140.
41. Andrews et al., 2010, p. 144.
42. Andrews et al., 2010, p. 139.
43. Andrews et al., 2010, p. 139.
44. Andrews et al., 2010, p. 137.
45. Andrews et al., 2010, p. 137.
46. Andrews et al., 2010, p. 135.
47. Andrews et al., 2010, p. 137.
48. Goodwin & Guze, 1996, p. 8.

CHAPTER 6
1. Mann, 1997; Dohrenwend, 1998.
2. Wing, Cooper, & Sartorius, 1974, p. 135.

3. Kessler, Koretz, Merikangas, & Wang, 2004.
4. First, 2002.
5. American Psychiatric Association, 1980, p. 225.
6. Kessler, Chiu, Demler, & Walters, 2005a; Kessler et al., 2005b.
7. Moffitt et al., 2009.
8. Wittchen & Jacobi, 2005.
9. Horwitz & Wakefield, 2006.
10. Grob, 1985.
11. Grob, 1985; Dohrenwend & Dohrenwend, 1982.
12. Dohrenwend & Dohrenwend, 1982.
13. Langner, 1962.
14. Murphy, 1990, p. 71.
15. American Psychiatric Association, 1968, p. 39.
16. Srole et al., 1978, p. 197.
17. E.g., Radloff. 1977; Papadatos, Nikou, & Potamianos, 1990.
18. Marks & Lader, 1973.
19. Weissman, Myers, & Harding, 1978.
20. Agras, Sylvester, & Oliveau, 1969.
21. American Psychiatric Association, 1980, p. 225.
22. Leaf, Myers, & McEvoy, 1991, p. 12.
23. Robins et al., 1984.
24. Robins et al., 1984, p. 294; Weissman & Merikangas, 1986, p. 15.
25. Marks, 1987, p. 305.
26. Barlow, 1988, p. 22.
27. Robins, 1992; Insel & Fenton, 2005.
28. Robins, 1992, p. 1.
29. Wittchen, 2000.
30. Wittchen, 2000, pp. 2–3.
31. http://www.uspreventivemedicine.com/About-Us/National-Advisory-Board/Ronald-Kessler.aspx.
32. Regier et al., 1998, p. 111.
33. Kessler et al., 2005b; Kessler, Chiu, Demler, & Walters, 2005a.
34. Kessler et al., 2005b; Kessler, Chiu, Demler, & Walters, 2005a.
35. WHO World Mental Health Survey Consortium, 2004.
36. Kessler et al., 2002, p. 960. Kessler assumes that clinical interviews are a "gold standard" for assessing the validity of the rates produced by the NCS questionnaires. However, clinicians as well as the NCS are using the same *DSM* criteria, which we have seen is itself flawed and prone to consider many kinds of natural anxieties as disordered.

37. Blazer, Hughes, George, Swartz, & Boyer, 1991.
38. American Psychiatric Association, 2000, p. 473.
39. Kessler, Walters, & Wittchen, 2004.
40. Kessler & Wittchen, 2002; Barlow, 1988; Brown, Barlow, & Liebowitz, 1994, p. 1273.
41. Breslau & Kessler, 2001.
42. Kessler, Brandenberg et al., 2005, p. 1080.
43. American Psychiatric Association, 1986, p. 252.
44. Greenberg, 2007, p. 44.
45. American Psychiatric Association, 1986, p. 252.
46. Wakefield & First, 2003.
47. Kessler, Koretz, Merikangas, & Wang, 2005.
48. The stance of the NCS researchers evokes psychiatrist's Lawrence Hartmann's (1991, p. 1132) observation that: "what is easiest to measure tends to get measured, published, and called 'real' or 'important'; what is harder to measure, even if as important or more important, gets measured far less and valued far less."
49. Ruscio et al., 2005, p. 1769.
50. Ruscio et al., 2007.
51. Kessler et al., 2005b.
52. Spitzer & Williams, 1984, p. 395.
53. Ruscio et al., 2007, p. 667. Conversely, if the duration requirement increases to 12 months, lifetime prevalence declines to 4.2%. See Kessler et al., 2005b, p. 1076.
54. Breslau & Davis, 1985.
55. Ruscio et al., 2005, p. 1762; Ruscio et al., 2007, p. 672.
56. Ruscio et al., 2005; Ruscio et al., 2007.
57. Horwitz & Wakefield, 2007.
58. Ruscio et al. 2005, p. 1769.
59. Kessler, Walters, & Wittchen, 2004, pp. 33–34.
60. Breslau, 1985.
61. Zimbardo, 1977.
62. Nesse, 1998.
63. Darwin, 1872/1998, p. 334.
64. Cicero, 1927, p. 355.
65. Wakefield, Horwitz, & Schmitz, 2005.
66. American Psychiatric Association, 1980, p. 228.
67. American Psychiatric Association, 1980, p. 228.
68. Eaton, Dryman, & Weissman, 1991.
69. Barlow, 1988, p. 536.

70. Kessler, Stein, & Berglund, 1998, pp. 613–619.
71. Ruscio et al., 2008, p. 18.
72. Studies using the criteria of the International Classification of Disease (ICD), which unlike the *DSM* does not consider anxiety over public speaking to be an anxiety disorder, find lower rates of social anxiety disorder. See Ballenger et al., 1998, p. 55.
73. Kessler, Stein, & Berglund, 1998, p. 618.
74. Pettus, 2006, p. 38.
75. American Psychiatric Association, 1980, p. 228.
76. Regier et al., 1998; Kessler et al., 2005a.
77. Magee, Eaton, Wittchen, McGonagle, & Kessler, 1996.
78. In another study, changing cut points from "a great deal of interference" to "a great deal of interference or distress" to "moderate interference or distress" resulted in increasing the prevalence of social anxiety disorder from 1.9% to 7.1% to 18.7%, respectively. See Stein, Waler, & Forde, 1994, p. 408. A European study using the same instrument as the NCS found that varying disorder criteria of avoidance, persistence, excessiveness, and impairment resulted in rates of disorder ranging from 0.9% to 67.1%! See Pelissolo, Andre, Moutard-Martin, Wittchen, & Lepine, 2000.
79. Kessler, Koretz, et al., 2004, p. 165.
80. Kessler, Koretz, et al., 2004, p. 168.
81. Darwin, 1877/1971, p. 5.
82. Freud, 1926/1959, pp. 778–79.
83. Marks, 1987.
84. The NCS studies also rely on the dubious assumption that people can accurately recall anxious symptoms that they experienced many years before they were interviewed.
85. Moffitt et al., 2009.
86. Wakefield, Horwitz, & Schmitz, 2005.
87. Kutchins & Kirk, 1997, p. 244.
88. Dohrenwend, 1973.
89. Dohrenwend, 1973, p. 167.
90. Galea et al., 2003.
91. Kessler et al., 2002; Kessler et al., 2003.
92. Galea et al., 2007.
93. Galea et al., 2007, p. 1427.
94. Wing, Cooper, & Sartorius, 1974, p. 147, italics added.
95. Wessely, 2005, pp. 548–49.
96. Rubin, Brewin, Greenberg, Simpson, & Wessely, 2005.

97. See Narrow, Rae, Robins, & Regier, 2002; Regier et al., 1998; Wakefield & Spitzer, 2002.

CHAPTER 7

1. Lerner & Micale, 2001, p. 3.
2. McHugh, 2008, p. 179.
3. McNally, 2003.
4. The work group for PTSD is also recommending significant changes in the diagnostic criteria for *DSM-5*. See Friedman, Resick, Bryant, & Brewin, 2010.
5. Mineka, 1992, p. 162.
6. Lees-Haley, Price, Williams, & Betz, 2001.
7. Mol et al., 2005; Gold, Marx, Soler-Baillo, & Sloan, 2005.
8. Dattilio, 2004.
9. Brazile, 2008.
10. Spitzer, First, & Wakefield, 2007.
11. Marks, & Nesse, 1994.
12. McHugh, 2008, p. 189.
13. Quoted in Wilson, 1993, p. 405.
14. Breslau & Davis, 1987.
15. Micale, 2008, p. 159.
16. Borch-Jacobsen, 2009, pp. 21–22.
17. Shephard, 2000.
18. Bodkin, Pope, Detke, & Hudson, 2007.
19. Breslau, Davis, Peterson, & Schultz. 2000.
20. Bracken, 2001.
21. Grinker & Spiegel, 1945a; Grinker & Spiegel, 1945b.
22. McHugh, 2008.
23. Young, 2007, p. 1031. See also Solnit, 2009.
24. Ward, 2002, pp. 207–210.
25. Boschen, 2008
26. Summerfield, 2001.
27. Boschen, 2008
28. Statistical Manual, 1942.
29. American Psychiatric Association, 1952.
30. American Psychiatric Association, 1952, p. 40.
31. American Psychiatric Association, 1952, p. 40.
32. American Psychiatric Association, 1952, p. 40.
33. American Psychiatric Association, 1952, p. 48.
34. American Psychiatric Association, 1968, p. 49.

35. E.g., Kolb, 1977; Goodwin & Guze, 1996.

36. Scott, 1990.

37. Scott, 1990, p. 300.

38. E.g., Andreasen, Norris, & Hartford, 1971; Andreasen & Norris, 1972.

39. E.g., Adler, 1943.

40. Scott, 1990.

41. Young, 1995.

42. American Psychiatric Association, 1980, p. 238.

43. Andreasen, 1980, p. 1518.

44. American Psychiatric Association, 1987, p. 250.

45. American Psychiatric Association, 1987, p. 250.

46. Herman, 1992, p. 1.

47. Ofshe & Watters, 1994; McNally, 2003.

48. McNally, 2003, p. 251.

49. American Psychiatric Association, 2000, p. 467.

50. American Psychiatric Association, 2000, p. 467.

51. Friedman, Rescik, Bryant, & Brewin, 2010.

52. Helzer, Robins, & McEvoy, 1987.

53. Davidson, Hughes, Blazer, & George, 1991.

54. Kessler, Sonnega, Bromet, Hughes, & Nelson, 1995.

55. Breslau, Davis, Andreski, Federman, & Anthony, 1991.

56. Young, 1995.

57. Breslau & Kessler, 2001.

58. Breslau & Kessler, 2001.

59. Schuster et al., 2001.

60. Schlenger et al., 2002.

61. Silver, Holman, McIntosh, Poulin, & Gil-Rivas, 2002.

62. Silver et al., 2002, p. 1237.

63. Schuster et al., 2001; Schlenger et al., 2002.

64. Schuster et al., p. 1510; Schlenger et al., 2002, p. 587.

65. Galea, Ahern, Resnick, & Vlahov, 2006; Galea et al., 2003.

66. Boscarino, Galea, Ahern, Resnick, & Vlahov, 2002.

67. Silver et al., 2002.

68. Norton et al., 1995, p. 82.

69. Seal, Bertenthal, Miner, Sen, & Marmar, 2007.

70. Hoge et al., 2004; See also Milliken, Aucherlonie, & Hoge, 2007.

71. Mental Health Advisory Team, 2009, p. 2.

72. McHugh, 2008, p. 189.

73. Tedeschi & Calhoun, 2004; See also Solnit, 2009.

74. Institute of Medicine and National Research Council, 2005.
75. Gladwell, 2004.
76. See Borch-Jacobsen, 2009, pp. 19–36.
77. Tanielian & Jaycox, 2008.
78. McHugh, 2008, pp. 194–195; McNally, 2003.
79. Hoge, 2011, p. 550.
80. Hoge, 2011, p. 549.
81. Hoge, 2011, p. 549.
82. Andreasen, 1995, p. 964.
83. Erichsen, 1866.
84. Quoted in Harrington, 2001, p. 45.
85. Quoted in Caplan, 2001, p. 61.
86. Shephard, 2001, p. 219.
87. Shephard, 2001, pp. 39–72; Jones & Wessely, 2007.
88. Young, 1995.
89. Keane & Penk, 1988, p. 1691.
90. Bourne, 1970a.
91. Bourne, 1970b, p. 296.
92. Borus, 1974.
93. McNally, 2003, p. 9; Grob, 1991b, p. 13.
94. Bourne, 1970a; Bourne, 1970b.
95. Shephard, 1991, pp. 339–353; Scott, 1990.
96. Lee, Vaillant, Torrey, & Elder, 1995.
97. Schnurr, Spiro, Vielhaer, Findler, & Hamblen, 2002.
98. McNally, 2003.
99. Centers for Disease Control, 1988a; Centers for Disease Control, 1988b.
100. Dohrenwend et al., 2006.
101. Young, 1995, p. 133.
102. Thompson, Gottesman, & Zalewski, 2006, p. 19.
103. Dohrenwend et al., 2006, p. 461.
104. McNally, 2006; McNally, 2007.
105. McNally, 2007, p. 483.
106. Schlenger et al., 2007, p. 469, 475.
107. Satel, 2007.
108. Schlenger et al., 2007, p. 476.
109. Breslau and McNally, 2006.
110. Marshall, 2006, pp. 626–627.
111. Marshall, Amsel, & Suh, 2008.
112. Rind, Tromovitch, & Bauserman, 1998.

113. American Psychological Association, 1999. http://www.apa.org/releases/childsexabuse.html.

114. Garrison & Kobor, 2002, p. 168.

115. Satel, 2003.

116. Wessely, 2005, p. 459.

CHAPTER 8

1. This chapter is a modified version of Allan V. Horwitz. 2010. "How an Age of Anxiety became an Age of Depression." *Milbank Quarterly*, 88, pp. 112-138. Used by permission.

2. Rosenberg, 2007.

3. Kessler, Chiu, Demler, & Walters, 2005.

4. Horwitz & Wakefield, 2007.

5. Selye, 1956.

6. Shorter, 1992.

7. Shorter, 1997.

8. Abbott, 1988, p. 285.

9. Harrington, 2008.

10. Abbott, 1990, p. 440.

11. Harrington, 2008.

12. Cannon, 1932/1963; Selye, 1956.

13. Shorter, 2009.

14. Blazer, 2005; Horwitz & Wakefield, 2007; Mojtabai & Olfson, 2008.

15. Tone, 2009; Herzberg, 2009.

16. Rickels, 1968, p. 10.

17. Blackwell, 1975, p. 29.

18. Herzberg, 2009, p. 260.

19. Murphy & Leighton, 2008, p. 1057.

20. Pincus, Henderson, Blackwood, & Dial, 1993.

21. Horwitz, 2002.

22. Healy, 1997, p. 65; Herzberg, 2009.

23. Smith, 1985, p. 316; Tone, 2009, p. 90.

24. Parry et al., 1973.

25. Shorter, 2009.

26. Murphy and Leighton, 2008, p. 1056.

27. Hirschbein, 2009, p. 59.

28. Ayd, 1961.

29. Herzberg, 2009, p. 260.

30. National Disease and Therapeutic Index, 1976, pp. 125–126.

31. Olfson et al., 2002a.
32. Olfson et al., 2002b.
33. Mojtabai & Olfson, 2008.
34. Pincus et al., 1999.
35. http://www.cdc.gov/nchs/fastats/mental.htm.
36. USDHHS, 2006.
37. Regier et al., 1998, p. 111; Kessler & Wang, 2008, p. 119.
38. Barber, 2008, p. 14.
39. Olfson & Klerman, 1993.
40. Zuvekas, 2005.
41. Mojtabai, 2008; Olfson & Marcus, 2009, p. 851.
42. Raofi & Schappert, 2006.
43. IMS Health, 2006.
44. Mojtabai & Olfson, 2008.
45. Rosenberg, 2007 p. 13.
46. Kessler et al., 2003, p. 3101.
47. Freud, 19261989, p. 101; Rycroft, 1988.
48. American Psychiatric Association, 1968, p. 39.
49. Szasz, 1974; Rosenhan, 1973.
50. Cooper et al., 1972.
51. Abbott, 1988.
52. Grob, 1991b, pp. 66–67; Kolb, Frazier, & Sirovatka, 2000, p. 213.
53. Baldessarini, 2000; Kirk, 1999; Schooler, 2007.
54. Kolb, Frazier, & Sirovatka, 2000, p. 221.
55. Kolb, Frazier, & Sirovatka, 2000, p. 223.
56. Healy, 1997.
57. Shapiro & Baron, 1961; Raynes, 1979; Cooperstock & Lennard, 1979.
58. Blackwell, 1973 p. 1638.
59. Herzberg, 2009.
60. Smith, 1985.
61. Bayer & Spitzer, 1985.
62. The important work of Donald Klein is an exception to this generalization (e.g., Klein & Fink, 1962).
63. Hirschbein, 2009, p. 28.
64. Herzberg, 2009, p. 163.
65. Brodie & Sabshin, 1973, p. 1314; Bunney & Davis, 1965; Schildkraut, 1965.
66. Shorter, 2009, p. 152.
67. Horwitz, 2002.
68. American Psychiatric Association, 1980.

69. American Psychiatric Association, 1980, pp. 225–239.
70. Norton, Cox, Asmundson, & Maser, 1995, p. 79; See also Cox et al., 1995, p. 536.
71. Boschen, 2008
72. American Psychiatric Association, 1980, p. 215.
73. Zimmerman & Spitzer, 1989.
74. Shorter, 2009.
75. American Psychiatric Association, 1980, p. 222.
76. Blazer, 2005, p. 28.
77. McPherson & Armstrong, 2006, p. 55.
78. American Psychiatric Association, 1980, pp. 213–214.
79. Murphy, 2006, p. 329.
80. American Psychiatric Association, 1980, p. 232.
81. Barlow, 1988, p. 567.
82. The GAD criteria, which required only one-month duration, were an exception. However, as noted above, the exclusion rules for this diagnosis insured that it could rarely be a stand alone diagnosis. In any case, the one-month duration for GAD was increased to six months in the *DSM-III-R*, which was issued in 1987.
83. American Psychiatric Association, 1980, p. 213.
84. American Psychiatric Association, 1980, pp. 227–230.
85. American Psychiatric Association, 1980, p. 230.
86. Swindle, Heller, Pescosolido, & Kikuzawa, 2009.
87. Quoted in Shorter, 2009, p. 164.
88. Healy, 2004.
89. Gabe, 1990.
90. Herzberg, 2009, p. 73.
91. Shorter, 2009, p. 116.
92. Shorter, 2009, p. 116.
93. Rickels, 1978; Piper, 1995.
94. Smith, 1985, p. 33.
95. Healy, 2004, p. 225.
96. Rickels & Hesbacher, 1977.
97. Rickels & Hesbacher, 1977.
98. Shorter, 2009, p. 149.
99. Kramer, 1992.
100. Healy, 1997; Hirshbein, 2009.
101. Druss, Marcus, Olfson, & Pincus, 2004.
102. Healy, 2008.

103. IMS Health, 2009.

104. Koerner, 2002.

105. Kessler et al., 2005c.

106. Quoted in Nikolas Rose, 2006, p. 471.

107. E.g., Kirsch, 2009; Bass, 2008; Shorter, 2009.

108. IMS Health, 2006.

109. http://www.dsm5.org/proposedrevision/pages/proposedrevision.aspx?rid=407.

110. Brown, 1995.

CHAPTER 9

1. Zerubavel, 1993.

2. Wakefield, 1998.

3. Quoted in Lane, 2007, p. 77.

4. Lebeau et al., 2010.

5. Herzberg, 2009; Tone, 2009.

6. Herzberg, 2009; Gabe, 1990.

7. *JAMA*, September 15, 1969. See Herzberg, 2009, pp. 70–71.

8. Smith, 1985.

9. Healy, 1997.

10. Shorter, 2009.

11. Smith, 1985, p. 187.

12. Smith, 1985, p. 188

13. Smith, 1985, p. 182.

14. Smith, 1985, p. 184.

15. Smith, 1985, p. 189.

16. Smith, 1985, p. 210.

17. Smith, 1985, p. 167.

18. Smith, 1985, p. 168.

19. Smith, 1985, p. 179.

20. Klerman, 1972.

21. Shorter, 2009.

22. Carey & Harris, 2008; Barber, 2008; Carlot, 2010; Greenberg, 2010.

23. Conrad & Leiter, 2008.

24. Donohue, Cevasco, & Rosenthal, 2007.

25. Barber, 2008, p. 49.

26. Ruscio et al., 2007.

27. Hawkins, 2007.

28. Rose, 2007. See also Stepnisky, 2007.

29. Wilkes, Bell, & Kravitz, 2000.
30. Tone, 2009, p. 217.
31. Zimbardo, 1977.
32. Moynihan & Cassells, 2005.
33. Williams later changed his tune and pronounced that marijuana "worked 10 times better for me than Paxil." See Tone, 2009, p. 220.
34. Greene & Herzberg, 2010.
35. http://allpsych.com/tests/diagnostic/anxiety.htm. Accessed June 29, 2009.
36. http://socialanxietydisorder.about.com/gi/dynamic/offsite.htm.
37. Kessler et al., 2001, p. 996.
38. Kessler et al., 2004, p. 168.
39. Kessler et al., 2004, p. 171.
40. New Freedom Commission on Mental Health, 2003.
41. Kessler & Wittchen, 2002.
42. Spitzer et al., 2006.
43. Spitzer et al., 2006, p. 1095.
44. American Psychiatric Association, 1994, p. 435.
45. Ballenger et al., 1998, p. 55.
46. Ballenger et al., 1998.
47. Kessler & Waters, 2002, pp. 348–349.
48. Kessler & Waters, 2002, p. 350.
49. Kessler & Walters, 2002.
50. Kessler, 2003, p. 566.
51. Dierker et al., p. 935.
52. March et al., 1997, p. 555.
53. Dierker et al., 2001, p, 932.
54. Horwitz & Wakefield, 2009.
55. Sommers & Satel, 2005.
56. Karp, 2006, p. 175.
57. Karp, 2006.
58. Wakefield, 1988.
59. See the many reports about the treatment of anxiety on the Cochrane Reviews website: www.cochrane.org. The general effectiveness of treatments for anxiety contrasts with the controversies over the benefits of treatments for depression (e.g., Kirsch, 2010; Greenberg, 2010).
60. Kirsch, 2010.
61. Conrad, 2007.
62. Karp, 2006, pp. 207–229.
63. Smith, 1985, p. 181.
64. Wakefield, Horwitz, & Schmitz, 2005.
65. Wakefield, 1988.
66. Rachman, 1978.

REFERENCES

Abbott, A. (1988). *The system of the professions*. Chicago: University of Chicago Press.

Abbott, A. (1990). Positivism and interpretation in sociology: Lessons for sociologists from the history of stress research. *Sociological Forum, 5*, 435–458.

Adler, A. (1943). Neuropsychiatric complications in victims of Boston's Coconut Grove disaster. *Journal of the American Medical Association, 123*, 1098–1101.

Agras, S., Sylvester, D., & Oliveau, D. (1969). The epidemiology of common fears and phobias. *Comprehensive Psychiatry, 10*, 1969, 151–156.

Akiskal, H.S. (1998). Toward a definition of generalized anxiety disorder as an anxious temperament type. *Acta Psychiatrica Scandivavia, 98* (suppl 393), 66–73.

Aldrich, T.K., Jackson G., Hall, C.B., Cohen, H.W., Mayris, P.H., Webber, P., Zeig-Owens, R., Cosenza, K., Christodoulou,V., Glass, L., Al-Othman, F., Weiden, M.D., Kelly, K.J., & Prezantet, D.J. (2010). Lung function in rescue workers at the World Trade Center after 7 years. *New England Journal of Medicine, 362*, April 8, 1263–1272.

American Psychiatric Association. (1952). *Diagnostic and statistical manual of mental disorders*. Washington, DC: Author.

American Psychiatric Association. (1968). *Diagnostic and statistical manual of mental disorders, 2nd ed.* Washington, DC: Author.

American Psychiatric Association. (1994). *Diagnostic and statistical manual of mental disorders, 4th ed.* Washington, DC: Author.

American Psychiatric Association. (1980). *Diagnostic and statistical manual of mental disorders, 3rd ed.* Washington DC: Author.

American Psychiatric Association. (1987). *Diagnostic and statistical manual of mental disorders, 3rd ed., Revised*. Washington DC: Author.

American Psychiatric Association. (2000). *Diagnostic and statistical manual of mental disorders, 4th ed., text rev.* Washington DC: Author.

American Psychological Association. 1999. Retrieved from http://www.apa.org/releases/childsexabuse.html

Andreasen, N.C. (1980). Posttraumatic stress disorder. In H.I. Kaplan, A.M. Freedman, & B.J. Saddock (Eds.), *Comprehensive textbook of psychiatry* (3rd ed., pp. 1517–1525). Baltimore: Williams and Wilkins.

Andreasen, N.C. (1984). *The broken brain: The biological revolution in psychiatry*. New York: HarperCollins.

Andreasen, N.C. (1995). Posttraumatic stress disorder: Psychology, biology, and the Manichean warfare between false dichotomies. *American Journal of Psychiatry, 152,* 963–965.

Andreason, N.J.C., & Norris, A.S. (1972). Long-term adjustment and adaptation mechanisms in severely burned adults. *Journal of Nervous and Mental Disorders, 154,* 352–362.

Andreason, N.J.C., Norris, A.S., & Hartford, C.E. (1971). Incidence of long-term psychiatric complications in severely burned adults. *Annals of Surgery, 174,* 785–795.

Andrews, G., Hobbs, M.J., Borkovec, T.D., Beesdo, K., Craske, M.G., Heimberg, R.G., Rapee, R.M., Ruscio, A.M., & Stanley, M.A. (2010). Generalized worry disorder: A review of DSM-IV generalized anxiety disorder and options for DSM-V. *Depression and Anxiety, 27,* 134–147.

Andrews, P.W., & Thomson, J.A. (2009). The bright side of being blue: Depression as an adaptation for analyzing complex problems. *Psychological Review, 116,* 620–654.

Aristotle. (1991). *The art of rhetoric* (H. Lawson-Tancred, Ed.). New York: Penguin.

Aristotle. (2009). *The Nichomachean ethics* (L. Brown & D. Ross, Eds). New York: Oxford.

Arnold, T. (1782). *Observations on the nature, kinds, causes, and prevention, of insanity.* London: Richard Phillips.

Ayd, F. (1961). *Recognizing the depressed patient.* New York: Grune and Stratton.

Baldessarini, R.J. (2000). American biological psychiatry and psychopharmacology, 1944–1994. In R.W. Menninger & J.C. Nemiah (Eds.), *American psychiatry after World War II* (pp. 371–412). Washington, DC: American Psychiatric Press.

Ballenger, J.C., Davidson, J.R.T., Lecrubier, Y., Nutt, D.J., Bobes, J., Beidel, D.C., Ono, Y., & Westenberg, H.G. (1998). Consensus statement on social anxiety disorder from the International Consensus Group on Depression and Anxiety. *Journal of Clinical Psychiatry, 59,* (suppl 17), 54–60.

Bandura, A. (1977). *Social learning theory.* Englewood Cliffs, NJ: Prentice Hall.

Barber, C. (2008). *Comfortably numb: How psychiatry is medicating a nation.* New York: Pantheon Books.

Barlow, D.H. (1988). *Anxiety and its disorders.* New York: The Guilford Press.

Bass, A. (2008). *Side effects: A prosecutor, a whistleblower, and a bestselling antidepressant on trial.* New York: Algonquin.

Bayer, R., & Spitzer, R.L. (1985). Neurosis, psychodynamics, and DSM-III: History of the controversy. *Archives of General Psychiatry, 42,* 187–196.

Beard, G. (1869). Neurasthenia, or nervous exhaustion. *Boston Medical and Surgical Journal, 3,* 217–221.

Bell, J. (2008). When anxiety is at the table. *New York Times*, February 6, E1.

Benedict, R. (1934). *Patterns of culture*. New York: Houghton Mifflin.

Black, D. (2011). *Moral time*. New York: Oxford University Press.

Blackwell, B. (1973). Psychotropic drugs in use today: The role of Diazepam in medical practice. *JAMA, 225*, 1637–1641.

Blackwell, B. (1975). Minor tranquilizers: Use, misuse or overuse? *Psychosomatics, 16*, 28–31.

Blazer, D. (2005). *The age of melancholy: Major depression and its social origins*. New York: Routledge.

Blazer, D.J., Hughes, D., George, L.K. Swartz, M., & Boyer, R. (1996). Generalized anxiety disorder. In L.N. Robins & D.A. Regier (Eds.), *Psychiatric disorders in America: The Epidemiologic Catchment Area Study* (pp. 180–203). New York: The Free Press.

Bloom, P. (2010). The moral life of babies. *The New York Times Magazine*, May 9, 65.

Bodkin, A., Pope, H.G., Detke, M.J., & Hudson, J.I. (2007). Is PTSD caused by traumatic stress? *Journal of Anxiety Disorders, 21*, 176–182.

Bolton, D. (2008). *What is mental disorder? An essay in philosophy, science, and values*. New York: Oxford University Press.

Borch-Jacobsen, M. (2009). *Making minds and madness: From hysteria to depression*. New York: Cambridge University Press.

Borus, J.F. (1974). Incidence of maladjustment in Vietnam returnees. *Archives of General Psychiatry, 30*, 554–557.

Boscarino, J.A, Galea, S., Ahern, J., Resnick, H., & Vlahov, D. (2002). Utilization of mental health services following the September 11th terrorist attacks in Manhattan, New York City. *International Journal of Emergency Mental Health, 4*, 143–156.

Boschen, M.J. (2008). Publication trends in individual anxiety disorders: 1980–2015. *Journal of Anxiety Disorders, 22*, 570–575.

Bourke, J. (2005). *Fear: A cultural history*. Emeryville, CA: Shoemaker & Hoard.

Bourne, P.G. (1970a). Military psychiatry and the Viet Nam experience. *American Journal of Psychiatry, 127*, 481–488.

Bourne, P.G. (1970b). *Men, stress, and Vietnam*. Boston: Little, Brown.

Bowlby, J. (1969). *Attachment and loss (Volume I. Attachment)*. New York: Basic Books.

Bowlby, J. (1970). Reasonable fear and natural fear. *International Journal of Psychiatry, 9*, 79–88.

Boyd, J.H., Burke, J.D., Gruenberg, E., Holzer, C.E., Rae, D.S., George, L.K., Karno, M., Stoltzman, R., McEyoy, L., & Nestadt, G. (1984). Exclusion criteria of DSM-III: A study of co-occurrence of hierarchy-free syndromes. *Archives of General Psychiatry, 41*, 983–989.

Bracken, P.J. (2001). Post-modernity and post-traumatic stress disorder. *Social Science and Medicine, 53*, 733–743.

Brazile, D. (2008). Commentary: A letter to the losers. *CNN Politics*. Retrieved from http://articles.cnn.com/2008-11-07/politics/brazile.losers

Breier, A., Charney, D.S., & Heninger, G.R. (1985). The diagnostic validity of anxiety disorders and their relationship to depressive illness. *American Journal of Psychiatry, 142*, 787–797.

Breslau, N. (1985). Depressive symptoms, major depression, and generalized anxiety: A comparison of self-reports on CES-D and results from diagnostic interviews. *Psychiatry Research, 15*, 219–229.

Breslau, N., & Davis, G.C. (1985). DSM-III generalized anxiety disorder: An empirical investigation of more stringent criteria. *Psychiatric Research, 15*, 231–238.

Breslau, N., & Davis, G. C. (1987). Posttraumatic stress disorder: The stressor criterion. *Journal of Nervous and Mental Disease, 175*, 255–264.

Breslau, N., & Kessler, R.C. (2001). The stressor criterion in DSM-IV posttraumatic stress disorder: An empirical investigation. *Biological Psychiatry, 50*, 699–704.

Breslau, N., & McNally, R. J. (2006). The epidemiology of 9-11: Technical advances and conceptual conundrums. In Y. Neria, R. Gross, R. Marshall, & E. Susser (Eds.), *9/11: Mental health in the wake of terrorist attacks* (pp. 521–528). Cambridge, UK: Cambridge University Press.

Breslau, N., Davis, G.C., Andreski, P., Federman, B., & Anthony, J.C. (1991). Traumatic events and post-traumatic stress disorder in an urban population of young adults. *Archives of General Psychiatry, 48*, 216–222.

Breslau, N., Davis, G.C., Peterson, E.L., & Schultz, L.R. (2000). A second look at comorbidity in victims of trauma: The posttraumatic stress disorder–major depression connection. *Biological Psychiatry, 48*, 902–909.

Brodie, H.K., & Sabshin, M. (1973). An overview of trends in psychiatric research: 1963–1972. *American Journal of Psychiatry, 130*, 1309–1318.

Brown, P. (1995). Naming and framing: The social construction of diagnosis and illness. *Journal of Health and Social Behavior, 36* (special issue), 34–52.

Brown, T.A., Barlow, D.H., & Liebowitz, M.R. (1994). The empirical basis of generalized anxiety disorder. *American Journal of Psychiatry, 151*, 1272–1280.

Buckley, T., McKinley, S., Tofler, G., & Bartrop, R. (2010). Cardiovascular risk in early bereavement: A literature review and proposed mechanisms. *International Journal of Nursing Studies, 47*, 229–238.

Buller, D.J. (2005). *Adapting minds: Evolutionary psychology and the persistent quest for human nature*. Cambridge: MIT Press.

Bulmer, M. (2003). *Francis Galton: Pioneer of heredity and biometry*. Baltimore: The Johns Hopkins University Press.

Bunney, W.E., & Davis, J.M. (1965). Norepinephrine in depressive reactions. *Archives of General Psychiatry, 13*, 483–494.

Burton, R. (1621/2001). *The anatomy of melancholy*. New York: New York Review Books.

Buss, D.M. (1995). Evolutionary psychology: A new paradigm for psychological science. *Psychological Inquiry, 6*, 1–30.

Buss, D.M. (2009). How can evolutionary psychology successfully explain personality and individual differences? *Perspectives on Psychological Science, 4*, 359–366.

Campbell-Sills, L., & Stein, M.B. (2005). Justifying the diagnostic status of social phobia: A reply to Wakefield and others. *Canadian Journal of Psychiatry, 50*, 320–323.

Cannon, W. (1932/1963). *The wisdom of the body*. New York: W. W. Norton.

Caplan, E. (2001). Trains and trauma in the American Gilded Age. In M.S. Micale & P. Lerner (Eds.), *Traumatic pasts* (pp. 57–77). New York: Cambridge University Press.

Caplan, P. (1996). *They say you're crazy: How the world's most powerful psychiatrists decide who's normal.* New York: De Capo Press.

Carey, B., & Harris, G. (2008). Psychiatric group faces scrutiny over drug industry ties. *The New York Times,* July 12, A1.

Carlot, D.J. (2010). *Unhinged: The trouble with psychiatry.* New York: Free Press.

Cates, D.F. (2009). *Aquinas on the emotions.* Washington, DC: Georgetown University Press.

Centers for Disease Control Vietnam Experience Study. (1988a). Health status of Vietnam veterans: I. Psychosocial characteristics. *Journal of the American Medical Association, 259,* 2701–2707.

Centers for Disease Control Vietnam Experience Study. (1988a). Health status of Vietnam veterans: II. Physical health. *Journal of the American Medical Association, 259,* 2708–2714.

Charlesworth, W.R., & Kreutzer, M.A. (1973). Facial expressions of infants and children. In P. Ekman (Ed.), *Darwin and facial expression: A century of research in review* (pp. 91–168). New York: Academic Press.

Cicero. (1927). Tusculan disputations (J.E. King, Trans.). London: William Heinemann.

Conrad, P. (2007). *The medicalization of society: The transformation of human conditions into treatable disorders.* Baltimore: Johns Hopkins University Press.

Conrad, P., & Leiter, V. (2008). From Lydia Pinkham to Queen Levitra: Direct-to-consumer advertising and medicalisation. *Sociology of Health and Illness, 30,* 825–838.

Cook, M., & Mineka, S. (1989). Observational conditioning of fear to fear-relevant versus fear—irrelevant stimuli in rhesus monkeys. *Journal of Abnormal Psychology, 98,* 448–459.

Cooper, D. (1967). *Psychiatry and anti-psychiatry.* London: Paladin.

Cooper, J. Rendell, R., Burfland, B., Sharpe, L., Copeland, J., & Simon R. (1972). *Psychiatric diagnosis in New York and London.* London: Oxford University Press.

Cooperstock, R., & Lennard, H. (1979). Some social meanings of tranquilizer use. *Sociology of Health and Illness, 1,* 331–347.

Cox, B.J., Wessel, I., Norton, G.R., Swinson, R.P., & Direnfeld, D.M. (1995). Publication trends in anxiety disorders research: 1990–92. *Journal of Anxiety Disorders, 9,* 531–538.

Crews, F. (1999). *Unauthorized Freud: Doubters confront a legend.* New York: Penguin.

Curtis, G.C., Magee, W.J., Eaton, W.W., Wittchen, H.-U., & Kessler, R.C. (1998). Specific fears and phobias: Epidemiology and classification. *British Journal of Psychiatry, 173,* 212–217.

Damasio, A. (1994). *Descartes' error: Emotion, reason, and the human brain.* New York: HarperCollins.

Darwin, C. (1872/1998). *The expression of emotions in man and animals, 3rd ed.* Minneapolis: Filiquarian Publishing.

Darwin, C. (1877/1971). A biographical sketch of an infant. *Developmental Medicine and Child Neurology, 13,* (suppl 24), 3–8 (originally in *Mind,* 1877, 7, 285–294).

Dattilio, F.M. (2004). Extramarital affairs: The much overlooked PTSD. *The Behavior Therapist, 27,* 76–78.

David, L.J. (2008). *Obsession: A history*. Chicago: University of Chicago Press.

Davidson, J.R., Hughes, D., Blazer, D.G., & George, L.K. (1991). Post-traumatic stress disorder in the community: An epidemiological study. *Psychological Medicine, 21,* 713–721.

Davidson, R.J. (2003). Darwin and the neural bases of emotion and affective style. *Annals of the New York Academy of Science, 1000,* 316–336.

Dierker, L.C., Albano, A.M., Clarke, G.N., Heimberg, R.G., Kendell, P.C., Merikangas, K.R., Lewinsohn, P.M., Offord, D.R., Kessler, R.C., & Kupfer, D.J. (2001). Screening for anxiety and depression in early adolescence. *Journal of the American Academy of Child and Adolescent Psychiatry, 40,* 929–936.

Dillon, S. (2008). Messages of exhortation, counsel, and congratulation. *New York Times,* June 15, A18.

Dohrenwend, B.P. (1998). A psychosocial perspective on the past and future of psychiatric epidemiology. *American Journal of Epidemiology, 147,* 222–231.

Dohrenwend, B.P., & Dohrenwend, B.S. (1982). Perspectives on the past and future of psychiatric epidemiology. *American Journal of Public Health, 72,* 1271–1279.

Dohrenwend, B.P., Turner, J.B., Turse, N.A., Adams, B.G., Koenen, K.C., & Marshall, R. (2006). The psychological risks of Vietnam for U.S. veterans: A revisit with new data and methods. *Science, 313,* 979–982.

Dohrenwend, B.S. (1973). Life events as stressors: A methodological inquiry. *Journal of Health and Social Behavior, 14,* 167–175.

Donohue, J.M., Cevasco, M., & Rosenthal, M.B. (2007). A decade of direct-to-consumer advertising of prescription drugs. *New England Journal of Medicine, 357,* 673–681.

Druss, B.G., Marcus, S.C., Olfson, M., & Pincus, H.A. (2004). Listening to generic Prozac: Winners, losers, and sideliners. *Health Affairs, 23,* 210–216.

Eaton, W.W., Dryman, A., & Weissman, M.M. (1991). Panic and phobia. In L. Robins & D. Regier (Eds.), *Psychiatric disorders in America* (pp. 155–179). New York: Free Press.

Ekman, P., & Friesen, W.V. (1971). Constants across cultures in the face and emotion. *Journal of Personality and Social Psychology, 17,* 124–129.

Erichsen, J.E. (1866). *On railway and other injuries of the nervous system*. London: Walton and Maberly.

Evans-Pritchard, E.E. (1937/1976). *Witchcraft, oracles and magic among the Azande.* New York: Oxford University Press.

Feighner, J.P., Robins, E., Guze, S.B., Woodruff, R.A., Winokur, G., & Munoz, R. (1972). Diagnostic criteria for use in psychiatric research. *Archives of General Psychiatry, 26,* 57–63.

Finlay-Jones, R., & Brown, G. W. (1981). Types of stressful life events and the onset of anxiety and depressive disorders. *Psychological Medicine, 11,* 803–815.

First, M.B. (2002). DSM-IV and psychiatric epidemiology. In M.T. Tsuang & M. Tohen (Eds.), *Textbook in psychiatric epidemiology* (2nd ed., pp. 333–342). New York: John Wiley & Sons.

Fisher, P. (2002). *The vehement passions*. Princeton: Princeton University Press.

Foderado, L.W. (2008). Children left at home, worriedly. *New York Times,* August 14, A18.

Fortenbaugh, W.W. (2002). *Aristotle on emotions (2nd ed.)*. London: Duckworth Publishers.

Frances, A. (2010). Good grief. *The New York Times*, August 14, A21.

Freud, S. (1909). Notes upon a case of obsessional neurosis. In *The standard edition of the complete psychological works of Sigmund Freud, Volume X (1909): Two case histories ("Little Hans" and the "Rat Man")*, 151–318.

Freud, S. (1894/1953). *The Neuro-psychoses of defence, standard edition*, volume 3. London: Hogarth Press.

Freud, S. (1916–17). *Introductory lectures on psycho-analysis, lecture XXV, standard edition, volume 15–16*. London: Hogarth Press.

Freud, S. (1926/1989). *Inhibitions, symptoms, and anxiety*. New York: W. W. Norton.

Freud, S. (1930). *Civilization and its discontents*. New York: Norton.

Freud, S. (1933/1965). *New introductory lectures on psycho-analysis,* lecture XXXII, *standard edition*, volume 22. New York: W.W. Norton.

Freud, S. (1957). *Collected papers, vol. 1*. London: Hogarth Press.

Friedman, M.J., Resick, P.A., Bryant, R.A., & Brewin, C. (2010). Considering PTSD for DSM-5. *Depression and Anxiety, 28*, 750–769.

Furedi, F. (2004). *Therapy culture*. New York: Routledge.

Gabe, J. (1990). Towards a sociology of tranquillizer prescribing. *British Journal of Addiction, 85*, 41–48.

Gajilan, C. (2008). Iraq vets and post-traumatic stress: No easy answers. Retrieved from http://www.cnn.com/2008/HEALTH/conditions/10/24/ptsd.struggle

Galea, S., Ahern, J., Resnick, H., & Vlahov, D. (2006). Post-traumatic stress symptoms in the general population after a disaster: Implications for public health. In Y. Neria, R. Gross, & R.D. Marshall (Eds.), *9/11: Mental health in the wake of terrorist attacks* (pp. 19–44). New York: Cambridge University Press.

Galea, S., Brewin, C.R., Gruber, M., Jones, R.T., King, D.W., King, L.A., McNally, R.J., Ursano, R.J, Petukhova, M., & Kessler, R.C. (2007). Exposure to hurricane-related stressors and mental illness after Hurricane Katrina. *Archives of General Psychiatry, 64*, 1427–1434.

Galea, S., Vlahov, D., Resnick, H., Ahern, J., Susser, E., Gold, J., Bucuvalas, M., & Kilpatrick, D. (2003). Trends of probable post-traumatic stress disorder in New York City after the September 11 terrorist attacks. *American Journal of Epidemiology, 158*, 514–524.

Garbowsky, M.M. (1989). *The house without the door*. Madison, NJ: Fairleigh Dickinson University Press.

Gardner, D. (2008). *The science of fear*. New York: Plume.

Garrison, E.G., & Kobor, P.C. (2002). Weathering a political storm: A contextual perspective on a psychological research controversy. *American Psychologist, 57*, 165–175.

Gay, P. (2002). *Schnitzler's century. The making of middle-class culture 1815–1914*. New York: W.W. Norton.

Gibson, E.J., & Walk, R.D. (1960). The "visual cliff." *Scientific American, 202*, 67–71.

Gilbert, P. (2001). Evolution and social anxiety: The role of attraction, social competition, and social hierarchies. *The Psychiatric Clinics of North America, 24*, 723–751.

Gladwell, M. (2004). Getting over it. *The New Yorker*, November 8, 75–79.

Glas, G. (1994). A conceptual history of anxiety and depression. In J.A. den Boer & J. M. Ad Sitsen (Eds.), *Handbook of depression and anxiety: A biological approach* (pp. 1–44). New York: Marcel Dekker.

Glassner, B. (1999). *The culture of fear: Why Americans are afraid of the wrong things.* New York: Basic Books.

Gold, S.D., Marx, B.P., Soler-Baillo, J.M., & Sloan, D.M. (2005). Is life stress more traumatic than traumatic stress? *Journal of Anxiety Disorders, 19,* 687–698.

Goldstein, K. (1963). *Human nature in the light of psychopathology.* New York: Schocken.

Goodall, J. (1990). *Through a window.* Boston: Houghton Mifflin.

Goodwin, D.W., & Guze, S.B. (1996). *Psychiatric diagnosis* (5th edition). New York: Oxford University Press.

Gould, S.J., & Lewontin, R.C. (1979). The spandrels of San Marco and the Panglossian paradigm: A critique of the adaptationist programme. *Proceedings of the Royal Society of London,* ser. B205, 581–598.

Graver, M.R. (2007). *Stoicism and emotion.* Chicago: University of Chicago Press.

Greenberg, G. (2010). *Manufacturing depression: The secret history of a modern disease.* New York: Simon & Shuster.

Greene, J.A., & Herzberg, D. (2010). Hidden in plain sight: Marketing prescription drugs to consumers in the twentieth century. *American Journal of Public Health, 100,* 793–803.

Griffiths, P.E. (1997). *What emotions really are: The problem of psychological categories.* Chicago: University of Chicago Press.

Grinker, R.R., & Spiegel, J.P. (1945a). *War neuroses.* Philadelphia: Blakiston.

Grinker, R.R., & Spiegel, J.P. (1945b). *Men under stress.* Philadelphia: Blakiston.

Grob, G. (1991a). Origins of DSM-I: A study of appearance and reality. *American Journal of Psychiatry, 148,* 421–431.

Grob, G. (1991b). *From asylum to community: Mental health policy in modern America.* Princeton: Princeton University Press.

Grob, G.N. (1985). The origins of American psychiatric epidemiology. *American Journal of Public Health, 75,* 229–236.

Gross, D.M. (2006). *The secret history of emotion: From Aristotle's rhetoric to modern brain science.* Chicago: University of Chicago Press.

Harrington, A. (2008). *The cure within: A history of mind-body medicine.* New York: W.W. Norton.

Harrington, R. (2001). The railway accident: Trains, trauma, and technological crises in nineteenth century Britain. In M.S. Micale & P. Lerner (Eds.), *Traumatic pasts* (pp. 31–56). New York: Cambridge University Press.

Hartmann, L. (1991). Response to the presidential address: Humane values and biopsychosocial integration. *American Journal of Psychiatry, 148,* 1130–1134.

Hawkins, B. (2007). Paxil is forever—can you quit?—marketing secrets. Retrieved from http://seroxatsecrets.wordpress.com/2007/12/30/paxil-is-forever-can-you-quit/

Healy, D. (1997). *The anti-depressant era.* Cambridge: Harvard University Press.

Healy, D. (2004). Shaping the intimate. *Social Studies of Science, 34,* 219–245.

Healy, D. (2008). *Mania: A short history of bipolar disorder.* Baltimore: Johns Hopkins University Press.

Hebb, D.O. (1968). Concerning imagery. *Psychological Review, 75*, 466–477.

Heckelman, L.R., & Schneier, F.R. (1995). Diagnostic issues. In R.G. Heimberg, M.R. Liebowitz, D.A. Hope, & F.R. Schneier (Eds), *Social phobia: diagnosis, assessment, and treatment* (pp. 3–20). New York: The Guilford Press.

Heidegger, M. (1977). What is metaphysics? In D.F. Krell (Ed.), *Basic writings*(pp. 95–138). New York: Harper and Row.

Helzer, J.E., Robins, L.N., & McEvoy, L. (1987). Post-traumatic stress disorder in the general population: Findings of the epidemiologic catchment area survey. *New England Journal of Medicine, 317*, 1630–1634.

Herman, J. (1992). *Trauma and recovery.* New York: Basic Books.

Herzberg, D. (2009). *Happy pills in America: From Miltown to Prozac.* Baltimore: Johns Hopkins University Press.

Higley, J.D., Mehlman, P.T., Higley, S.B., Fernald, B., Vickers, J., Lindell, S.G., Taub, D.M., Suomi, S.J., Linnoila, M. (1996). Excessive mortality in young free-ranging male nonhuman primates with low cerebrospinal fluid 5-hydroxyindoleacetic acid concentrations. *Archives of General Psychiatry, 53*, 537–543.

Hirschbein, L. (2009). *American melancholy.* New Brunswick: Rutgers University Press.

Hobbes, T. (1651/2009). *The leviathan.* New York: Oxford World Classics.

Hoge, C.W. (2011). Interventions for war-related posttraumatic stress disorder: Meeting veterans where they are. *JAMA, 306*, 549–551.

Hoge, C.W., Castro, C.A., Messer, S.C., McGurk, D., Cotting, D.I., & Koffman, R.L. (2004). Combat duty in Iraq and Afghanistan, mental health problems, and barriers to care. *The New England Journal of Medicine, 351*, 13–22.

Horney, K. (1937). *The neurotic personality of our time.* New York: W.W. Norton.

Horwitz, A.V. (2002). *Creating mental illness.* Chicago: University of Chicago Press.

Horwitz, A.V., & Wakefield, J.C. (2006). The epidemic in mental illness: Clinical fact or survey artifact? *Contexts, 5*, 19–23.

Horwitz, A.V., & Wakefield, J.C. (2007). *The loss of sadness: How psychiatry transformed normal sorrow into depressive disorder.* New York: Oxford University Press.

Horwitz, A.V., & Wakefield, J.C. (2009). Should screening for depression among children and adolescents be demedicalized? Placing screening in the context of normal intense adolescent emotion. *Journal of the Academy of Child and Adolescent Psychiatry, 48*, 683–687.

Huizinga, J. (1924). *The waning of the Middle Ages.* New York: St. Martin's Press.

Hume, D. (1740/1967). *A treatise of human nature.* New York: Oxford University Press.

IMS Health. (2006). Top 10 therapeutic classes by U.S. dispensed prescriptions. Retrieved from www.imshealth.com

IMS Health. (2009). Top therapeutic classes by U.S. sales. Retrieved from http://www.imshealth.com/portal/site/imshealth/menuitem

Insel, T.R., & Cuthbert, B.N. (2009). Endophenotypes: Bridging genomic complexity and disorder heterogeneity. *Biological Psychiatry, 66*, 988–989.

Insel, T.R., & Fenton, W.S. (2005). Psychiatric epidemiology: It's not just about counting anymore. *Archives of General Psychiatry, 62*, 590–592.

Institute of Medicine and National Research Council. (2005). *PTSD compensation and military service.* Washington DC: National Academics Press.

Jackson, S. (1986). *Melancholia and depression: From Hippocratic times to modern times.* New Haven: Yale University Press.

James, W. (1884). What is an emotion? *Mind, 9,* 188–205.

James, W. (1900). *Psychology (American Science Series, briefer course).* New York: Henry Holt and Company.

Janet, P. (1903/1976). *Les obsessions et la psychasthénie.* New York: Arno Press.

John, Enid M. (1941). A study of the effects of evacuation and air raids on children of pre-school age. *British Journal of Educational Psychology, 11,* 173–182.

Jones, E., & Wessely, S. (2007). A paradigm shift in the conceptualization of psychological trauma in the 20th century. *Journal of Anxiety Disorders, 21,* 64–175.

Kagan, J. (1976). Emergent themes in human development. *American Scientist, 64,* 186–196.

Kagan, J. (2007). *What is emotion? History, measures, and meanings.* New Haven: Yale University Press.

Kagan, J., Kearsley, R.B., & Zelazo, P.R. (1978). *Infancy: Its place in human development.* Cambridge, MA: Harvard University Press.

Kaiser, S.H. (2003). The world should know what he did to my family. *The Washington Post,* May 18, B02.

Kakutani, M. (2008). When fear and chaos are normal, peace and safety become unimaginable. *The New York Times,* September 2, E4.

Kandel, E.R. (1998). A new intellectual framework for psychiatry. *American Journal of Psychiatry, 155,* 457–469.

Karp, D. (2006). *Is it me or my meds? Living with antidepressants.* Cambridge: Harvard University Press.

Kaufman, M.R. (1947). Ill health as an expression of anxiety in a combat unit. *Psychosomatic Medicine, 9,* 104–109.

Kazdin, A.E. (1978). *History of behavioral modification.* Baltimore: University Park Press.

Keane, T.M., & Penk, W.E. (1988). The prevalence of post-traumatic stress disorder. *New England Journal of Medicine, 318,* 1691.

Kendler, K.S. (2008). Book review, Loss of Sadness. *Psychological Medicine, 38,* 148–150.

Kessler, D. (2009). *The end of overeating.* New York: Rodale Press.

Kessler, R.C. (2003). The impairments caused by social phobia in the general population: Implications for intervention. *Acta Psychiatrica Scandivavica, 108* (suppl 417), 19–27.

Kessler, R.C., & Wang, P.S. (2008). The descriptive epidemiology of commonly occurring mental disorders in the United States. *Annual Review of Public Health, 29,* 115–129.

Kessler, R.C., & Waters, E.E. (2002). The National Comorbidity Survey. In M.T. Tsaung & M. Tohen (Eds.), *Textbook in psychiatric epidemiology* (pp. 343–362). New York: John Wiley & Sons.

Kessler, R.C., & Wittchen, H.-U. (2002). Patterns and correlates of generalized anxiety disorder in community samples. *Journal of Clinical Psychiatry, 63* (suppl 8), 4–10.

Kessler, R.C., Andrews, G., Colpe, L.J., Hiripi, E., Mroczek, D.K., Normand, S.L., Walters, E.E., & Zaslavsky, A.M. (2002). Short screening scales to monitor population prevalences and trends in non-specific psychological distress. *Psychological Medicine,* *32,* 959–976.

Kessler, R.C., Barker, P.R., Colpe, L.J., Epstein, J.F., Gfroerer, J.C., Hiripi, E., Howes, M.J, Normand, S.-L.T., Manderscheid, R.W., Walters, E.E., & Zaslavsky, A.M. (2003). Screening for serious mental illness in the general population. *Archives of General Psychiatry, 60,* 184–189.

Kessler, R.C., Berglund, P.A., Bruce, M.L., Koch, J.R., Laska, E.M., Leaf, P.J., Manderscheid, R.W., Rosenheck, R.A., Walters, E.E., & Wang, P.S. (2001). The prevalence and correlates of untreated serious mental illness. *Health Services Research, 36,* 987–1007.

Kessler, R.C., Berglund, P.A., Foster, C.L., Saunders, W.B., Stang, P.E., & Walters, E.E. (1997). The social consequences of psychiatric disorders: II. Teenage childbearing. *American Journal of Psychiatry, 154,* 1405–1411.

Kessler, R.C., Berglund, P., Demler, O., Jin, R., Koretz, D., Merikangas, K.R., Rush, A.J., Walters, E.E., & Wang, P.S. (2003). The epidemiology of major depressive disorder: Results from the National Comorbidity Survey Replication. *JAMA, 289,* 3095–3105.

Kessler, R.C., Berglund, P., Demler, O., Jin, R., Merikangas, K.R., & Walters, E.E. (2005a). Lifetime prevalence and age-of-onset distributions of DSM-IV disorders in the National Comorbidity Survey replication. *Archives of General Psychiatry, 62,* 593–602.

Kessler, R.C., Brandenburg, N., Lane, M., Roy-Byrne, P., Stang, P.D., Stein, D.J., & Wittchen, H.-U. (2005b). Rethinking the duration requirement for generalized anxiety disorder: Evidence from the National Comorbidity Survey Replication. *Psychological Medicine, 35,* 1073–1082.

Kessler, R.C., Chiu, W.T, Demler, O., & Walters, E.E. (2005c). Prevalence, severity, and comorbidity of 12-month DSM-IV disorders in the National Comorbidity Survey Replication. *Archives of General Psychiatry, 62,* 617–627.

Kessler, R.C., Foster, C.L., Saunders, W.B., & Stang, P.E. (1995). The social consequences of psychiatric disorders: I. Education attainment. *American Journal of Psychiatry, 54,* 313–321.

Kessler, R.C., Koretz, D., Merikangas, K.R., & Wang, P.S. (2004). The epidemiology of adult mental disorders. In B.L. Levin, J. Petrilice, & K.D. Hennessey (Eds.), *Mental health services: A public health perspective* (2nd ed., pp. 157–176). New York: Oxford University Press.

Kessler, R.C., Merikangas, K.R., Beglund, P., Eaton, W.W., Koretz, D.S., & Walters, E.E. (2003). Mild disorders should not be eliminated from the *DSM-V. Archives of General Psychiatry, 60,* 1117–1122.

Kessler, R.C., Sonnega, A., Bromet, E., Hughes, M., & Nelson, C.B. (1995). Posttraumatic stress disorder in the National Comorbidity Survey. *Archives of General Psychiatry, 52,* 1048–1060.

Kessler, R.C., Stang, P., Wittchen H.-U., Stein, M., Walters, E.E. (1999). Lifetime comorbidities between social phobia and mood disorders in the U.S. National Comorbidity Survey. *Psychological Medicine, 29,* 555–567.

Kessler, R.C., Stein, M.B., & Berglund, P. (1998). Social phobia subtypes in the National Comorbidity Survey. *American Journal of Psychiatry, 155,* 613–619.

Kessler, R.C., Walters, E.E., & Wittchen, H.-U. (2004). Epidemiology. In R.G. Heimberg, C.L. Turk, & D.S. Mennin (Eds.), *Generalized anxiety disorder: Advances in research and practice* (pp. 77–108). New York: Guilford Press.

Kessler, R.C., Zhao, S., Katz, S.J., Kouzis, A.C., Frank, R.G., Edlund, M., & Leaf, P. (1999). Past-year use of outpatient services for psychiatric problems in the National Comorbidity Survey. *American Journal of Psychiatry, 156,* 115–123.

Kierkegaard, S. 1844/1980. *The concept of anxiety* (R. Thomte, Trans.). Princeton: Princeton University Press.

Kirk, S.A. (1999). Instituting madness: The evolution of a federal agency. In C.A. Aneshensel & J.C. Phelan (Eds.), *Handbook of the sociology of mental health* (pp. 539–562). New York: Plenum.

Kirk, S.A., & Kutchins, H. (1992). *The selling of DSM-III: The rhetoric of science in psychiatry.* New York: Aldine de Gruyter.

Kirsch, I. (2010). *The emperor's new drugs: Exploding the antidepressant myth.* New York: Basic Books.

Klein, D.F. (1981). Anxiety reconceptualized. In D.F. Klein & J. Rabkin (Eds.), *Anxiety: New research and changing concepts* (pp. 159–260). New York: Raven.

Klein, D.F., & Fink, M. (1962). Psychiatric reaction patterns to imipramine. *American Journal of Psychiatry, 119,* 432–438.

Kleinman, A. (1986). *Social origins of disease and distress: Depression, neurasthenia and pain in modern China.* New Haven: Yale University Press.

Klerman, G.L. (1972). Psychotropic hedonism vs. pharmacological Calvinism. Hastings Center Report, 2, 1–3.

Klerman, G.R. (1985). Controversies in research on psychopathology of anxiety and anxiety disorders. In A.H. Tuma & J. Maser (Eds.), *Anxiety and the anxiety disorders* (pp. 775–781). Mahwah, NJ: Lawrence Erlbaum Associates.

Klerman, G.R. (1987). Overview. In G. Tischler (Ed.), *Diagnosis and classification in psychiatry* (pp. 260–265). New York: Cambridge University Press.

Koerner, B.I. (2002). Disorders made to order. *Mother Jones,* July 31, 58–63.

Kolb, L.C. (1977). *Modern clinical psychiatry.* Philadelphia: Saunders.

Kolb, L.C., Frazier, S.H., & Sirovatka, P. (2000). The National Institute of Mental Health: Its influence on psychiatry and the nation's mental health. In R.W. Menninger & J.C. Nemiah (Eds.), *American psychiatry after World War II: 1944–1994* (pp. 207–231). Washington DC: American Psychiatric Press.

Konstan, D. (2006). *The emotions of the Ancient Greeks: Studies in Aristotle and classical literature.* Toronto: University of Toronto Press.

Kraepelin, E. (1896). *Psychiatrie. ein kurzes lehrbuch fur studirende und aerzte,* 5th ed. (Leipzig: Abel).

Kramer, P.D. (1992). *Listening to Prozac: A psychiatrist explores antidepressant drugs and the remaking of the self.* New York: Viking.

Krueger, R. (1999). The structure of common mental disorders. *Archives of General Psychiatry, 56,* 921–926.

Kutchins, H., & Kirk, S. (1997). *Making us crazy: DSM: The psychiatric bible and the creation of mental disorders.* New York: Free Press.

Lane, C. (2007). *Shyness: How normal behavior became a sickness.* New Haven: Yale University Press.

Langner, T.S. (1962). A twenty-two item screening score of psychiatric symptoms indicating impairment. *Journal of Health and Social Behavior, 3,* 269–276.

Lantz, P.M., Lichtenstein, R.L., & Pollack, H.A. (2007). Health policy approaches to population health: The limits of medicalization. *Health Affairs, 26,* 1253–1256.

Lazarus, R. (1994a). *Emotion and adaptation.* New York: Oxford.

Lazarus, R. (1994b). *Passion and reason: Making sense of our emotions.* New York: Oxford University Press.

LeBeau, R.T., Glenn, D., Liao, B., Wittchen, H.-U., Beesdo-Baum, K., Ollendick, T., & Craske, M.G. (2010). Specific phobia: A review of DSM-IV specific phobia and preliminary recommendations for DSM-V. *Depression and Anxiety, 27,* 148–167.

LeDoux, J. (1996). *The emotional brain: The mysterious underpinnings of emotional life.* New York: Simon & Schuster.

LeDoux, J. 2002. *Synaptic self: How our brains become who we are.* New York: Penguin.

Leaf, P.J., Myers, J.K., & McEvoy, L.T. (1991). Procedures used in the Epidemiological Catchment Area Study. In L. Robins & D. Regier (Eds.), *Psychiatric disorders in America* (pp. 11–32). New York: Free Press.

Lee, K.A., Vaillant, G.E., Torrey, W.C., & Elder, G.H. (1995). A 50-year prospective study of the psychological sequelae of World War II combat. *American Journal of Psychiatry, 152,* 516–522.

Lee, W.E., Wadsworth, M.E.J., & Hotopf, A. (2006). The protective role of trait anxiety: A longitudinal cohort study. *Psychological Medicine, 36,* 345–351.

Lees-Haley, P., Price, J.R., Williams, C.W., & Betz, B.P. (2001). Use of the impact of events scale in the assessment of emotional distress and PTSD may produce misleading results. *Journal of Forensic Neuropsychology, 2,* 45–52.

Lerner, P., & Micale, M.S. (2001). Trauma, psychiatry, and history: A conceptual and historiographical introduction. In M. Micale & P. Lerner (Eds.), *Traumatic pasts: History, psychiatry, and trauma in the modern age, 1870–1930* (pp. 1–27). New York: Cambridge University Press.

Lewis, A. (1970). The ambiguous word "Anxiety." *International Journal of Psychiatry, 9,* 62–79.

Lewis, A. (1976). A note on classifying phobia. *Psychological Medicine, 6,* 21–22

Lutz, T. (1991). *American nervousness: 1903.* Ithaca: Cornell University Press.

MacDonald, M. (1981). *Mystical bedlam: Madness, anxiety, and healing in seventeenth-century England.* New York: Cambridge University Press.

Magee, W.J., Eaton, W.W., Wittchen, H.-U., McGonagle, K.A., & Kessler, R.C. (1996). Agoraphobia, simple phobia, and social phobia in the National Comorbidity Survey. *Archives of General Psychiatry, 53,* 159–168.

Mann, A. (1997). The evolving face of psychiatric epidemiology. *British Journal of Psychiatry, 171,* 314–318.

March, J.S., Parker, J.D.A., Sullivan, K., Stallings, P., & Conners, C.K. (1997). The Multidimensional Anxiety Scale for Children (MASC): Factor structure, reliability, and validity. *Journal of the American Academy of Child and Adolescent Psychiatry, 36,* 554–565.

Marks, I.M. (1987). *Fears, phobias, and rituals: Panic, anxiety, and their disorders.* New York: Oxford University Press.

Marks, I.M., & Lader, M.H. (1973). Anxiety states (anxiety neurosis): A review. *Journal of Nervous and Mental Disorders, 156,* 3–18.

Marks, I.M., & R.M. Nesse. (1994). Fear and fitness: An evolutionary analysis of anxiety disorders. *Ethology and Sociobiology, 15,* 247–261.

Marmot, M., & Wilkerson, R. (Eds.). (1999). *Social determinants of health.* New York: Oxford University Press.

Marshall, R. (2006). Learning from 9/11: Implications for disaster research and public health. In Y. Neira, R. Gross, R. Marshall, & E. Susser (Eds.), *9/11: Mental health in the wake of terrorist attacks* (pp. 617–630). Cambridge: Cambridge University Press.

Marshall, R.D., Amsel, L., & Suh, E.J. (2008). Response to McNally and Breslau. *American Psychologist, 63,* 283–285.

Maudsley, H. (1879). *Pathology of mind* (3rd ed.). London: MacMillan.

May, R. (1977). *The meaning of anxiety.* New York: Pocket Books.

Mayberg, H.S., Liotti, M., Brannan, S.K., McGinnis, S., Mahurin, R.K., Jerabek, P.A., et al. (1999). Reciprocal limbic-cortical function and negative mood: Converging PET findings in depression and normal sadness. *American Journal of Psychiatry, 156,* 675–682 *mind.* New York: Dana Press.

McNally, R.J. (2003). *Remembering trauma.* Cambridge: Harvard University Press.

McNally, R.J. (2006). Psychiatric casualties of war. *Science, 313,* 923–924.

McNally, R.J. (2007). Revisiting Dohrenwend et al.'s Revisit of the National Vietnam Veterans Readjustment Study. *Journal of Traumatic Stress, 20,* 481–486.

McPherson, S., & Armstrong, D. (2006). Social determinants of diagnostic labels in depression. *Social Science and Medicine, 62,* 50–58.

McReynolds, P. (1985). Changing conceptions of anxiety: A historical review and a proposed integration. *Issues in Mental Health Nursing, 7,* 131–158.

Mechanic, D. (2006). *The truth about health care: Why reform is not working in America.* New Brunswick: Rutgers University Press.

Mental Health Advisory Team. (2009). *Operation Iraqi Freedom.* Washington DC: Office of the Surgeon General. Multi-National Corps-Iraq and Office of the Surgeon General United States Army Medical Command.

Menzies, R.G., & Clarke, J.C. (1995). The etiology of phobias: A nonassociative account. *Clinical Psychology Review, 15,* 23–48.

Micale, M.S. (1994). *Approaching hysteria: Disease and its interpretations.* Princeton: Princeton University Press.

Micale, M.S. (2008). *Hysterical men: The hidden history of male nervous illness.* Cambridge: Harvard University Press.

Michels, R., Frances, A., & Shear, M.K. (1985). Psychodynamic models of anxiety. In A.H. Tuma & J. Maser (Eds.), *Anxiety and the anxiety disorders* (pp. 595–618). Mahwah, NJ: Lawrence Erlbaum Associates.

Milliken, C.S., Auchterlonie, J.L., & Hoge, C.W. (2007). Longitudinal assessment of mental health problems among active and reserve component soldiers returning from the Iraq War. *Journal of the American Medical Association, 298,* 2141–2148.

Mineka, S. (1992). Evolutionary memories, emotional processing, and the emotional disorders. *The Psychology of Learning and Motivation, 28,* 161–206.

Mineka, S., Davidson, M., Cook, M., & Keir, R. (1984). Observational conditioning of snake fear in rhesus monkeys. *Journal of Abnormal Psychology, 93,* 355–372.

Mirowsky, J., & Ross, C.E. (1989). Psychiatric diagnosis as reified measurement. *Journal of Health and Social Behavior, 30,* 11–24.

Mitchell, S.W. (1867). *Fat and blood, and how to make them.* Philadelphia: J.B. Lippincott.

Moffitt, T.E. Caspi, A., Taylor, A., Kokaua, J., Milne, B.J., Polanczyk, G., & Poulton, R. (2009). How common are common mental disorders? Evidence that lifetime prevalence rates are doubled by prospective versus retrospective ascertainment. *Psychological Medicine, 40,* 899–909.

Mojtabai, R. (2008). Increase in antidepressant medication in the US adult population between 1990 and 2003. *Psychotherapy and Psychosomatics, 77,* 83–92.

Mojtabai, R., & Olfson, M. (2008). National trends in psychotherapy by office-based psychiatrists. *Archives of General Psychiatry, 65,* 965.

Mol, S., Arntz, A., Metsemakers, F.M., Dinant, G.-J., Vilters-Van Montfort, P., & Knottnerus, J.A. (2005). Symptoms of post-traumatic stress disorder after non-traumatic events: Evidence from an open population study. *British Journal of Psychiatry, 186,* 494–499.

Montaigne, M. (1955). *The complete essays of Montaigne* (D.M. Frame, Trans.). Stanford: Stanford University Press.

Moynihan, R., & Cassells, A. (2005). *Selling sickness.* New York: Nation Books.

Murphy, D.(2006). *Psychiatry in the scientific image.* Cambridge: MIT Press.

Murphy, J. (1990). Depression screening instruments: History and issues. In C.C. Attkisson & J.M. Zich (Eds.), *Depression in primary care: Screening and detection* (pp. 65–83). New York: Routledge.

Murphy, J.M., & Leighton, A.H. (2008). Anxiety: Its role in the history of psychiatric epidemiology. *Psychological Medicine, 39,* 1055–1064.

Nance, J. (1976). *The gentle Tasaday.* New York: Harcourt, Brace, Jovanovich.

Narrow, W.E., Rae, D.S., Robins, L.N., & Degier, D.A. (2002). Revised prevalence estimates of mental disorders in the United States: Using a clinical significance criterion to reconcile 2 surveys' estimates. *American Journal of Psychiatry, 59,* 115–123.

National Disease and Therapeutic Index. (1976). Ambler, PA: IMS America.

Nesse, R.M. (1990). Evolutionary explanations of emotions. *Human Nature, 1,* 261–289.

Nesse, R.M. (1998). Emotional disorders in evolutionary perspective. *British Journal of Medical Psychology, 71,* 397–415.

Nesse, R.M. (2005). Natural selection and the regulation of defenses: A signal detection analysis of the smoke detector principle. *Evolution and Human Behavior, 26,* 88–105.

Nesse, R.M., & Jackson, E.D. (2006). Evolution: Psychiatric nosology's missing biological foundation. *Clinical Neuropsychiatry, 3,* 121–131.

Nettle, D. (2006). The evolution of personality variation in humans and other animals. *American Psychologist, 61,* 622–631.

Pinned climber cuts off arm to get free. (2003). *New York Times*, May 3, A15.

Norton, G.R., Cox, B.J., Asmundson, G.J.G., & Maser, J.D. (1995). The growth of research on anxiety disorders during the 1980s. *Journal of Anxiety Disorders, 9*, 75–85.

Ofshe, R., & Watters, E. (1994). *Making monsters: False memories, psychotherapy, and sexual hysteria*. Berkeley: University of California Press.

Ohman, A. (1986). Face the best and fear the face: Animal and social fears as prototypes for evolutionary analyses of emotion. *Psychophysiology, 23*, 123–145.

Ohman, A. (2001). Fears, phobias, and preparedness: Toward an evolved module of fear and fear learning. *Psychological Review, 108*, 483–522.

Ohman, A., & Mineka, S. (2001). Fears, phobias, and preparedness: Toward an evolved module of fear and fear learning. *Psychological Review, 108*, 483–522.

Okano, K. (1994). Shame and social phobia: A transcultural viewpoint. *Bulletin of the Menninger Clinic, 58*, 323–328.

Olfson, M., & Klerman, G.L. (1993). Trends in the prescription of psychotropic medications: The role of physician specialty. *Medical Care, 31*, 559–564.

Olfson, M., & Marcus, S.C. (2009). National patterns in antidepressant medication treatment. *Archives of General Psychiatry, 66*, 848–856.

Olfson, M., Marcus, S.C., Druss, B., & Pincus, H.A. (2002a). National trends in the outpatient treatment of depression. *JAMA, 287*, 203–209.

Olfson, M., Marcus, S.C., Druss, B., Elinson, L., Tanielian, T., & Pincus, H.A. (2002b). National trends in the use of outpatient psychotherapy. *American Journal of Psychiatry, 158*, 1914–1920.

Olfson, M., Marcus, S.C., Wan, G.J., & Geissler, E.C. (2004). National trends in the outpatient treatment of anxiety disorders. *Journal of Clinical Psychiatry, 65*, 1166–1173.

Papadatos, Y., Nikou, K., & Potamianos, G. (1990). Evaluation of psychiatric morbidity following an earthquake. *International Journal of Social Psychiatry, 36*, 131–136.

Parry, H., Balter, M.M., Mellinger, G., Cisin, I., & Manheimer, D. (1973). National patterns of psychotherapeutic drug use. *Archives of General Psychiatry, 28*, 769–783.

Pelissolo, A., Andre, C., Moutard-Martin, F., Wittchen, H.-U., & Lepine, J.P. (2000). Social phobia in the community: Relationship between diagnostic threshold and prevalence. *European Psychiatry, 15*, 25–28.

Pescosolido, B.A., Martin, J.K., Link, B.G., Kikuzawa, S., Burgos, G., Swindle, R., et al. (2000). *Americans' views of mental health and illness at century's end: Continuity and change*. Bloomington: Indiana Consortium for Mental Health Services Research.

Pettus, A. (2006). Psychiatry by prescription. *Harvard Magazine*, July–August, 38–44.

Phillips, K.A. (2009). Report of the DSM-5 anxiety, obsessive-compulsive spectrum, posttraumatic, and dissociative disorders work group. Retrieved from http://www.dsm5.org/progressreports

Pincus, H.A., Henderson, B., Blackwood, D., & Dial, T. (1993). Trends in research in two general psychiatric journals in 1969–1990: Research on research. *American Journal of Psychiatry, 150*, 135–142.

Pincus, H.A., Zarin, D.A., Tanielian, T.L., Johnson, J.L., West, J.C., Pettit, A.R., Marcus, S.C., Kessler, R.C., & McIntyre, J.S. (1999). Psychiatric patients and treatments in

1997: Findings from the American Psychiatric Practice Research Network. *Archives of General Psychiatry, 56,* 441–449.

Pinker, S. (1999). *How the mind works.* New York: W.W. Norton & Co.

Piper, A. (1995). Addiction to benzodiazepines—How common? *Archives of Family Medicine, 4,* 964–970.

Plato. (1974). *The republic* (G.M.A. Grube, Trans.). Indianapolis: Hackett.

Plato. (1992). *Laches and Charmides* (R. Sprague, Trans.). Indianapolis: Hackett Publishing.

Plato. (2005). *Dialogues* (L. Cooper, Trans.). Princeton: Princeton University Press.

Poulton, R., & Menzies, R.G. (2002). Non-associative fear acquisition: A review of the evidence from retrospective and longitudinal research. *Behaviour Research and Therapy, 40,* 127–149.

Poulton, R., Thomson, W.M., Davies, S., Kruger, E., Brown, R.H., & Silva, P.A. (1997). Good teeth, bad teeth and fear of the dentist. *Behaviour Research and Therapy, 35,* 327–334.

Poulton, R., Waldie, K.E., Thomson, W.M., & Locker, D. (2001). Determinants of early-versus late-onset dental fear in a longitudinal-epidemiological study. *Behaviour Research and Therapy, 39,* 777–785.

Rachman, S.J. (1978). *Fear and courage: Their birth, life, death.* New York: W. H. Freeman.

Rachman, S.J. (2004). Fear and courage: A psychological perspective. *Social Research, 71,* 149–176.

Radloff, L. (1977). The CES-D scale: A self-report depression scale for research in the general population. *Applied Psychological Measurement, 3,* 249–265.

Raofi, S., & Schappert, S.H. (2006). Medication therapy in ambulatory medical care: United States, 2003–04. *Vital Health Statistics, 163,* 1–40.

Raynes, N.V. (1979). Factors affecting the prescribing of psychotropic drugs in general practice consultations. *Psychological Medicine, 9,* 671–679.

Regier, D.A., Kaelber, C.T., Rae, D.S., Farmer, M.E., Knauper, B., Kessler, R.C., & Norquist, G.S. (1998). Limitations of diagnostic criteria and assessment instruments for mental disorders. *Archives of General Psychiatry, 55,* 109–115.

Reznek, L. (1987). *The nature of disease.* London: Routledge and Kegan Paul.

Richardson, R.C. (2007). *Evolutionary psychology as maladapted psychology.* Cambridge: MIT Press.

Rickels, K. (1968). Drug use in outpatient treatment. *American Journal of Psychiatry, 125* (suppl 124), 20–31.

Rickels, K. (1978). Use of antianxiety agents in anxious outpatients. *Psychopharmacology, 58,* 1–17.

Rickels, K., & Hesbacher, P. (1977). Psychopharmacologic agents: Prescription patterns of non-psychiatrists. *Psychosomatics, 18,* 37–40.

Rickels, K., & Rynn, M. (2001). Overview and clinical presentation of generalized anxiety disorder. *Psychiatric Clinics of North America, 24,* 1–17.

Rind, B., Tromovitch, P., & Bauserman, R. (1998). A meta-analytic examination of assumed properties of child sexual abuse using college samples. *Psychological Bulletin, 124,* 22–53.

Robins, L.N. (1992). The future of psychiatric epidemiology. *International Journal of Methods in Psychiatric Research, 2,* 1–3.

Robins, L.N., Helzer, J.E., Weissman, M.M., Orvaschel, H., Gruenberg, E., Burke, J.D., & Regier, D.A. (1984). Lifetime prevalence of specific psychiatric disorders in three sites. *Archives of General Psychiatry, 41,* 1984, 949–956.

Roccatagliata, G. 1986. *A history of ancient psychiatry.* New York: Greenwood Press.

Rose, N. (2006). Disorders without borders? The expanding scope of psychiatric practice. *BioSocieties, 1,* 465–484.

Rose, N. (2007). *The politics of life itself: Biomedicine, power, and subjectivity in the twenty-first century.* Princeton: Princeton University Press.

Rosenberg, C. (2007). *Our present complaint: American medicine, then and now.* Baltimore: Johns Hopkins University Press.

Rosenhan, D.L. (1973). On being sane in insane places. *Science, 179,* 250–258.

Routtenberg, A., & Glickman, S.E. (1964). Visual cliff behavior in undomesticated rodents, land and aquatic turtles, and cats (Panthera). *Journal of Comparative and Physiological Psychology, 58,* 143–146.

Rubin, G.J., Brewin, C.R., Greenberg, N., Simpson, J., & Wessely, S. (2005). Psychological and behavioral reactions to the bombings in London on 7 July 2005: Cross sectional survey of a representative sample of Londoners. *British Medical Journal, 331,* 606–612.

Ruprecht, T. (2010). High school redux. *New York Times Magazine,* April 4, 50.

Ruscio, A.M., Brown, T.A., Chiu, W.T., Sareen, J., Stein, M.B., & Kessler, R.C. (2008). Social fears and social phobia in the USA: Results from the National Comorbidity Survey Replication. *Psychological Medicine, 38,* 15–28.

Ruscio, A.M., Lane, M., Roy-Byrne, P., Stang, P.E., Stein, D.J., Wittchen, H.-U., & Kessler R.C. (2005). Should excessive worry be required for a diagnosis of generalized anxiety disorder? Results from US National Comorbidity Survey Replication." *Psychological Medicine, 35,* 1761–1772.

Ruscio, A.V., Chiu, W.T., Roy-Byrne, P., Stang, P.E., Stein, D.J., Wittchen, H-U., & Kessler, R.C. (2007). Broadening the definition of generalized anxiety disorder: Effects on prevalence and associations with other disorders in the National Comorbidity Survey Replication. *Journal of Anxiety Disorders, 21,* 662–676.

Rycroft, C. (1988). *Anxiety and neurosis.* London: Maresfield Library.

Sapolsky, R.M. (2004). *Why zebras don't get ulcers* (3rd ed.). New York: Henry Holt and Company.

Sareen, J., Cox, B.J., Afifi, T.O., de Graaf, R., Asmundson, G.J.G., ten Have, M., & Stein, M.B. (2005). Anxiety disorders and risk for suicidal ideation and suicide attempts: A population-based longitudinal study of adults. *Archives of General Psychiatry, 62,* 1249–1257.

Satel, S. (2003). The trauma society. *The New Republic,* May 19, 32–37.

Satel, S. (2007). The trouble with traumatology: Is it advocacy or is it science? *The Weekly Standard,* February 12, A15.

Saul, H. (2001). *Phobias: Fighting the fear.* New York: Arcade.

Schildkraut, J.J. (1965). The catecholamine hypothesis of affective disorders: A review of supporting evidence. *American Journal of Psychiatry, 122,* 509–522.

Schlenger, W.E., Caddell, J.M., Ebert, L., Jordan, B.K., Rourke, K.M., Wilson, D., Thalji, L., Dennis, J.M., Fairbank, J.A., & Kulka, R.A. (2002). Psychological reactions to terrorist attacks: Findings from the National Study of Americans' Reactions to September 11. *JAMA, 288,* 581–588.

Scheff, T.J. (1966). *Being Mentally Ill.* Chicago: Aldine.

Schlenger, W.E., Kulka, R.A., Fairbank, J.A., Hough, R.L., Jordan, B.K., Marmar, C.R., & Weiss, D.S. (2007). The psychological risks of Vietnam: The NVVRS perspective. *Journal of Traumatic Stress, 20,* 467–479.

Schnurr, P.P., Spiro, A., Vielhaer, M.J., Findler, M.N., & Hamblen, J.L. (2002). Trauma in the lives of older men: Findings from the Normative Aging Study. *Journal of Clinical Geropsychology, 8,* 175–187.

Schooler, C. (2007). The changing role(s) of sociology (and psychology) in the National Institute of Mental Health Intramural Research Program. In W.R. Avison, J.D. McLeod, & B.A. Pescosolido (Eds.), *Mental health, social mirror* (pp. 55–66). New York: Springer.

Schuster, M.A., Stein, B.D., Jaycox, L.H., Collins, R.L., Marshall, G.N., Elliott, M.N., Zhou, A.J., Kanouse, D.E., Morrison, J.L., & Berry, S.H. (2001). A national survey of stress reactions after the September 11, 2001, terrorist attacks. *New England Journal of Medicine, 345,* 1507–1512.

Schweder, R.A., & Haidt, J. 2000. The cultural psychology of the emotions: Ancient and new. In M. Lewis & J.M. Haviland-Jones (Eds.), *Handbook of emotions* (pp. 397–414). New York: Guilford Press.

Scott, S. (2007). *Shyness and society: The illusion of competence.* New York: Palgrave Macmillan.

Scott, W.J. (1990). PTSD in DSM-III: A case in the politics of diagnosis and disease. *Social Problems, 37,* 294–310.

Seal, K.H., Bertenthal, D., Miner, C.R., Sen, S., & Marmar, C. (2007). Bringing the war back home: Mental health disorders among 103,788 US veterans returning from Iraq and Afghanistan seen at Department of Veterans Affairs Facilities. *Archives of Internal Medicine, 167,* 476–482.

Sedgwick, P. (1973) Illness, mental and otherwise. *Hastings Center Studies, 1,* 19–40.

Seligman, M, (1971). Phobias and preparedness. *Behavior Therapy, 2,* 307–321.

Seligman, M.E.P., & Hager, J.L. (1972). Biological boundaries of learning: The sauce-bearnaise syndrome. *Psychology Today, 6,* 59–61, 84–87.

Selye, H. (1956). *The stress of life.* New York: McGraw-Hill.

Shapiro, S., & Baron, S. (1961). Prescriptions for psychotropic drugs in a noninstitutional population. *Public Health Reports, 76,* 481–488.

Shephard, B. (2001). *A war of nerves: Soldiers and psychiatrists in the twentieth century.* Cambridge: Harvard University Press.

Shorter, E. (1992). *From paralysis to fatigue: A history of psychosomatic illness in the modern era.* New York: The Free Press.

Shorter, E. (1994). *From the mind into the body: The cultural origins of psychosomatic symptoms.* New York: Free Press.

Shorter, E. (1997). *A history of psychiatry: From the era of the asylum to the age of Prozac.* New York: Wiley.

Shorter, E. (2009). *Before Prozac: The troubled history of mood disorders in psychiatry*. New York: Oxford University Press.

Silver, R.C., Holman, E.A., McIntosh, D.N., Poulin, M., & Gil-Rivas, V. (2002). Nationwide longitudinal study of psychological responses to September 11, *JAMA, 288*, 1235–1244.

Simon, B. (1978). *Mind and madness in ancient Greece: The classical roots of modern psychiatry*. Ithaca: Cornell University Press.

Smith, M.C. (1985). *A social history of the minor tranquillizers*. New York: Pharmaceutical Products Press.

Solnit, R. (2009). *A paradise built in hell: The extraordinary communities that arise in disaster*. New York: Viking.

Solomon, A. (2008). Depression, too, is a thing with feathers. *Contemporary Psychoanalysis, 44*, 509–530.

Sommers, C.H., & Satel, S. (2005). *One nation under therapy: How the helping culture is eroding self-reliance*. New York: St. Martin's Press.

Spiegel, H.X. (1943). Psychiatric observations in the Tunisian campaign. *American Journal of Orthopsychiatry, 14*, 381–385.

Spitzer, R.L. (1978). The data-oriented revolution in psychiatry. *Man and Medicine, 3*, 193–194.

Spitzer, R.L., & Williams, J.B.W. (1984). Diagnostic issues in the DSM-III classification of the anxiety disorders. In L. Grinspoon (Ed.), *Psychiatry updates* (vol. III, pp. 395–425). Washington, DC: American Psychiatric Association.

Spitzer, R.L., First, M.B., & Wakefield, J.C. (2007). Saving PTSD from itself in DSM-V. *Journal of Anxiety Disorders, 21*, 233–241.

Spitzer, R.L., Gibbon, M., Skodol, A.E., Williams, J.B.W., First, M.B. (1994). *DSM-IV casebook: A learning companion to the diagnostic and statistical manual of mental disorders*. Washington, DC: American Psychiatric Publishing.

Spitzer, R.L., Kroenke, K., Williams, J.B.W., & Lowe, B. (2006). A brief measure for assessing generalized anxiety disorder: The GAD-7. *Archives of Internal Medicine, 166*, 1092–1097.

Spitzer, R.L., Williams, J.B.W., & Skodol, A.E. (1980). DSM-III: The major achievements and an overview. *American Journal of Psychiatry, 137*, 151–164.

Srole, L., Langner, T.S., Michael, S.T., Kirkpatrick, P., Opler, M.K., & Rennie, T.A.C. (1978). *Mental health in the metropolis: The Midtown Manhattan Study* (Rev. ed. Enlarged). New York: McGraw Hill.

Stagnitti, M.N. (2005). *Trends in antidepressant use by the U.S. civilian non-institutionalized population, 1997 and 2002*. Rockville, MD: Agency for Healthcare Research and Quality.

Statistical Manual for the Use of Hospitals for Mental Diseases Prepared by the Committee on Statistics of the American Psychiatric Association in Collaboration with the National Committee for Mental Hygiene (10th ed.). (1942). Utica, NY: State Hospitals Press.

Stein, D.J., & Bouwer, C. (1997). A neuron-evolutionary approach to the anxiety disorders. *Journal of Anxiety Disorders, 11*, 409–429.

Stein, M.B., Waler, J.R., & Forde, D.R. (1994). Setting diagnostic thresholds for social phobia: Considerations from a community survey of social anxiety. *American Journal of Psychiatry, 151*, 408–412.

Stepnisky, J.N. (2007). Narrative magic and the construction of selfhood in antidepressant advertising. *Bulletin of Science, Technology & Society, 27*, 24–36.

Stern, H. (1995). *Miss America*. New York: Harper.

Sulzberger, A.G., & Wald, M.L. (2009). Jet flyover frightens New Yorkers. *New York Times*, April 28, A1.

Summerfield, D. (2001). The invention of post-traumatic stress disorder and the social usefulness of a psychiatric category. *British Medical Journal, 322*, 95.

Super, C.M., & Harkness, S. (2011, in press). Culture and infancy. In G. Bremner & T.D. Wachs (Eds.), *Blackwell handbook of infant development* (vol.1). Oxford, England: Blackwell.

Swindle, R., Heller, K., Bescosolido, B., & Kikuzawa, S. (2009). Responses to nervous breakdown in America over a 40-year period. *American Psychologist, 55*, 740–749.

Szasz, T. (1974). *The myth of mental illness: Foundations of a theory of personal conduct*. New York: Harper & Row.

Tanielian, T., & Jaycox, L.H. (Eds.). 2008. *Invisible wounds of war: Psychological and cognitive injuries, their consequences, and services to assist recovery*. Santa Monica: RAND.

Taylor, S.E., & Brown, J.D, (1988). Illusion and well-being: A social psychological perspective on mental health. *Psychological Bulletin, 103*, 193–210.

Tedeschi, R.G., & Calhoun, L.G. (2004). Posttraumatic growth: Conceptual foundations and empirical evidence. *Psychological Inquiry, 15*, 1–18.

Thirlwell, A. (2011). Visionary naturalism. *The New Republic*, June 9, 27–32.

Thompson, W.W., Gottesman, I.I., & Zalewski, C. (2006). Reconciling disparate prevalence rates of PTSD in large samples of US male Vietnam veterans and their controls. *BMC Psychiatry, 6*, 19.

Tien, Y.-F. (1979). *Landscapes of fear*. New York: Pantheon.

Tone, A. (2009). *The age of anxiety: A history of America's turbulent affair with tranquilizers*. New York: Basic Books.

Tooby, J., & Cosmides, L. (1990). On the universality of human nature and the uniqueness of the individual: The role of genetics and adaptation. *Journal of Personality, 58*, 17–67.

Tooby, J., & Cosmides, L. (1990). The past explains the present: Emotional adaptations and the structure of ancestral environments. *Ethology and Sociobiology, 11*, 375–424.

Treffers, P.D.A., & Silverman, W.K. (2001). Anxiety and its disorders in children and adolescents before the twentieth century. In P.D.A. Treffers & W.K. Silverman (Eds.), *Anxiety disorders in children and adolescents: Research, assessment, and intervention* (pp. 1–22). New York: Cambridge University Press.

Trower, P., & Gilbert, P. (1989). New theoretical conceptions of social anxiety and social phobia. *Clinical Psychology Review, 9*, 19–35.

Turner, J. (2000). *On the origins of human emotions: A sociological inquiry into the evolution of human affect.* Palo Alto: Stanford University Press.

Twenge, J.M. (2000). The age of anxiety? Birth cohort change in anxiety and neuroticism, 1952–1993. *Journal of Personality and Social Psychology, 79,* 1007–1021.

Tyrer, P. (1984). Classification of anxiety. *British Journal of Psychiatry, 144,* 78–83.

USDHHS. (1999). *Mental health: A report of the Surgeon General.* Rockville: Author.

USDHHS. (2006). *Ambulatory care visits to physician offices, hospital outpatient departments, and emergency departments: United States, 2001–02.* Washington, DC: Center for Disease Control, National Center for Health Statistics.

Valentine, C.W. (1930). The innate bases of fear. *Journal of Genetic Psychology, 37,* 394–420.

WHO World Mental Health Survey Consortium. (2004). Prevalence, severity, and unmet need for treatment of mental disorders in the World Health Organization World Mental Health Surveys. *JAMA, 291,* 2581–2590.

Wakefield, J.C. (1988). Psychotherapy, distributive justice, and social work: Part 1: Distributive justice as a conceptual framework for social work. *Social Service Review, 62,* 187–210.

Wakefield, J.C. (1992a). The concept of mental disorder: On the boundary between biological facts and social values. *American Psychologist, 47,* 373–388.

Wakefield, J. C. (1992b). Disorder as harmful dysfunction: A conceptual critique of DSM-III-R's definition of mental disorder. *Psychological Review, 99,* 232–247.

Wakefield, J.C. (1999). Evolutionary versus prototype analyses of the concept of disorder. *Journal of Abnormal Psychology, 108,* 374–399.

Wakefield, J.C. (2000). Aristotle as sociobiologist: The "function of a human being" argument, black box essentialism, and the concept of mental disorder. *Philosophy, Psychiatry, and Psychology, 7,* 17–44.

Wakefield, J.C. (2001). The myth of DSM's invention of new categories of disorder: Houts's diagnostic discontinuity thesis disconfirmed. *Behavior Research and Therapy, 39,* 575–624.

Wakefield, J.C., & First, M.B. (2003). Clarifying the distinction between disorder and non-disorder: confronting the overdiagnosis ("false positives") problem in DSM-V. In K. Phillips, M. First, & H. Pincus (Eds.), *Advancing DSM: Dilemmas in psychiatric diagnosis* (pp. 23–56). Washington: American Psychiatric Publishing.

Wakefield, J.C., & Spitzer, R.L. (2002). Lowered estimates—but of what? *Archives of General Psychiatry, 59,* 129–130.

Wakefield, J.C., Horwitz, A.V., & Schmitz, M.F. (2005). Are we overpathologizing the socially anxious? Social phobia from a harmful dysfunction perspective. *Canadian Journal of Psychiatry, 50,* 317–319.

Wakefield, J.C., Horwitz, A.V., & Schmitz, M.F. (2005). Social disadvantage is not mental disorder: Response to Campbell-Sills and Stein. *Canadian Journal of Psychiatry, 50,* 324–326.

Wakefield, J.C., Pottick, K.J., & Kirk, S.A. (2002). Should the DSM-IV diagnostic criteria for conduct disorder consider social context? *American Journal of Psychiatry, 159,* 380–386.

Wald, M.L. (2008). Flight's first fatal trip. *New York Times,* July 27, K5.

Wald, M.L. (2010). For no signs of trouble, kill the alarm. *The New York Times*, August 1, E2.

Walk, R.D., & Gibson, E.J. (1961). A comparative and analytical study of visual depth perception. *Psychological Monographs, 75*, Whole No. 519.

Wang, P.S., Lane, M., Olfson, M., Pincus, H.A., Wells, K.B., & Kessler, R.C. (2005a). Twelve-month use of mental health services in the United States. *Archives of General Psychiatry, 62*, 629–640.

Ward, S.C. (2002). *Modernizing the mind: Psychological knowledge and the remaking of society*. Westport: Praeger.

Watson, J.B. (1924). *Behaviorism*. New York: J.B. Lippincott.

Watson, J.B., & Raynor, R. (1920). Conditioned emotional reactions. *Journal of Experimental Psychology, 3*, 1–14.

Weiss, M., Seifman, D., & Olshan, J. (2009). Air heads in DC terrorize city. *New York Post*, April 28, 1.

Weissman, M.M., & Merikangas, K.R. (1986). The epidemiology of anxiety and panic disorders: An update. *Journal of Clinical Psychiatry, 47* (suppl 6), 11–17.

Weissman, M.M., Myers, J.K., & Harding, P.S. (1978). Psychiatric disorders in a US urban community. *American Journal of Psychiatry, 135*, 459–462.

Wessely, S. (2005). Victimhood and resilience. *New England Journal of Medicine, 353*, 548–550.

Westphal, C. (1871–72). Die agoraphobie, eine neuropathische erscheinung. *Archiv für Psychiatrie und Nervenkrankheiten, 3*, 138–161.

Whitaker, R. (2011). *Anatomy of an epidemic: Magic bullets, psychiatric drugs, and the astonishing rise of mental illness in America*. New York: Broadway.

Wierzbicka, A. (1999). *Emotions across languages and cultures*. New York: Cambridge University Press.

Wilkes, M., Bell, R., & Kravitz, R. (2000). Drug research and development: Direct-to-consumer prescription drug advertising. *Health Affairs, 19*, 110–128.

Wilson, M. (1993). DSM-III and the transformation of American psychiatry: A history. *American Journal of Psychiatry, 150*, 399–410.

Wing, J.K., Cooper, J.E., & Sartorius, N. (1974). *Measurement and classification of psychiatric symptoms*. New York: Cambridge University Press.

Wittchen, H.-U., & Jacobi, F. (2005). Size and burden of mental disorders in Europe—A critical review and appraisal of 27 studies. *European Neuropsychopharmacology, 15*, 357–376.

Witttchen, H.-U. (2000). Epidemiological research in mental disorders: Lessons for the next decade of research—the NAPE lecture 1999. *Acta Psychiatrica Scandinavica, 101*, 2–10.

Wolpe, J. (1969). *The practice of behavioral therapy*. New York: Pergamon Press.

Young, A. (1995). *The harmony of illusions: Inventing post-traumatic stress disorder*. Princeton: Princeton University Press.

Young, A. (2007). Mental health in the wake of terrorist attacks. *Journal of Nervous and Mental Diseases, 195*, 1030–1032.

Zerubavel, E. (1993). *The fine line*. Chicago: University of Chicago Press.

Zimbardo, P. (1977). *Shyness: What it is: What to do about it.* Reading MA: Addison Wesley.

Zimmerman, M., & Spitzer, R.L. (1989). Melancholia: From *DSM-III* to *DSM-III*-R. *American Journal of Psychiatry, 146,* 20–28.

Zuvekas, S.H. (2005). Prescription drugs and the changing patterns of treatment for mental disorders, 1996–2001. *Health Affairs, 24,* 195–205.

INDEX

anxiety. *See also* fear; *specific anxieties*
  absence of, 62–63, 64
  age of, 199, 215
  ambiguity of, 18, 52–53, 62, 77, 100–101,
      103, 145–46, 221, 222–23, 225
  atypical, 100
  behavioral model of, 26–28
  biological markers for, 24
  in body, 82, 88
  in brain, viii–ix, 24–25, 54, 58, 72, 99,
      247n6
  chronic, 52, 98, 99, 113, 114
  conditioning for, 26, 27–28, 123
  as continuum, 90
  with decision-making, 31, 38
  definitions of, 19, 20, 21, 22, 33, 94
  depression and, 6–7, 88, 94, 101, 137,
      199–200, 202, 204–5, 209,
      211–18
  expression of, 44, 53
  fatigue and, 85–86
  fear and, 20, 21, 90, 94–95, 97, 103–4
  free-floating, 21, 89, 94, 98, 101
  by gender, 68–69
  Hippocrates on, 80
  inexplicable, 7
  in infants, viii
  through inferences, 27
  instantaneous activation, 53–54
  intensity of, 25, 30–31, 32, 52, 62, 77,
      111–12, 113–14, 117–18, 139, 225
  as irrational, 58
  medication for, 202, 203, 207–8, 213–16,
      218, 225–28, 232
  in melancholia, 81
  memory and, 2, 28, 57
  philosophers on, 20–21
  as primitive instinct, viii
  in psychiatry, 86, 87, 89–90, 217, 218
  rarity of, 30–31
  repression and, 88
  social values and, 28–30, 72, 199
  as spiritual problem, 87
  statistical distribution of, 30–31
  suppression of, 62
  threshold with, 56, 58
  uncertainty and, 59

  unconscious causes of, 91, 92, 93, 95, 99
  universality of, 38, 47–48, 90
anxiety, normal, 3
  for adolescents, 233
  advertisements for, 19, 207–8, 226, 226f,
      227, 229–31
  after disasters, 164–68
  in brain, 24
  causes of, 4–5, 7, 27, 38–39, 59, 71–72
  as contextual, 22, 34–35, 227, 229–30,
      231, 232–33, 241
  cultural variation with, 13–14, 18, 44–46,
      72, 223
  definition of, 17–19, 33, 113, 145–46
  in *DSM*, 163, 164
  evolutionary, 8–11, 13–14, 18, 22, 34–35,
      36, 40, 41, 64–67, 68, 69–70,
      74–75, 119–20, 141, 162–63,
      221–22, 239–40
  existential, 20–21
  functions of, 37, 38
  impairment with, 13–14, 70, 71, 72, 241
  intensity of, 139, 225
  memory in, 172–73
  in NCS, 153, 154–55, 163
  PTSD and, 169–70
  rates of, 164
  social values with, 148–49
  trauma and, 179, 180, 186
  treatment for, 19, 121–22
anxiety disorder not otherwise specified
      (NOS), 111
anxiety disorders. *See also specific disorders*
  in adolescents, 236–37
  after September 11, 2001, 3–5
  Burton on, 81–83
  categories of, 100
  causes of, 60–61, 110
  compulsive, 5–6
  criteria for, 10, 13, 14–17, 18, 22, 23–24,
      52–53, 59–60, 71, 74–75, 76, 79,
      81, 84, 93–94, 95–96, 97–107,
      109–41, 215–16, 239
  definition of, 21
  in *DSM*, 14–16, 18, 93–94, 97–107,
      109–41, 143–44, 147, 151, 210,
      215–16

Environment of Evolutionary Adaptation
(EEA), 35
Epictetus, 54, 80
Epidemiological Catchment Area Study
(ECA), 1, 149–50, 161, 182
epidemiological studies, 18–19, 144
after disasters, 164–68
depression in, 202
interviews for, 149, 154, 155
NCS, 150–68, 160*t*, 236, 255n36, 257n78
self-report in, 147–48
Erichsen, John, 188
eye contact, 68

facial expressions, viii, 63
falling, 43
fathers, 92
fatigue, 85–86
FDA. *See* Food and Drug Administration
fear. *See also* anxiety
absence of, 63, 64
in animals, 27, 38–39, 43, 56, 122
of animals, 8–9, 10, 27, 39, 40, 65–66, 92,
100, 101, 122, 123–24
anxiety and, 20, 21, 90, 94–95, 97, 103–4
as anxiety disorder, 10, 13, 61
avoidance of, 125–26
of being buried alive, 13
of being lost, 40
biology of, 54–55, 57–58, 61
in body, 39, 73
in brain, 54–55, 57–58
of castration, 91, 92
in children, 26, 27, 40–41, 42*f*, 43–44, 46,
46*f*, 47, 48, 64, 65–66, 69, 91–92,
100, 101, 162
chronic, 125
of closed spaces, 9, 10
conditioning for, 26, 27–28, 39, 40, 48,
63, 122
consciousness of, 54
cues for, 38–39, 58, 82
cultural conditioning for, 44–46, 46*f*, 47
of darkness, 27, 65, 82–83
definition of, 20
dental, 26
etiology of, 143

as evolutionary, 8–11, 13–14, 18, 22,
34–36, 40–42, 42*f*, 43–44, 49–50,
52, 64–71, 74–77, 90–92, 121–25,
128, 129, 222, 224, 247n3
expression of, 39, 40–41
of flying, 9–10, 69, 74, 75–76
of food allergies, 13, 45
Freud on, 90–92
function of, 37
as future-oriented, 57
of heights, 11, 40, 41–42, 42*f*, 43–44, 48,
64, 76
impairment from, 103, 104, 114, 115,
127, 142–43
intensity of, 76, 143
irrational, viii, ix, 5–6, 18, 58, 75–77, 82,
83, 98, 104, 106, 119–24, 129, 134,
143, 222
of isolation, 67
of kidnapping, 69
from others, 26
over time, 75
pathological, 10, 13, 61, 70
performance, 80
phobias and, 86
photographs of, 41
with PTSD, 56
of public speaking, 14, 67, 68, 131,
160, 161
rational, 122, 154
response mechanisms of, 38, 54–58,
61–62, 65, 69
of separation, 40, 65, 101
of snakes, 8–9, 10, 27, 39, 65, 122,
123–24
in soldiers, 30, 58–59, 177
of strangers, 45, 46, 46*f*, 47, 65–67
suppression of, 13, 48, 55
as temporal, 20, 57
threshold for, 55–56
uncertainty and, 57, 59
universality of, 39–41, 45, 76–77
variations in, 10–11, 12*f*, 47–49, 76,
222–23
of violence, 69
of witchcraft, 13, 45
fear disorders, 21

humiliation, 80, 131, 132–33
humoralism, 83–84
Hurricane Katrina, 4, 165–66
hypervigilance, 62
hypochondria, 83, 84, 209
hysteria, 84, 209

ICD. *See* International Classification of
    Disease
illness, 28–29
imipramine, 99
impairment principle, 70, 71, 72–73
India, 41
industrial society, 85
infants
    anxiety in, viii
    fear in, 40
    stranger fear in, 46, 46*f*, 47, 67
    sudden infant death syndrome, 65
International Classification of Disease
    (ICD), 257n72
Internet, 232
Iraq, 7
Iraq War, 184–85
isolation, 67

Jackson, Stanley, 81
JAMA. *See* Journal of the American Medical
    Association
James, William, 35, 55
Janet, Pierre, 86, 87
Japan, 41
Jelzer, John, 189
Job, 41
Journal of the American Medical Association
    (JAMA), 226*f*

K6 scale, 164–66, 168
Kagan, Jerome, 160–61
Karp, David, 237–38
Keane, Terence, 189
Kendler, Kenneth, 3, 25
Kessler, Robert, 150, 151, 161–62, 236, 255n36
kibbutzim, 46*f*, 47
kidnappings, 69
Kierkegaard, Soren, 20–21, 38
Kirk, Stuart, 163

Klein, Donald, 99, 212–13
Konstan, David, 44
Korean War, 190, 191
Kraepelin, Emil, 86, 87
Kramer, Peter, 214
!Kung San, 46*f*, 47
Kutchins, Herb, 163

labeling, 71
Ladinos, 46*f*, 47
Langner scale, 148
LeBeau, R.T., 128
LeDoux, Joseph, 28, 58, 247n6
Leighton, Alexander, 203
Lerner, Paul, 169
Levine, Michael, 9
Lewis, Aubrey, 87, 119
Lexapro, 230
Librium, 202, 226, 226*f*, 228
Lifton, Robert Jay, 178, 179
*Listening to Prozac: A Psychiatrist Explores
    Antidepressant Drugs and the Remaking
    of the Self* (Kramer), 214
Little Hans, 27, 92, 100, 101
lobotomies, 63
Loftus, Elizabeth, 196
London, 26
loss
    depression and, 57, 94, 129
    Freud on, 88, 91, 101
The Loss of Sadness (Horwitz and Spitzer), 129
lost, fear of being, 40
loud noises, 38
love, 82
lungs, 36

Madden, John, 9, 74–76
major depressive disorder (MDD), 106, 158,
    210–11, 212, 217
manic depression, 86
MAOIs. *See* monoamine oxidase inhibitors
marijuana, 265n33
Marks, Isaac, 40, 162
Marshall, Randall, 193, 194
MASC. *See* Multidimensional Anxiety Scale
    for Children
masturbation, 30, 45

Maudsley, Henry, 87
Mayans, 46f, 47
McHugh, Paul, 185
McNally, Richard, 192, 193
MDD. *See* major depressive disorder
Mead, Margaret, 239
Meade, Robin, 130–31
meaninglessness, 21
medical care, primary, 235–36
medication, 95, 99
    for adolescents, 237–38
    advertisements for, 19, 207–8, 215, 216,
        226, 226f, 227, 229–32
    antidepressants, 204, 213–15, 216, 218
    antipsychotic, 215
    for anxiety, 202, 203, 207–8, 213–16,
        218, 225–28, 232
    anxiolytic, 213–14, 216, 226, 227–28
    backlash against, 213
    benzodiazepines, 207, 213–14, 216,
        227–28
    for depression, 202–3, 204, 213–15,
        216, 218
    Effexor, 216
    gender and, 213
    generic, 215
    imipramine, 99
    Lexapro, 230
    Librium, 226, 226f, 228
    meprobamate, 202, 226
    Miltown, 202, 226
    Paxil, 216, 230–32
    profit from, 228–29
    Prozac, 214
    Serentil, 227
    for social phobia, 216, 231–32
    SSRI, 204, 213, 214, 218
    tranquilizers, 202, 203, 207–8, 214, 226,
        227, 228
    Valium, 202
    Zoloft, 216
melancholia, 81–82, 83, 84, 210
melancholic depression, 210
Melanesia, 45
memory
    anxiety and, 2, 28, 57
    in normal anxiety, 172–73

in PTSD, 172–73, 180–81
    of trauma, 180–81
mental asylums, 86
mental disorders, 24
    anxiety disorders and, viii, ix, 86
    as dysfunction, 34, 74, 77
    etiology of, 95–96
    HD analysis for, 73, 224–25
    morality and, 240
    normality and, 33, 164–68
    social control and, 72
    in social norms, 28–30
    statistical distribution of, 30–31
    stigmatization with, 237–38
    in U.S., 147
meprobamate, 202, 226
Micale, Marc, 169
Middle Ages, 45
Midtown Manhattan Study, 148
Miltown, 202, 226
Miss California USA contest, 73
monkeys, 27, 39
monoamine oxidase inhibitors (MAOIs), 203
monogamy, 73
Montaigne, Michel, 6
mood disorders, 137, 139, 166, 203, 210, 217
morality
    mental disorder and, 240
    PTSD and, 170, 179, 187–89, 192, 193,
        196–97
    trauma and, 188, 195–96
mothers
    fear from, 26, 27
    with GAD, 158
    Oedipal conflict with, 92
    separation from, 40, 65, 101
Multidimensional Anxiety Scale for Children
    (MASC), 236–37
murder, 69
Murphy, Jane, 148, 203

National Alliance for the Mentally Ill, 207
National Comorbidity Study (NCS),
    150–51, 167, 255n36, 257n78
    anxiety disorder rates in, 160t, 236
    excessiveness criterion in, 154–55, 156–59
    GAD in, 152–59

memory in, 172–73, 180–81
morality and, 170, 179, 187–89, 192,
     193, 196–97
in NCS, 182
normal anxiety and, 169–70
normalizing, 187
onset of, 179
persistence in, 62
qualifiers for, 104
rates of, 182, 185, 189–91, 192–93, 196
recovery from, 185
stressor criterion for, 180
symptoms of, 170, 171–74, 175–76, 180,
     183–84
trauma in, 170, 173–75
treatment for, 197
in U.S., 183
predators, 38–39, 63
Prejean, Carrie, 73
Present State Examination, 97, 167
primary anxiety, 20
primates, viii
Prozac, 214
Psychiatric Diagnosis (Goodwin and Guze), 142
psychiatry
     anxiety in, 86, 87, 89–90, 217, 218
     biological perspective in, 208–9
     depression in, 208–9, 216–17, 218
     diagnosis in, 23, 93
     diagnostic specificity in, 205–6, 218
     hierarchy in, 89–90, 98–99, 105
     as social control, 72, 73
     in World War II, 93
psychoanalysis, 95
psychogenic theory, 85, 87
Psychological Bulletin, 194–95
psychoneuroses, 88, 93, 96, 99, 202,
     205–6, 209
psychosis, 83
PTSD. *See* post-traumatic stress disorder
public speaking, 14, 67, 68, 131, 160, 161

Quartzsite, 9
Quechua Indians, 174

Rachman, Stanley, 13
railway spine, 188–89

rape, 69
Rasadhyaya, 41
"Rat Man," 6, 20
rattlesnakes, 8–9
Raynor, Rosalie, 26
Reagan, Ronald, 228
reason, 120
recklessness, 62, 64
relationships, 75, 82
repression, 88
reproduction, 73
Research Domain Criteria Project, 24
Reznek, Laurie, 28
Rickels, Karl, 201–2
Rind, Bruce, 194
risk, 49, 63, 64
Robins, Lee, 150, 189
Robinson, Nicholas, 83
role impairment, 31–32, 114, 115, 127,
     142, 241
Rosenberg, Charles, 205
Rosenhan, D. L., 206
Rowling, J. K., 31
runaways, 69
Rush, Benjamin, 86, 121

SAD. *See* social anxiety disorder
sadness, 25, 83
Sandoz Pharmaceutical, 227
Sartorius, Norman, 145–46
schizophrenia, 86
Schlessinger, Laura, 195
schools, 236
Schrekneurose, 86
science fiction, 70–71
screening, 233, 234–36
Sears Tower, 11, 12*f*
Sedgwick, Peter, 28–29
selective serotonin reuptake inhibitor
     (SSRI), 204, 213, 214, 218
self-report, 23
     in *DSM*, 98, 99–100, 117, 142
     in epidemiological studies, 147–48
     in NCS, 257n84
     treatment and, 146
Seligman, Martin, 27, 122–23
Selye, Hans, 200

for Freud, 100
of GAD, 138
multiplicity of, 141
non-specificity of, 138
of OCD, 60–61, 97–98, 99, 104
of PTSD, 170, 171–74, 175–76, 180,
183–84
treatment for, 238
Szasz, Thomas, 206

Tasaday, 45
taste, 35, 73, 122–23
technology, 72
teenagers, 233, 236
temperament, 48–49, 80, 159, 161
for emotions, 13, 14, 248n11
trauma and, 181–82
testosterone, 74
thalamus, 55
Thomas Aquinas, 55
Time, 228
Tooby, John, 35
torture, 6
tranquilizers, 202, 203, 207–8, 214, 226,
227, 228
Transient Situational Personality Disorders,
177–78
trauma, 170, 173
from CSA, 195
definitions of, 174–75, 182–83
effects of, 178
exposure to, 184
memory of, 180–81
morality and, 188, 195–96
normal anxiety and, 179, 180, 186
for soldiers, 7, 174–78, 184–85
temperament and, 181–82
treatment. *See also* medication
for anxiety disorders, 19, 121–22, 215,
216, 231
for depression, 202–3, 204, 213–15
diagnosis in, 93
encouragement for, 229, 233–34
informed consent for, 241
in mental hospitals, 93
for neurasthenia, 85
for normal anxiety, 19, 121–22

outpatient, 93
payment for, 93, 206, 208, 239
for PTSD, 197
rates of, 145
self-report and, 146
for symptoms, 238
Tromovitch, Philip, 194
Tuan, Yi-Fu, 67
Tyrer, Peter, 100

uncertainty, 57, 59
unconscious, 91, 92, 93, 95, 99
United Kingdom, 13, 26
United States (U.S.), 13, 41
anxiety disorders in, 151
Congress, 190
mental disorders in, 147
PTSD in, 183
shyness in, 231
social phobia in, 44
stranger fear in, 46f, 47
U.S.–U.K. Diagnostic Project, 206

Valium, 202
values theory, 28–30
VES. *See* Vietnam Experience Study
veterans, 7, 178, 184–85, 187. *See also*
post-traumatic stress disorder
Veterans Administration, 177, 178
Victorian era, 30
Vietnam Experience Study (VES), 191, 192
Vietnam Veterans Against the War
(VVAW), 178
Vietnam War, 175, 178, 190, 191
violence, 69
virtue, 240
visual cliff, 41–42, 42f, 43
VVAW. *See* Vietnam Veterans Against the War

Walk, Richard, 41, 42
war neuroses, 149, 176–77, 189. *See also*
post-traumatic stress disorder
wars
Afghanistan War, 184–85
Iraq War, 184–85
Korean War, 190, 191
Vietnam War, 175, 178, 190, 191

wars (*Continued*)
    World War I, 175
    World War II, 26, 30, 58, 93, 190–91
Washington University, 97
Waters, E.E., 236
Watson, John, 26, 27
websites, 232–33
Wessely, Simon, 167, 196
Westphal, Carl, 86
Whytt, Robert, 84
Williams, Janet, 157
Williams, Ricky, 232
Willis Tower, 11, 12*f*
Wing, John, 145–46
witchcraft, 13, 45

withdrawal method, 88
Wittchen, Hans-Ulrich, 150
World Trade Center, 3–5, 36
World War I, 175
World War II, 26, 30, 58
    psychiatry in, 93
    PTSD after, 190–91
worry, 145–46
    causes of, 154
    in GAD, 136–40, 154, 155–56

Yolles, Stanley, 228
Young, Allan, 176

Zoloft, 216